Plastic Reconstructive Surgery: Essential Concepts

Plastic Reconstructive Surgery: Essential Concepts

Edited by **Adam Bachman**

FOSTER
ACADEMICS

New Jersey

Published by Foster Academics,
61 Van Reypen Street,
Jersey City, NJ 07306, USA
www.fosteracademics.com

Plastic Reconstructive Surgery: Essential Concepts
Edited by Adam Bachman

International Standard Book Number: 978-1-63242-324-5 (Hardback)

Contents

Preface

This book presents all the major aspects associated with the procedure of plastic surgery. Plastic Surgery is a surgical specialty which is developing at a fast pace. It is not just limited to cosmetic applications but also includes aesthetic and reconstructive procedures which attempt to restore functionality and normal appearance of organs damaged due to neoplasm, ageing, trauma or iatrogenesis. More than three thousand years ago, Indian surgeons were able to reconstruct nasal deformities inflicted as punishment using reconstructive procedures. Advances in research and technology have led to significant developments in reconstructive surgery although some age-old procedures like Indian forehead flap for nasal reconstruction continue to be used due to their effective outcomes.

This book is a result of research of several months to collate the most relevant data in the field.

When I was approached with the idea of this book and the proposal to edit it, I was overwhelmed. It gave me an opportunity to reach out to all those who share a common interest with me in this field. I had 3 main parameters for editing this text:

1. Accuracy – The data and information provided in this book should be up-to-date and valuable to the readers.
2. Structure – The data must be presented in a structured format for easy understanding and better grasping of the readers.
3. Universal Approach – This book not only targets students but also experts and innovators in the field, thus my aim was to present topics which are of use to all.

Thus, it took me a couple of months to finish the editing of this book.

I would like to make a special mention of my publisher who considered me worthy of this opportunity and also supported me throughout the editing process. I would also like to thank the editing team at the back-end who extended their help whenever required.

Editor

Part 1

Basic Topics in Reconstructive Surgery

Scar Revision and Secondary Reconstruction for Skin Cancer

Michael J. Brenner[1,2] and Jennifer L. Nelson[2]
[1]Director of Facial Plastic & Reconstructive Surgery
[2]Division of Otolaryngology, Department of Surgery
Southern Illinois University School of Medicine
USA

1. Introduction

Late wound management requires not only mastery of the techniques involved in scar revision, but a thorough understanding of facial anatomy, wound healing, and the psychological factors associated with traumatic injury. Treatment of a patient for scar revision requires the surgeon to understand that a patient's perception of a scar is often influenced by emotionally charged circumstances and possible self-critical evaluation. This chapter addresses the etiology, evaluation, and treatment of traumatic wounds in the delayed setting with emphasis on scar revision.

2. Pathogenesis of scar formation

Unsightly scar formation and impaired wound healing may arise from a variety of factors related to trauma, surgery, or inflammation.(1) While the stigmata of trauma often appear isolated to the skin, many deformities also involve deeper injury to muscle, bone, or other underlying deep tissues. This distinction is of paramount importance because failure to appropriately identify a structural defect in the scaffolding and supporting tissue that is deep to the skin will almost certainly result in an unfruitful attempt at revision. Furthermore certain types of injuries, such as gunshot wounds, avulsions, and full thickness burns are associated with significant tissue loss.

Several additional factors also adversely affect healing. Infection in the wound bed will exacerbate the degree of injury and will likely to cause added delay in revision. Infected wounds are characterized by greater tissue loss and destruction, as well as increased collagen deposition, impaired vascular supply, and worse scarring. Blunt injuries tend to cause more diffuse soft tissue injury than sharp injuries. Crush injuries that produce stellate tears, irregular lacerations, and diffuse underlying soft tissue destruction may result in particularly severe scarring. Host factors, such as skin thickness, predisposition to keloid formation or hypertrophic scars, skin pigmentation, prior injury, poor nutritional status, sun exposure, and smoking history will all also affect healing and scar formation.

The initial management of a traumatic wound heavily impacts the need for revision.(2) Wound closure is often performed by personnel with limited experience in plastic surgical technique and wound management. As a result, wounds may be inadequately cleansed, with devitalized tissue and foreign body contamination predisposing to infection and inflammation. Conversely, overzealous debridement may result in an uneven or irregular wound. The wound closure may be inadequate or traumatic, and widened scars occur over sites of excess tension. Depressed scars occur if wound edges are not appropriately everted. When wounds are not covered with an occlusive dressing or appropriate ointment, desiccation will impair wound healing. Last, those, wounds that are situated at sites of repeated motion are prone to widening and delayed repair.

3. Evaluation of late wounds

Successful late wound management is predicated upon a thorough history and evaluation of the patient considering both the location and characteristics of the wound as well as the goals and expectations of the patient.(3) Preoperative photography plays an important role in documenting the extent of disfigurement. Patients need to be reminded that while treatments may camouflage pathologic wound healing, most interventions will exchange one type of scar or deformity for another, lesser one.(4) The indications for delayed wound management relate to an unacceptable appearance or a functionally problematic healing outcome.(5) Evaluation is influenced by anatomic site, mechanism of injury, extent of the deformity, and likelihood of pathologic healing.

3.1 Characteristics of disfiguring scars

Scars are perceived as unsightly when their surface characteristics differ markedly from the surrounding skin such that they are poorly camouflaged by the surrounding surface skin anatomy. Whereas scars that fall into shadows generally appear hidden, scars that traverse a smooth convexity such as the chin or malar eminence will be readily noticeable. Abnormal color, contour, and texture make scars more conspicuous and unsightly. Scars that are widened, long, and linear will similarly draw attention, particularly when they are unfavorably oriented relative to relaxed skin tension lines or disrupt an aesthetic subunit. Not uncommonly, cosmetically disfiguring scars are also associated with functional problems, such as contracture, distortion, stenosis, or fistula formation. Some examples are ectropion, entropion, or webbing of the eyelids; disruption of salivary ducts; and deformity of the nasal alae, ears, or lips.

3.1.1 Scar color, contour, and texture

Poor color match results from hyperpigmentation or hypopigmentation. Hyperpigmented scars have a deep red hue from inflammation or have darkening from increased melanin. Hypopigmentation reflects a loss of melanocytes and tend to be irreversible. Traumatic tattooing occurs when dirt, asphalt, graphite, or other foreign material is embedded within the skin. These particles can be particularly difficult to remove because they tend to be distributed across several different skin layers. Scars that are hypertrophied, elevated, depressed, or that have other poor contour are also difficult to mask, especially when accompanied by webbing or pin cushioned appearance. Unacceptable appearance also results from poor texture, such as a scar that is too shiny or too smooth.

3.1.2 Scar length

Long, linear scars are usually more problematic than shorter scars with more segments because their regular appearance is readily discerned. The human eye has more difficulty detecting a scar's full extent if there is intervening normal tissue or irregularity to the scar. In addition, it is common for long scars to have a bowstring effect over sites such as the medial canthus or mandible to the neck, where webbing can occur due to concavity of these areas. In addition, muscle action can exaggerate a linear deformity, as in the example of curved scars that form a trapdoor deformity.

3.1.3 Scar depth

Deeper injuries induce greater scar formation than shallow injuries as a result of the correspondingly greater soft tissue contracture and volume loss. The underlying mechanism involves the melding of superficial and deep scar, resulting in tethering and visible depression. Multiple depths of injury will multiply the extent of scaring, with stellate or crushing injuries resulting in worse injury. Avulsion of tissue will further complicate healing, making it impossible to align skin edges at time of initial injury. Deep, beveled injuries maximize the amount of dermal trauma due to the correspondingly greater area of tissue traversed and the tendency of oblique contracture of the dermis to cause one skin edge to slide over the other. This pattern of scarring may cause either a pin cushioned appearance or a heaped appearance. In such cases, the surgeon may either debulk the elevated skin and place bolster sutures or fully excise the affected area.

3.1.4 Relation to relaxed skin tension lines (RSTLs)

Relaxed skin tension lines (RSTLs) run perpendicular to the direction of maximal underlying tension within the skin (Figure 1). Those scars that are unfavorably positioned relative to RSTLs are most likely to require revision. Often the approach to scar revision is based upon how the scar can be reoriented to fall within these lines. The ability to align scars in this manner is often the difference between an excellent and mediocre result because placement within RSTLs improves camouflage and enables the contractile forces on the skin to approximate wound edges, rather than distracting the edges apart. The lines of maximum extensibility (LMEs) run perpendicular to the RSTLs and are usually parallel to muscle fibers. Lines of maximum extensibility are important to consider when recruiting tissue from adjacent areas for flap reconstruction.

Relaxed skin tension lines generally lie perpendicular to the underlying muscle fibers; but, this rule is not absolute. The RSTLs reflect tension on the skin that arises not only from muscle forces but also from stretch by soft tissue or rigid bone/cartilage. Similarly, wrinkle lines do not always accurately reflect the positions of the RSTLs. For example, the lines between the lower lip and mentum run parallel to the orbicularis oris muscle. Most of the RSTLs are parallel to 4 main facial lines: the facial median, the nasolabial, the facial marginal, and the palpebral lines. The facial median line spans from the alar facial groove to the columella and lip and then inferiorly to the mentum. The nasolabial line runs from the alar facial groove inferolaterally to form the nasolabial fold, traverses lateral to the oral commissure, and then extends inferiorly to form marionette lines. The facial marginal line starts at the hairline, travels anterior to the tragus, and descends along the posterior margin of the mandible, across the submandibular triangle, and to the hyoid. The palpebral line extends from the superolateral dorsum to the medial canthus and then proceeds to the lateral canthus to the cheek and submental area.

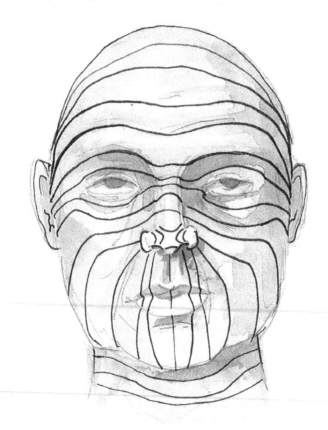

Fig. 1. Relaxed Skin Tension Lines.

3.2 Relative contraindications to scar revision

While many patients will benefit from surgical scar revision, several considerations must be taken into account including medical co-morbidities and the prospects for achieving a favorable visible outcome. It is preferable to avoid operating on immature scar, and the surgeon must use judgment when a patient presses for an inappropriately timed surgical intervention. Consideration must also be given to the psychological preparedness of the patient with attention to any unrealistic expectations that the patient may not have disclosed initially. Cigarette smoking should be discontinued at least 2 weeks prior to surgery. Use of nonsteroidal anti-inflammatory agents, Vitamin E, and herbal preparations that may impair wound healing should also be discontinued perioperatively.

3.3 Timing and psychological considerations

The time course of scar maturation is approximately 12 to 18 months, during which a complex sequence of histological changes associated with wound healing occurs.(6) A general guideline is that scar revision is considered appropriate after 6 to 12 months, when type I collagen has largely replaced type III collagen and the general extent of scar formation is apparent.(7) Earlier scar revision may be considered in unfavorable scars in order to positively influence aesthetic and functional outcomes while also alleviating the patient's psychological distress. Unfavorable scars typically cross cosmetic subunits, do not fall within relaxed skin tension lines, and have more conspicuously disfiguring appearance. In contrast, scars that do not disrupt cosmetic subunits and that have favorable orientation relative to relaxed skin tension lines may have a satisfactory appearance at 1 year without any surgery, despite initial erythema and discoloration.

Patients who opt to pursue scar revision often have persistent psychological trauma associated with the original traumatic event, even if a significant period of time has elapsed between the original injury and the time of surgical consultation. The surgeon must therefore be attentive to the patient's concerns and ensure that the patient has realistic goals. The surgeon should impress upon the patient that complete elimination of scars is seldom, if ever, achieved, although improvement is often possible.(8) It is also important to stress the role for planned secondary procedures as part of the treatment. For example, scar revision with excision is often followed by steroid injection or contour correction with dermabrasion. Similarly, scar revision by serial excision involves sequential procedures.

In cases of significant psychological trauma, a specialist with relevant expertise may be consulted. When domestic violence has occurred, camouflaging may be particularly helpful as an interim strategy prior to definitive surgical therapy. Inquiring about the patient's social support system may afford the surgeon insights regarding potential factors that might adversely affect postoperative care. The patient should also understand the significant period of time required for healing.

4. Surgical treatment

A wide range of techniques are available for scar revision. Among these approaches are simple or serial excision, either with or without tissue expansion; irregularization through z-plasty, w-plasty, m-plasty, or broken line closure; resurfacing with dermabrasion and lasers; minimally invasive approaches such as fillers and paralytic agents; and adjunctive techniques involving steroids, silicone sheeting, and cosmetics.(9) Each of these approaches is discussed in detail in the following section.

4.1 General principles

Atraumatic tissue handling, always important in surgery, assumes critical importance in revision surgery, where the wound edges are likely to have baseline vascular compromise. Toothed tissue forceps should be used, and tissue handling should be minimized. Use of skin hooks may diminish the need for traumatic tissue manipulation. Damp sponges may be used to help hydrate the skin edges, an approach that is of special value when using more labor intensive approaches, such as geometric broken line closures. Subdermal undermining lateral to wound margins is essential to achieving a tension free closure. Skin flap undermining is performed sharply, while elevating the flap atraumatically with skin hooks or toothed forceps. Layered closure is performed with tension placed upon the deep sutures to facilitate hypereversion.(10)

Adequate hemostasis is a prerequisite for successful scar revision. Collections of blood under a flap will predispose to infection and more visible scar. A bipolar cautery is preferred to monopolar cautery due to decreased thermal injury. Meticulous subcutaneous closure minimizes dead space and ensures a stable foundation for the overlying skin surface. Beveling of the skin incision can be used to improve wound margin eversion. For deep tissue and deep dermal closure on the face, 5-0 and 6-0 absorbable sutures are preferred (PDS or vicryl). For the skin, non-absorbable sutures (6-0 or 7-0 prolene or ethilon) are best due to their low tissue bioreactivity; however, these may be cumbersome to remove in hair-bearing areas. Absorbable suture, such as fast absorbing gut, is an acceptable alternative. Of note, the needle on ethilon suture can be too rough for use on delicate tissues such as eyelids or facial tissue in infants

4.2 Surgical methods of irregularization

A variety of methods are available for irregularization of scars, so as to camouflage scars. The eye is naturally attracted to straight lines, as such lines seldom appear in nature. Therefore, introducing irregularity affords significant benefit in making scars less conspicuous.

4.2.1 Z-plasty

The classic Z-plasty involves the transposition of two adjacent undermined triangle flaps, usually with angles of the Z measuring approximately 60 degrees. Classic Z-plasty and its variations are used for a variety of purposes, including to:

- Reorient a scar to lie parallel to RSTLs
- Increase scar length to lengthen a site of contracture
- Reorient a scar to lie in a more favorable position relative to cosmetic subunits
- Irregularize a scar by breaking a single line into segments
- Orient a skin incision away from an underlying scar to avoid a depressed scar

The simple Z-plasty is composed of 3 limbs, as shown in Figure 2. After transposition of the two triangle flaps, the middle limb is reoriented approximately 90 degrees if the Z-plasty is 60 degrees. The extent of rotation and the lengthening both diminish with tighter Z-plasty configurations, as shown in Figure 3. The lengthening in one axis corresponds to shortening in the other axis with associated tissue distortion. As shown, a 30 degree Z-plasty results in a 25% increase in length; a 45 degree Z-plasty results in a 50% increase in length; and a 60 degree Z-plasty results in a 75% increase in length. A Z-plasty with a higher angle tends to create a standing cone deformity, whereas a Z-plasty with <30 degree angles has more risk of necrosis of the tips. The use of serial Z-plasty or compound Z-plasty can achieve effective scar lengthening with less tissue distortion and improved camouflage. The compound Z-plasty minimizes the number of incisions required for scar revision. Because a given scar can be reoriented in either of 2 directions, the surgeon must choose both the angle and the orientation for the Z-plasty that will most effectively align the scar with the RSTLs.

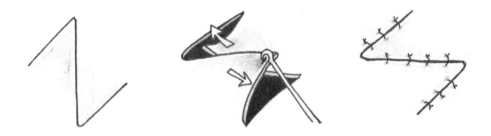

Fig. 2. Depiction of Z-plasty.

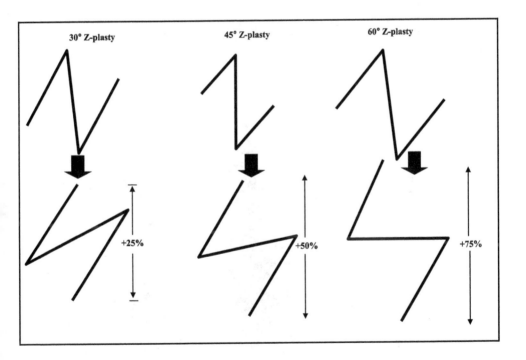

Fig. 3. With wider angle Z-plasty configurations, rotation and the lengthening both increase

The double-opposing Z-plasty, unequal triangle Z-plasty, and planimetric Z-plasty are other variants of the basic Z-plasty. The double opposing Z-plasty involves use of overlying Zplasties in reverse orientation. This method can be used to redistribute volume and avoid placing multiple layers of closure over a single line of tension. This approach has been most widely applied in cleft palate surgery, although it has also found application for treatment of cervical webs, using the platysma for the deep Z-plasty and the skin and subcutaneous fat for the superficial opposing Z-plasty. The unequal triangle Z-plasty involves a Z with non-parallel limbs and is useful when it is desirable to transpose unequal tissue areas. Planimetric Z-plasty entails excising the excess elevated tissue (dog ears) that is produced with standard Z-plasty on a flat surface. It is used for scar irregularization and limited skin elongation on planar surfaces.

4.2.2 W-plasty

The W-plasty (Figure 4) is most useful in changing a linear scar into an irregular scar .(11) It can also be useful in converting a curvilinear scar into an irregular scar that might otherwise be predisposed to a trap-door type deformity. The length of the limbs in W-plasty should be less than 6 mm. When using a curved W-plasty, the triangles of the outer limb must be wider than those of the inner limb in order that the tissue edges interlock properly. One advantage of the W-plasty is that it avoids the scar lengthening seen with Z-plasty. In addition, this W-plasty may be more amenable to orientation of the scar within RSTLs. However, the repetitive zig-zag pattern of W-plasty is often more readily discernible to the eye than more irregular Z-plasty. Figure 5 compares a curved serial Z-plasty against a curved W-plasty.

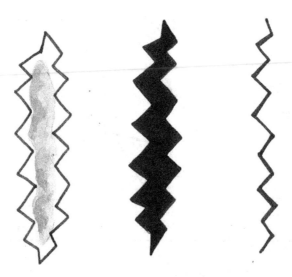

Fig. 4. W-plasty

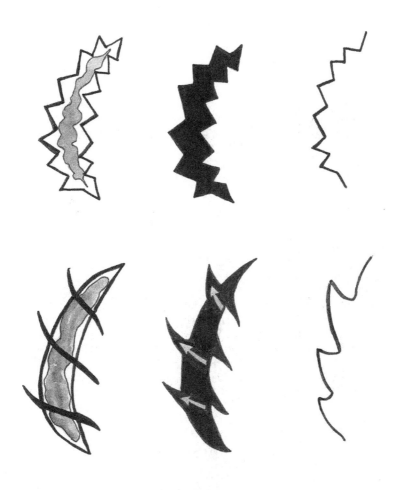

Fig. 5. Comparison of W-plasty versus serial Z-plasty

4.2.3 Geometric broken line closure

The geometric broken line closure is a variant of the W-plasty, in which a linear scar is rendered irregular by use of a mixture of triangles, squares, rectangles, and/or circles (Figure 6).(12) The geometric broken line closure is more labor intensive to construct than the W-plasty given its varied design but yields a less visually perceptible result. The geometric shapes are intended to have a random sequence that interlocks on upper and lower sides. When the rectangles or squares within the geometric broken line closure are perpendicular to RSTLs, use of extra triangles may minimize any unfavorable appearance.

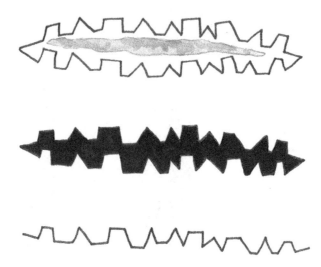

Fig. 6. Geometric Broken Line Closure

4.2.4 M-plasty

The M-plasty (Figure 7) minimizes the loss of surrounding healthy tissue at the site of a scar and also can minimize the length of the scar. When compared to the simple ellipse excision, the loss of healthy, normal tissue is decreased by approximately 50%. The price paid for this preservation of healthy tissue is having two limbs at each pole of the M-plasty. The M-plasty is constructed by diminishing the distance from the midpoint of the wound to the lateral extents of the excision. By advancing the lateral triangles of tissue into the wound in a V-Y advancement fashion, the scar is shortened.

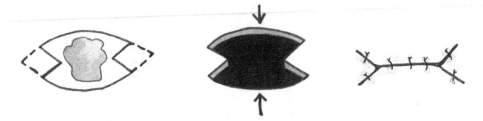

Fig. 7. M-plasty

4.3 Other surgical methods of scar revision

A variety of other surgical approaches are also useful in scar revision. Serial excision of scar is a logical extension of simple excision of ellipses in RSTLs. In this approach, a wound that would not readily close following complete excision is excised in multiple separate sittings to avoid undue stretch on the skin. Tissue expansion followed by excision may circumvent the need for serial excision if a sufficient area of skin for closure is created by the expander.

Usually 2 expanders are required to achieve the desired degree of skin expansion. The major risks of tissue expanders are infection and unintended trauma to the skin from distention.(13) A V to Y advancement flap (Figure 8) allows for recruitment of excess tissue from laterally and proximally into an area that has been shortened by contracture. This method is also useful when a soft tissue defect needs to be reconstructed. It is sometimes preferable to excise an entire cosmetic subunit before proceeding with reconstruction using a local flap.(14)

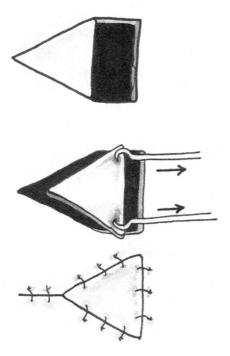

Fig. 8. V to Y advancement

4.4 Special considerations related to subsite

Each area of the head and neck has distinctive features with corresponding implications for the approach to scar revision. The various facial subsites differ in terms of RSTL orientation, solar exposure, skin thickness, pilosebaceous density, and muscle movement. The forehead, eyebrows, cheeks, nasolabial fold, and mentum are discussed below because of the special considerations that come into play for these areas.

4.4.1 Forehead

While simple fusiform excision yield favorable results in the upper forehead, at the junction of the forehead and glabella the RSTLs are virtually perpendicular. This orientation corresponds to the perpendicular orientation of corrugator and frontalis fibers. Scar revision in this area may require a combination a Z-plasty to reorient scars and irregularization with W-plasty. Botulinum toxin may attenuate the wrinkles of this area.

4.4.2 Eyebrow

The eyebrow region is a frequent area of unfavorable scarring that also warrants special consideration. Due to the prominence of the supraorbital rim, this site is prone to trauma in continuity with the forehead. Blunt trauma to this area may results in the underlying bone cutting the skin from beneath, as when the impact of a boxer's glove causes skin to shear against the underlying bone. This extensive soft tissue trauma predisposes to a significantly widened scar. While vertical incisions are commonly used elsewhere in scar revision, a beveled incision is needed in the eyebrow. The shafts of hair follicles are oriented obliquely; therefore, incisions made perpendicular to the skin are more likely to result in alopecia than beveled incisions that run parallel to the hair follicles. W-plasty is useful in camouflaging long, linear scars. Care must be taken to align the hairs when the eyebrow is divided by a scar.

4.4.3 Cheek, nasolabial fold, and mentum

The cheek, nasolabial fold, and mentum are also important areas in scar revision. The RSTLs of the cheek run from the zygoma to the mandible in a curved fashion. Many scars in this area run opposite the RSTLs and therefore require the use of a serial Z-plasty approach. When scars run parallel to the direction of RSTLs, a W-plasty will achieve excellent cosmesis. A terminal Z-plasty may achieve further irregularization.

The nasolabial fold is extremely useful in scar camouflage, and Z-plasty can be used to excellent advantage to reorient scars along the RSTLs. Only one of the two possible combinations of Z-plasty will yield an optimal cosmetic result, with the lateral limbs nearest the direction of the RSTLs. Scars along the mentum are effectively managed with W-plasty or Z-plasty for scars running parallel and oblique to RSTLs, respectively.

4.5 Adjunctive treatments

A variety of adjunctive techniques are available to assist in late wound management and scar camouflage. Many of these approaches are most effective when used as part of a surgical regimen, although some may prove useful alone. An important aspect of scar minimization is optimal postoperative care. This includes wound compression immediately following the procedure (such as using silicone sheets or micropore tape), UV protection (especially important in the first year after the procedure), and smoking cessation.

4.5.1 Dermabrasion and lasers

Dermabrasion and Laser skin resurfacing can be used to correct skin contour irregularities. Dermabrasion is useful to level a scar, to modify the texture of a scar, or to improve camouflage through blending with surrounding skin. It is typically performed approximately 6 to 8 weeks after W-plasty, Z-plasty, or geometric broken line closure.(15) Preoperative treatment with Retin-A will alleviate scarring, and antiviral therapy is indicated for patients with a history of herpetic infection. Care must be taken to avoid deep penetration into the reticular dermis, as excessive depth of dermabrasion is associated with risk of melanocyte loss and resulting permanent hypopigmentation. The adverse effects of dermabrasion on pigmentation are less significant in individuals with fairer skin. An occlusive dressing and moist ointment with regular cleansing will facilitate reepithelization. Hyperpigmented areas can be addressed with depigmentation agents, including hydroquinone, which blocks the production of melanin. This is available in 2%

concentrations over the counter or 4% concentrations by prescription, with stronger concentrations being more effective but more prone to local skin irritation. Azelaic acid and kojic acid are two other effective depigmentation agents. Depressed scars may be ameliorated with use of fat/dermis grafts or allograft dermal matrix grafts. CO_2 and Erbium lasers are also used for resurfacing. Lasers induce collagen reorganization and can thereby enhance camouflage, although variable depth of thermal damage and the potential for hypopigmentation are risks.(16) Intense pulsed light, KTP laser, and ND:YAG are among the techniques that have been used for vascular and pigmentary irregularities.(17;18)

4.5.2 Minimally invasive treatments

Noninvasive resurfacing can be achieved using fillers. Improved symmetry can be achieved with administration of botulinum toxin to weaken one side of the face if the contralateral side is weak or paralyzed. Plucking of brows may also camouflage irregularities. Cosmetics, hairstyling, and hair replacement have all been used to enhance results. Makeup, tattoos, and prosthetics also can find useful application. Aestheticians are particularly helpful in the postoperative period, both to improve appearance during healing and to prevent erythema from sun exposure. Aestheticians also may treat irregularities that are not amenable to surgical revision.

5. Special considerations: Hypertrophic and keloid scars

Hypertrophic scars and keloids are generally accepted to occur more commonly in young, darkly pigmented individuals. Clinically, hypertrophic scars exhibit excessive deposition within the scar, whereas keloid scars overgrow the original margins of an incision to involve adjacent tissues. Ultrastructurally, hypertrophic scars have parallel alignment of collagen sheets, whereas keloids have disorganized sheets. Keloids also demonstrate a greater increase in collagenase and proline hydroxylase than do hypetrophic scars.

Although a variety of nonsurgical treatments have been investigated for management of hypertophic scars and keloids, the most common approach is primary excision with serial injection of steroid. Other approaches have included serial excision, carbon dioxide laser excision, and use of skin grafting. Topical application of silicone sheeting over sites of keloid formation has been shown to be beneficial in some series, although the mechanism by which sheeting may improve scar outcomes remains uncertain.(19) Benefit may be related to the improved hydration of tissues associated with this approach, as nonsilicone gel dressings may have similar efficacy.(20) Pulsed-dye lasers have been found effective for hypertrophic scars.(21) Other methods, including creams/vitamins, pressure dressings, and interferons have also been suggested. Thus there are a variety of options for treatment of scars. The role of compression garments, silicone sheets, scar massage and ultrasound should also be considered.

6. Concluding remarks

Late wound management after trauma includes surgical camouflaging of the aesthetically unacceptable scar and correction of functional impairments related to aberrant wound healing. The surgeon must remember that patients undergoing these procedures may harbor a significant emotional component to their injury. Optimal results are achieved through an in depth understanding of the mechanisms of scar formation and application of the optimal surgical technique, taking into consideration the characteristics of the site.

7. References

[1] Kaplan B, Potter T, Moy RL, Kaplan B, Potter T, Moy RL. Scar revision. Dermatologic Surgery 1997; 23(6):435-442.

[2] Zakkak TB, Griffin JE, Jr., Max DP, Zakkak TB, Griffin JEJ, Max DP. Posttraumatic scar revision: a review and case presentation. Journal of Cranio-Maxillofacial Trauma 1998; 4(1):35-41.

[3] Thomas JR, Ehlert TK, Thomas JR, Ehlert TK. Scar revision and camouflage. Otolaryngologic Clinics of North America 1990; 23(5):963-973.

[4] Kokoska MS, Thomas JR. Scar Revision. In: Papel ID, editor. Facial Plastic and Reconstructive Surgery. New York: Thieme, 2002: 55-60.

[5] Schweinfurth JM, Fedok F, Schweinfurth JM, Fedok F. Avoiding pitfalls and unfavorable outcomes in scar revision. Facial Plastic Surgery 2001; 17(4):273-278.

[6] Goslen JB, Goslen JB. Wound healing for the dermatologic surgeon. Journal of Dermatologic Surgery & Oncology 1988; 14(9):959-972.

[7] Thomas JR, Prendiville S, Thomas JR, Prendiville S. Update in scar revision. Facial Plastic Surgery Clinics of North America 2002; 10(1):103-111.

[8] Moran ML, Moran ML. Scar revision. Otolaryngologic Clinics of North America 2001; 34(4):767-780.

[9] Thomas JR, Mobley SR. Scar Revision and Camouflage. In: Cummings CW, Flint PW, Harker LA, Haughey BH, Richardson MA, Robbins KT et al., editors. Cummings Otolaryngology Head & Neck Surgery. Philadelphia: Elsevier, 2005: 572-581.

[10] Zide MF, Zide MF. Scar revision with hypereversion. Journal of Oral & Maxillofacial Surgery 1996; 54(9):1061-1067.

[11] Kelleher JC, Kelleher JC. W-plasty scar revision and its extended use. Clinics in Plastic Surgery 1977; 4(2):247-254.

[12] Harnick DB, Harnick DB. Broken geometrical pattern used for facial scar revision. Laryngoscope 1984; 94(6):841-842.

[13] Mostafapour SP, Murakami CS, Mostafapour SP, Murakami CS. Tissue expansion and serial excision in scar revision. Facial Plastic Surgery 2001; 17(4):245-252.

[14] Clark JM, Wang TD, Clark JM, Wang TD. Local flaps in scar revision. [Facial Plastic Surgery 2001; 17(4):295-308.

[15] Harmon CB, Zelickson BD, Roenigk RK, Wayner EA, Hoffstrom B, Pittelkow MR et al. Dermabrasive scar revision. Immunohistochemical and ultrastructural evaluation. Dermatologic Surgery 1995; 21(6):503-508.

[16] Alster T, Zaulyanov-Scanlon L, Alster T, Zaulyanov-Scanlon L. Laser scar revision: a review. [Review] [46 refs]. Dermatologic Surgery 2007; 33(2):131-140.

[17] Cassuto D, Emanuelli G, Cassuto D, Emanuelli G. Non-ablative scar revision using a long pulsed frequency doubled Nd:YAG laser. Journal of Cosmetic & Laser Therapy 2003; 5(3-4):135-139.

[18] Westine JG, Lopez MA, Thomas JR, Westine JG, Lopez MA, Thomas JR. Scar revision. Facial Plastic Surgery Clinics of North America 2005; 13(2):325-331.

[19] Katz BE, Katz BE. Silicone gel sheeting in scar therapy. Cutis 1995; 56(1):65-67.

[20] de Oliveira GV, Nunes TA, Magna LA, Cintra ML, Kitten GT, Zarpellon S et al. Silicone versus nonsilicone gel dressings: a controlled trial. Dermatologic Surgery 2001; 27(8):721-726.

[21] Bradley DT, Park SS, Bradley DT, Park SS. Scar revision via resurfacing. Facial Plastic Surgery 2001; 17(4):253-262.

2

The Social Limits of Reconstructive Surgery: Stigma in Facially Disfigured Cancer Patients

Alessandro Bonanno

Texas State University System Regents Professor of Sociology
Department of Sociology, Sam Houston State University
USA

1. Introduction

The last few decades have been particularly significant in terms of advancements of scientific knowledge and medical knowledge in particular. Within medicine, reconstructive surgical procedures have achieved spectacular results. While the popularity of elective cosmetic procedures has reached unprecedented – and in some instances socially concerning – proportions, the beneficial effects of reconstructive surgery for trauma and/or disease generated cases have been significant. This is also the instance of patients affected by cancer of the head and neck. The multiplicity and frequencies of these forms of cancers now generate a large enough group of patients who face the condition of survivors with an added social problem: The stigma of being facially disfigured.

This chapter probes the issue of the limits of reconstructive surgery as a form of intervention that while addresses relevant medical problems, it also opens up new social problems. In this case, the issue studied is the social consequences of reconstructive surgery on head and neck cancer patients. In particular, this chapter investigates the manner in which social stigma is generated as cancer survivors re-enter society after reconstructive surgery and associated treatments concluded their cancer therapies.

Developments recorded in medicine increasingly generate the long term survival of cancer patients (American Cancer Society, 2009; Mood 1997; Davis, Wingo and Parker 1998). These medical improvements have also had beneficial results for head and neck patients (Davis, Roumanas and Nishimura 1997; Dropkin 1999). In the instance of this particular group of patients, needed surgical intervention signifies the removal of portions of the face that are affected by the malignancy. One of the common consequences of this type of intervention is the alteration of the patient's face and the permanent facial disfigurement that it entails (American Cancer Society, 2009). Surgical procedures to restore the original facial appearance are common. Similarly common is the availability of increasingly sophisticated – albeit often costly and difficult to use – prostheses (Davis, Roumanas and Nishimura 1997). Reconstructive surgery is central in the processes and its success is evident. However, the severity of the alterations caused by the removal of the malignancy, make a restoration of the normal shape of the face virtually impossible. The result is that the survival of the patient and the success of the surgical interventions and medical treatments translate into a social problem: patients remain facially disfigured. Survivors typically live the rest of their lives with facial disfigurement.

Because of the importance of the face in social relations –a central element of communication (Kish and Lansdown, 2000; Macgregor, 1990), and an item employed to attribute both "normality" and ownership of socially desirable characteristics (Furness, Garrud, Faulder, Swift 2006; Goffman, 1963; Hawkesworth, 2001; Hughes, 1998; Ishii, Carey, Byrne, Zee and Ishii. 2009; Macgregor, 1974) –individuals with the abnormal face experience stigma and are treated differently than the rest of the members of society. They are labeled as different and treated as such (Bull and Stevens 1981; Callahan 2004:75; Furness et al. 2006; Hawkesworth 2001; Hughes 1998; Kent 2000; Macgregor 1951; 1974; 1990; Millstone 2008). According to available literature, facially disfigured patients' interaction with acquaintances and strangers – these are members of secondary social groups – is viewed as a constant source of stigma. Acquaintances and strangers are seen as exercising prejudice (negative feelings and/or beliefs) and/or discrimination (actual differential treatment) against patients. However, the characteristics of the interaction process have not been clearly mapped out leaving a gap in the available knowledge on the manner in which stigma is actually created (Hughes, 1998; Macgregor 1990; van Doorne, van Waas and Bergsma 1994). The knowledge obtained from this study contributes to the reduction of this gap and can be employed to inform caregivers as they deal with disfigured patients and their families.

2. Methods

This is a qualitative research based on in-depth interviews with a purposive sample fifteen cancer patients who underwent surgery to treat head and neck malignancies that affected their facial appearance. Patients were selected through the review of records at a major cancer center located in the Southwest of the United States of America. Eligibility criteria excluded persons under the age of 18, those who had surgery six month prior to the interview, those who were receiving active cancer therapy at the time of the interview, and those who could not express themselves in English. In-depth individual interviews were conducted between January 2008 and February 2010. Twenty potential participants were contacted. Two of them could not participate for scheduling problems and three refused to be part of the project. Finally, a total of eight men and seven women were interviewed. The median age of these patients was 66 years and the youngest patient was 31 and the oldest 81. The patients included in the study all underwent orbital exenteration. At the time of the interview, the post-surgical period ranged from ten months to thirty five years and the median was five years. Some patients underwent additional reconstructive and plastic surgical procedures. While the extent of disfigurement varied, all of the patients were left with significant alterations in their facial appearance. An illustration of the degree of disfigurement can be seen through the photos accompanying this chapter. Photos 1 and 2 are illustration of severe cases of disfigurement after ablative surgery. Photo 3 illustrates a case in which surgery allowed the use of a prosthesis that adequately concealed the disfigurement (Photo 4). One family member for each of the participating patients was also interviewed.

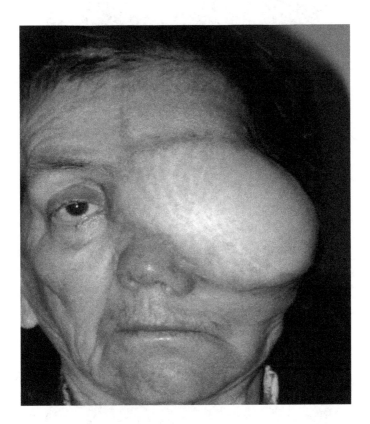

Photo 1

In the course of the interviews both patients and family members were asked to reconstruct instances of encounters with strangers and acquaintances. The interviews were audio recorded with the participants' and family members' consent and the transcribed texts were analyzed employing the qualitative methodology Grounded Theory (Charmaz 2006). The guiding assumption of the study was to develop analytical categories (variables) that would identify patterns of interaction between facially disfigured cancer patients and members of secondary groups. These categories were created to illustrate the collective action process leading to stigma rather than the manner in which patients felt in the interaction process itself. Analytical categories were constructed through line-by-line coding and constant comparative analysis (Charmaz 2006). Once developed, codes were grouped in relevant categories that were saturated as no new relevant properties of these categories emerged. Along with saturation, the negative cases technique was employed to validate categories and their properties (Charmaz 2006; Holton 2007). In this case, there was a deliberate search for situations that would contradict the analysis. Their absence was employed to validate the conclusions (Charmaz 2006).

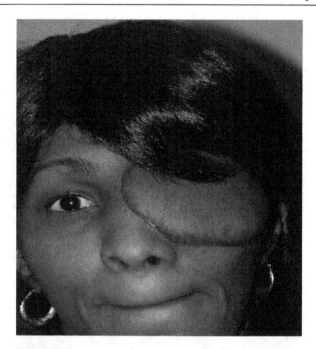

Photo 2

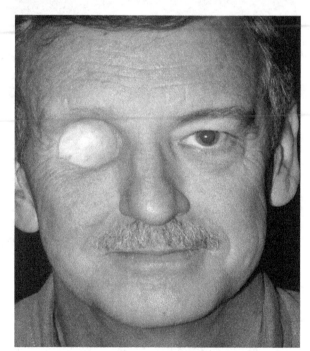

Photo 3.

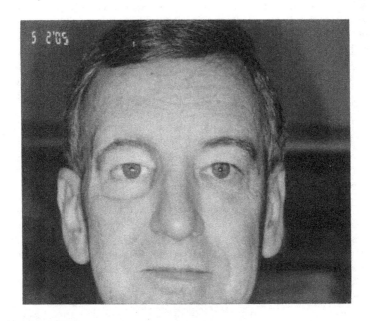

Photo 4.

Three primary analytical categories were generated to illustrate patients' interaction with secondary groups leading to stigmatization: Intrusion, sympathy and benign neglect. Intrusion indicates interaction based on unsolicited attention paid to patients. Strangers and acquaintances ask unwanted questions, make unwelcome remarks, stare and/or make their unspoken curiosity felt. Sympathy refers to unsolicited comments and/or actions showing support to patients and the desire to be of assistance, while benign neglect denotes a situation in which interaction is characterized by people not paying particular attention to patients. Additionally, small and large groups also emerged as relevant categories as differences exist in interaction within these groups. Intrusion, sympathy and benign neglect describe conditions that are decreasingly favorable to the creation of stigma. As intrusion fosters stigma, benign neglect defines patterns on interaction in which patients are granted that kind indifference that is "normally" given to strangers and/or distant attention granted to acquaintances.

3. Brief review of salient literature on cancer generated facial disfigurement

Stigma is defined as the "social disgrace" associated with people who are considered different (Goffman 1963). Difference is socially constructed and is the outcome of discrepancies between an individual virtual social identity (expectations about what that individual ought to be) and his/her actual social identity (the attributes he/she actually posses) (Goffman 1963:2). When the actual social identity is perceived as departing from normality, the individual is stigmatized. Stigma is attached to an individual's feature "that is deeply discrediting" and that separates that person from the group of the "normals." However, its actual genesis is relational as he/she is constantly compared to other members of society. Therefore, some specific individual characteristics generate stigma in some instances but not in others (de-stigmatization). Stigma is generated by the existence of a number of blemishes. There are those of individual character such as homosexuality, dishonesty, imprisonment, radical political behavior, and addiction. There are those of tribal stigma that are related to a person's group of reference such as religion, ethnicity or race. And there are those of "abominations of the body" that refer to physical abnormalities. Facial disfigurement pertains to this last category.

Stigma has been widely studied and this production includes works such as those on stigma generated from diseases (i.e., cancer and AIDS) (Fife and Wright, 2000), physical disabilities (Cahill and Eggleston, 1995; Susman 1994 Link and Phelan 2001:365-66; Jacobi 1994), and mental health (Angermeyer and Matschinger 1994; Corrigan and Penn 1999; Cahill and Eggleston, 1995). Despite this wealth of contributions, stigma caused by facial disfigurement has been the subject of only a relatively small number of works (Clarke 1999; Clarke et al. 2003; Kent, 2000; Kish and Lansdown 2000; Hughes, 1998; Pruizinsky et al. 2006). These analyses stress the social importance of the face, the problems that affect those who display visible facial blemishes and indicate that the face represents one of the most notable physical attributes and a significant source of social information prior to, and during, social interaction (Anderson and Franke 2002; Cole 1998; Furness et al. 2006; Goffman 1963; Hawkesworth 2001; Hughes, 1998; Macgregor 1974) Accordingly, people possessing an attractive face are not only considered physically pleasing, but they are often viewed as endowed with intellectual and emotional characteristics such as intelligence, kindness, and high morality and better treated by others than less attractive individuals (Bull and Rumsey 1998; Cash and Pruzinsky 2002; Feingold 1992; Kish and Lansdown 2000; Macgregor 1990). Facially disfigured individuals commonly engender negative responses by other members of society (Callahan, 2004; Hagedoorm and Molleman, 2006: Kish and Lansdown 2000). Stigma is further divided into felt stigma and enacted stigma (Jacobi 1994). Felt stigma refers to situations in which the individual perceive that he/she is viewed as different. Enacted stigma refers to explicit actions that result in stigma. In both instances, stigma is a relational process as it involves at least two interacting parties.

Facially disfigured cancer patients are primarily concerned with surviving cancer. Yet, as their survival becomes apparent, they become concerned with disfigurement: a situation that affects both patients and their family members (Bonanno 2009; van Doorne, van Waas and Bergsma 1994). The association of cancer and disfigurement is persistent. Therapy almost inevitably mandates surgical removal of cancer-affected parts of the face making it an undesirable consequence of successful medical intervention (Callahan 2004; Millsopp, Brandom, Humphris, and Lowe 2006; Valente 2004).

Among the limits of this otherwise important literature, is the lack of attention paid to the social process that generates stigma (Kent 2000:199; Clarke 1999; Furness et al., 2006; Thompson and Kent 2001). In particular, limited attention has been paid to the fact that disfigurement and stigma are socially constructed and generated through processes of interaction that involve multiple actors and take different forms according to the settings in which they unfold (Kent 2000). Accordingly, it is important to recognize that attention paid to the adaptation of patients to their condition of facially disfigured is only one component of an otherwise much more complex process in which "others" are often the source of stigma. In this respect, and while evidence indicates that society as a whole is the primary source of stigma (Callahan, 2004; Hagedoorm and Molleman, 2006; Kish and Lansdown 2000; Pruzinsky et al. 2006; van Doorne et al. 1994:325), the manners through which stigma emerges in interaction between the patients and "others" requires further investigation (Bonanno, Choi and Esmaeli 2008). More specifically, because stigma does not occur homogeneously, it is important to identify the circumstances in which it appears in interaction and the ways in which interaction can be directed to avoid the occurrence of stigma. Van Doorne et al. (1994), for instance, indicate that interaction with strangers almost certainly leads to the creation of stigma. They, however, stress that interaction with acquaintances requires additional investigation. The present study addresses this gap in current knowledge.

4. Results

A model of interaction patterns between facially disfigured cancer patients and members of secondary groups was generated through the application of Grounded theory (Charmaz 2006; Holton 2007). Figure 1 graphically synthesizes this model.

In the case of the interaction of patients with members of secondary groups, three fundamental analytical categories were developed. *Intrusion* indicates interaction based on unsolicited attention paid to patients by strangers and acquaintances. People ask unwanted questions, make unwelcome remarks, stare and make their unspoken curiosity felt. *Sympathy* refers to unsolicited comments and/or actions showing support to patients and the desire to be of assistance. Finally, *benign neglect* denotes a situation in which interaction is characterized by people not paying particular attention to patients and giving them that "civil inattention" and/or distant attention that characterizes everyday interaction among strangers. Benign neglect is the desired form of interaction as it does not generate stigma.

Interaction patterns change in regard to the size of interacting groups. Interaction characterized by intrusion in large and small groups generates stigma. These are *felt* and *enacted* forms of stigma. Sympathy produces enacted stigma in interaction in small groups and enacted and felt stigma in interaction within large groups. As by definition, benign neglect does not produce stigma in interaction within all groups. Following are more detailed illustrations of these patterns.

Intrusion – This is a situation that engenders stigma in interaction within small and large groups alike. Members of interacting groups grant disfigured individuals the particular status of "different" through the construction of actions based on unwanted attention. Strangers and acquaintances' questions, stares, remarks constitute elements that transform disfigurement into stigma. Of particular importance are situations in which patients remain for relatively long periods of time in a relatively still position in full view of others. Because of this *immobility*, patients tend to feel uncomfortable. This felt stigma, however, can translate into enacted stigma as stares, comments, or questions characterized the behavior of others. The unusual shape of patient's face makes strangers and acquaintances curious. As this *curiosity* is made explicit, stigma occurs. This is the case even when interacting individuals attempt to conceal their intrusive behavior. This *concealed enacted stigma* refers to actions of intrusions accompanied by attempts to hide them from patients. Patients tend to feel *resentment* to intrusive actions. They resent the unwanted attention of others and often express this resentment by defining these actions as "rude" and "inconsiderate." Simultaneously, patients display *unconcerned awareness*. This is a pattern in which patients remain aware of stigmatizing actions but simultaneously indicate that are not affected by them.

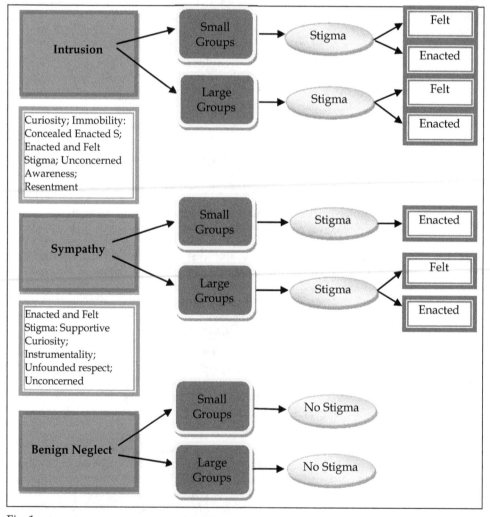

Fig. 1.

Sympathy – It refers to intrusive patterns of interaction in which individuals provide and/or manifest support to facially disfigured patients. It creates enacted stigma in small group interaction and felt and enacted stigma in large group interaction. In the case of small group interaction, *supportive curiosity* occurs. It refers to questions that people ask about patients' appearance that are accompanied by actions and expressions that are supportive of patients. It is a form of enacted stigma. The expression "everybody is nice," frequently reported by patients, captures this pattern of interaction. Patients do not experience felt stigma as they feel comfortable with the support that strangers and acquaintances offer. In large group interaction, patients may use this offered support to their advantage even when it is not necessary. This *instrumentality* is not exercised in small groups. Interaction in large groups, however, leads to stigma when offered assistance is viewed as unnecessary and/or exaggerated in relation to the actual physical conditions of patients. Simultaneously, when sympathy guided action transcends established expectations and creates *unfounded attention* enacted stigma occurs in small and large groups. Because of their status of cancer survivors and facially disfigured individuals, patients are granted what they perceive as undeserved respect. These actions create felt stigma.

Benign Neglect – refers to interaction in which strangers and acquaintances do not pay particular attention to disfigured individuals. It is that common pattern that characterizes interaction among people who are not familiar with each other. While people are aware of the presence of others, they do not focus on, nor pay particular attention to, their actions. As Macgregor (1974: 60) put it, "it is that civil inattention normally granted to others in society." Because of its "normality," interaction characterized by benign neglect becomes particularly important in situations in which difference is present. Facially disfigured individuals not only feel comfortable during these interactions, but also acknowledge the fact that they are treated normally without any particular emphasis placed on their physical appearance.

5. Relevance of these findings for surgeons and other caregivers

This study demonstrates the ways in which interaction between facially disfigure cancer patients and secondary groups creates stigma. Because only limited knowledge is available on this topic, caregivers should use these results to assist patients and provide needed information and assistance to patients' family members. Through a grounded theory analysis, the study identifies key types of interaction patterns related to social stigma. These findings add to existing knowledge in a variety of ways. First, they point out that interaction between facially disfigure cancer patients and secondary groups is not a uniform process but it varies according to different settings and groups. It follows that current knowledge that indicates that "the reaction of people on the streets or in the neighborhood is …. consistent: they stare at most patient with facial defect" (van Doorne at al 1994:325; see also Hughes 1998; Macgregor 1990), while overall accurate, requires to be specified. This research demonstrates that the behavior of members of secondary groups consists of three distinct interaction patterns.

Benign neglect is the only type of interaction that does not create stigma. It refers to "normal" interaction as individuals are aware of the presence of others but do not pay particular attention to them. Accordingly, patients and their family members should be informed on the importance of creating conditions that lead to this type of interaction. In particular, patients and family members should be instructed on the tendency of people to pay unwanted attention to patients. This is a situation that should be addressed through action planning and education whereby patients ought to plan their social activities carefully. Similarly, the general public should receive education on the conditions of these patients[1].

Interaction characterized by intrusion consistently generates felt and enacted stigma. Episodes of felt and enacted stigma occur in small and large group settings, making it the most difficult type of interaction for patients and family members. Patients and their families should be advised of the difficulties that episodes of intrusion generate. Strangers and acquaintances alike will ask questions, make comments, stare and make other intrusive actions. A number of additional elements characterize this type of interaction. The categories of curiosity; immobility; unconcerned awareness and resentment discussed above frequently accompany intrusion. As indicated above, educational efforts should be made to sensitize the general public on episodes of intrusion. It is also important to inform patients and their family members that these conditions may or may not be alleviated by reconstructive surgery.

In the case of interaction characterized by sympathy, stigma develops in different ways in small groups than in large groups. In small groups stigma takes the form of enacted stigma. In large groups it takes the forms of both enacted and felt stigma. While sympathy indicates that interacting individuals either provide or manifest support to facially disfigured patients, it also refers to the fact that this interaction ultimately creates stigma. The categories of supportive curiosity, instrumentality and unfounded respect characterize this type of interaction. Caregivers should make clear to patients and family members that the desire of strangers and acquaintances to assist patients does not necessarily translate into a non-stigmatized interaction. Accordingly, efforts to educate interested parties on this contradictory situation can be beneficial.

Second, this study indicates that acquaintances' interaction with patients does not differ significantly from that recorded for strangers. Both strangers and acquaintances contribute to the creation of stigma when intrusion and sympathy occur. Both groups are capable, however, to establish interaction based on benign neglect. These findings add to existing knowledge by clarifying patterns of interaction between patients and acquaintances.

Third, this research underscores the importance of approaching the creation of stigma for facially disfigured cancer patients in relational terms. Stigma emerges as the product of interaction. As such, it involves facially disfigured patients and other segments of society as they interact in varying ways and with varying results. While the study of the manner through which individuals respond to disfigurement remains important, an enhanced understanding of the construction of stigma is achieved by considering the collective dimension of this process. Caregivers should be aware of this aspect and avoid the

---

[1] The patterns of actions needed to address stigma are not the topic of this chapter. However, it is important to note that both education of the public and action planning are to be considered two of the most important strategies to address this problem.

presentation of stigma as an issue that pertains exclusively to the patients' individual sphere. Stigma is a collective process that involves a multiplicity of actors.

Finally, the issue of stigma associated to cancer generated facial disfigurement is the byproduct of advancements in medicine and surgical techniques. It is a situation that is the outcome of the success of scientific advancements. However, it is a state of affairs that cannot be address exclusively by medicine in general and surgical actions in particular. It requires a multidisciplinary effort and the cooperation of multiple actors in the medical sciences as well as the social and behavioral sciences. Accordingly, it is important that surgeons become aware of this and similar conditions and that these situations become integrated into training protocols. Surgeons as well as other caregivers should be exposed to knowledge about the creation of pertinent social problems and to the boundaries that surgical intervention entails for the overall quality of life of patients.

6. References

Angermeyer M. & Matschinger H. (1994). Lay beliefs about schizophrenic disorder: the results of a population study in Germany.*Acta Psychiatrica Scandinavica*. 89, 39-45.

American Cancer Society. (2009). Detailed guide: Eye cancer. Retrieved July 5, 2009 from www.cancer.org.

Anderson, R.C. & Franke, K.A. (2002). Psychological and psychosocial implications of head and neck cancer. *Internet Journal of Mental Health*, 1 (2), 55-64.

Berremberg, J.L. (1989). Attitudes towards cancer as a function of experience with the disease: A test of three models. *Psychology and Health*, 3,233-243.

Bloom, J. & Kessler, L. (1994). Emotional support following cancer: A test of the stigma and social activity hypothesis. *Journal of Health and Social Behavior*, 35,118-133.

Bonanno, A. & Choi J.Y. (2009). Psychosocial aspects of orbitofacial disfigurement in cancer patients. In B. Esmaeli, (ed.) *Ophthalmic Oncology* (pp. 311-319). Norwell, MA: Springer.

Bonanno, A., Choi, J.Y., & Esmaeli, B. (2008, March). The contradictions of medical sociology understanding of stigma in facially disfigured individuals. Paper presented at the Annual Meeting of the Southwest Social Science Association. Las Vegas, NV.

Bull, R. & Rumsey, N. (1988). *The social psychology of facial appearance*. New York: Springer Vale.

Bull, R. & Stevens. J. (1981). The effects of facial disfigurement on helping behavior. *The Italian Journal of Psychology*, 8 (1) April.

Cahill, S., and Eggleston, R. (1995). Reconsidering the stigma of physical disability: wheelchair use and public kindness. *The Sociological Quarterly*, 36(4), 681-698.

Callahan, C. (2004). Facial disfigurement and sense of self in head and neck cancer. *Social Work in Health Care*, 40(2),73-87.

Cash T.F., & Pruzinsky, T. (eds.) (2002). *Body image. A handbook of theory, research, and clinical practice*. New York: The Guilford Press.

Charmaz, K. (2006). *Constructing grounded theory. A practical guide though qualitative analysis*. London: Sage.

Clarke, A. (1999). Psychosocial aspects of facial disfigurement: problems, management and the role of a lay-led organization. *Psychology, Health and Medicine,* 4(2),127-142.

Clarke, A., Rumsey, N., Collin, JRO & Wyn-Williams M.. (2003). Psychological distress associated with disfiguring eye conditions. *Eye,* 17,35-40.

Cole, J. (1998). *About face.* Cambridge: The MIT Press.

Corrigan, P.W. & Penn, D. L. (1999). Lessons from social psychology on discrediting psychiatric stigma. *American Psychologist,* 54,765-76.

Davis, K., Wingo, P., & Parker S. (1998). Cancer statistics by race and ethnicity. *CA Cancer J Clin* 1,31-47.

Davis, K., Roumanas E.D., & Nishimura R.D. (1997). Prosthetic-surgical collaboration in the rehabilitation of patients with head and neck defects. *Otolaryngologic Clinics of North America,* 30 (4), 631-645.

Dropkin, M.J. (1999). Body image and quality of life after head and neck cancer surgery. *Cancer, Practice* November/December 7(6), 309-313.

Esmaeli, B. (2009) (ed.). *Ophthalmic Oncology.* Norwell, MA: Springer.

Fife, B. L., & Wright, E. R. (2000). The dimensionality of stigma: A comparison of its impact on the self of persons with HIV/AIDS and cancer. *Journal of Health Social Behavior,* 42, 50-67.

Feingold, A. (1992). Good looking people are not what we think. *Psychological Bulletin,* 111, 304-341.

Furness, P., Garrud, P., Faulder, A., & Swift, J. (2006). Coming to terms. A grounded theory of adaptation to facial surgery in adulthood. *Journal of Health Psychology,* 11 (3), 453-466.

Goffman, E. (1963). *Stigma. Notes on the management of spoiled identity.* New York: Simon & Shuster.

Hagedoorn, M. & Molleman, E., (2006). Facial disfigurement in patients with head and neck cancer: The role of social self-efficiency. *Health Psychology,* 25(5), 643-647

Hawkesworth, M. (2001). "Disabling spatialities and the regulation of a visible secret." *Urban Studies,* 38(2),299-318.

Hughes, M. (1998). *The social consequences of facial disfigurement.* Aldershot: Ashgate.

Holton. J.A. (2007). The Coding Process and its Challenges. in A, Bryant and K. Charmaz, *The SAGE handbook of grounded theory* (pp. 265-289). Los Angeles: SAGE Publications.

Ishii, L., Carey, J. Byrne, P. Zee, D.S., and Ishii, M. (2009). "Measuring attention bias to peripheral facial deformities" *The American Laryngological,* 119, 459-465.

Jackson, L. A. (2002). Physical attractiveness: A sociostructural perspective. In Cash, T.F. and Pruzinsky, T. (Eds.) *Body image. A handbook of theory, research, and clinical practice* (pp. 13-21). New York: The Guilford Press.

Jacobi, A. (1994). Felt versus enacted stigma: A concept revisited. *Social Science and Medicine,* 38(2), 269-274.

Kent, G. (2000). Understanding the experiences of people with disfigurements: An integration of four models of social and psychological functioning. *Psychology, Health & Medicine,* 5(2),117-129.

Kish, V. & Lansdown, R. (2000). Meeting the psychosocial impact of facial disfigurement: developing a clinical service for children and families. *Clinical Child Psychology and Psychiatry*, 5(4), 497-512.

Link, B.G. and Phelan, J.C.. (2001). Conceptualizing stigma. *Annual Review of Sociology*, 27,363-85.

Macgregor, F. (1990). Facial disfigurement: problems and management of social interaction and implication for mental health. *Aesthetic and Plastic Surgery*, 14 (4), 249-257. (1974). *Transformation and Identity: The Face and Plastic Surgery*. New Your: Quadrangle/The New York Times Book Co.

Millsopp, L. Brandom, L., Humphris G., & Lowe D., (2006). Facial appearance after operations for oral and oropharyngeal cancer: A comparison of casenotes and patient-completed questionnaire. *British Journal of Oral and Maxillofacial Surgery*, 44, 358-363.

Millstone, S. (2008). Facial Discrimination. *Therapy Today*, 19, 35-38.

Mood, D. W. (1997). Cancers of the head and neck. In C. Varricchio (ed.) *A Cancer Source Book for Nurses* (pp. 271-283). Sudbury, MA: Jones and Bartlett Publishers.

Mosher, C. $ Danoff-Burg, S. (2007). Death anxiety and cancer related stigma: A terror management analysis *Death Studies*, 31,855-907.

Newell, R. J. (1999). Altered body image: A fear-avoidance model of psycho-social difficulties following disfigurement. *Journal of Advanced Nursing*, 30 (5),1230-38.

Partridge, J. (1998). Changing faces: taking up Macgregor' s challenge. *Journal of Burn Care and Rehabilitation*, 19,174-180.

Pruzinsky, T.; Levine, E., Persing J.A., Barth, J.T., & Obrecht, R.. (2006). "Facial trauma and facial cancer." in Sarwer, D.B., Pruzinsky, T. F., T., Goldwyn, R.M., & Persing, J.A. *Psychological Aspects of Reconstructive and Cosmetic Plastic Surgery: Clinical, Empirical and Ethical Perspectives* (pp.125-143). Philadelphia PA: Lippincott Williams.

Rybarczyk B.D, & Behel, J.M. (2002). Rehabilitation medicine and body image. In Cash T.F. & Pruzinsky, T. (eds.) *Body image. A handbook of theory, research, and clinical practice* (pp. 387-393). New York: The Guilford Press.

Susman, J. (1994). Disability, stigma and deviance. *Social Science and Medicine*, 38, 15-22.

Synnott, A. (1989). Truth and Goodness, Mirrors and Masks – Part I: A sociology of beauty and the face. *The British Journal of Sociology*, 40 (4): 607-636.

Thompson, A. & Kent, G., (2001). Adjusting to disfigurement: process involved in dealing with being visibly different. *Clinical Psychology Review*, 21(5):663-682.

Valente, S. (2004). "Visual disfigurement and depression." *Plastic Surgical Nursing*, 24 (4) 14-146.

van Doorne J.M., van Waas, M.A., & Bergsma, J. (1994). Facial disfigurement after cancer resection: a problem with an extra dimension. *Journal of Investigative Surgery*, 7 (4):321-326.

Vickery, LE; Latchford, G., Hewinson, J., Bellew, M., & Faber, T. (2003). The impact of head and neck cancer and facial disfigurement on the quality of life of patients and their partners. *Head & Neck* 25 (4):289-96.

Weiner, B., Perry, R.P., & Magnusson, J. (1988). "An attributional analysis of reaction to stigma." *Journal of Social Issues*, 35 (1):120-55.

3

Local Antibiotic Therapy in the Treatment of Bone and Soft Tissue Infections

Stefanos Tsourvakas
Orthopedic Department, General Hospital of Trikala
Greece

1. Introduction

Bone and soft tissue infections are serious problems in orthopedic and reconstructive surgery. Especially, chronic osteomyelitis is a difficult infection to treat and eradicate. Long term parenteral antibiotics with multiple surgical debridements are often required for effective therapy (Cierny & Mader, 1984). Therefore, it is understandable that continuous efforts are being made and complete one or other element in the treatment of bone and soft tissue infections.

There is a long history of local antibiotic use for the treatment of bone and soft tissue infections. During World War I, Alexander Fleming observed that locally applied antiseptics failed to sterilize chronically infected wounds, but they did reduce the burden of bacteria (Fleming, 1920). In 1939, the instillation of sulfanilamide crystals, along with thorough debridement, hemostasis, primary closure and immobilization, resulted in a reduced infection rate for open fractures (Jensen et al, 1939). As additional systemic antimicrobial agents became available, interest in the topical treatment of wounds waned, but the management of established osteomyelitis remained problematic. In the 1960s, the method of closed wound irrigation-suction was popularized as a method which could be used to deliver high concentrations of an antibiotic after debridement (Dombrowski & Dunn, 1965). An alternative method for delivering high concentrations of an antibiotic to sites of lower extremity osteomyelitis was isolation and perfusion (Organ, 1971).

The delivery of local antibiotics for the treatment of musculoskeletal infection has become increasingly popular for a variety of reasons. The basis for developing and using local antibiotic delivery systems in the treatment of bone and soft tissue infection is either to supplement or to replace the use of systemic antibiotics. High local levels of antibiotics facilitate delivery of antibiotics by diffusion to avascular areas of wounds that are inaccessible by systemic antibiotics and in many circumstances the organisms that are resistant to drug concentrations achieved by systemic antibiotic are susceptible to the extremely high local drug concentrations provided by local antibiotic delivery.

The local use of antibiotics to prevent and treat bone and soft tissue infections was revived in Germany with the widespread use of prosthetic joint replacement, a situation in which infections were not anticipated consequence of trauma or sepsis but a devastating complication of elective surgery (Buchholz & Engelbrecht, 1970). However, it is from the year 2000 that research on local delivery of antibiotics to bone has gained considerable attention. Note that the numbers of publications in the last five years are double and decuple published in earlier decades (Soundrapandian et al, 2009).

Bacterial infection in orthopedic and reconstructive surgery can be devastating, and is associated with significant morbidity and poor functional outcomes (Haddad et al, 2004). Operative treatments (excision of infected and devascularized tissues, obliteration of dead space, restoration of blood supply and soft tissue coverage, stabilization and reconstruction of the damaged bone), removal of all foreign bodies and systemic antimicrobial therapy are three crucial components of the treatment of these cases (Lazzarini et al, 2004). A long-term course of systemic antibiotherapy has been considered essential, but these prolonged therapies can result in side effects or toxicity. In order to achieve therapeutic drug concentration in the affected area, high systemic doses are generally required which can further worsen toxic side effects (Nandi et al, 2009). Antibiotic treatment may be inadequate or ineffective in patients with poorly vascularized infected tissues and osteonecrosis, which is often present in cases of osteomyelitis. Moreover, normal doses of systemic antibiotics may be insufficient to breach the glycocalyx or biofilm produced by the infecting bacteria (El-Husseiny et al, 2011). Despite intensive therapy, advances in surgical techniques, and development of new antimicrobials, relapse rate are still significant and treatment of bone and soft tissue infections remain challenging.

New methods such as local delivery of antibiotics have evolved in an attempt to improve the prognosis of patients with musculoskeletal infections. The use of local antibiotic delivery system has become an accepted treatment method that continues to evolve for a variety of reasons. There has been an explosion of new technologies that are designed to facilitate the delivery of local antibiotics in new and creative ways. The primary reason for using these local antibiotic delivery vehicles is the ability to achieve very high local concentrations of antibiotics without associated systemic toxicity. In the typical infected wound environment, which frequently has zones of avascularity, the ability to achieve high levels of antibiotics in these otherwise inaccessible areas is highly desirable (Cierny, 1999). Additional reasons for use of these delivery vehicles include the desire to treat remaining plactonic organisms and sessile organisms in biofilms more effectively with high concentrations of antibiotics (Hanssen et al, 2005). Because bone regeneration often is required as a part of the treatment plan, a recent trend has been simultaneously to provide a frame work of osteoinductive and osteoconductive materials along with antibiotics (Gitelis & Brebach, 2002).

Despite the rapid acceptance of these antibiotic delivery vehicles, there are many unanswered questions related to their use, particularly when viewed within the environment of biofilms. Considerable investigation and development still are required to develop the necessary data to help determine a number of unknown variables associated with the use of local antibiotic delivery systems. In the application of a local antibiotic therapy for bone and soft tissue infections the following aspects should be considered: a) delivery technique; b) type of antibiotic that can be used; c) pharmacokinetics; d) possibility of application to a coating and to fillers; e) possibility of combination with osteoconductive and osteoinductive factors; f) use as prophylaxis and/or therapy; g) drawbacks.

This review introduces bone and soft tissue infection-its present options for drug delivery systems and their limitations, and the wide range of carrier materials and effective drug choices. Also, I will describe and contrast the different local antibiotic delivery vehicles to provide a context for their current clinical use and to discuss the emerging investigate and developmental directions of these biomaterials.

2. Criteria for the production of a local delivery system for antimicrobial agents

Despite the reduction in the risk of contamination due to improved material, implant, and clean room technique as well as peri-operative antibiotic prophylaxis, infections still remain a feared complication in orthopedic and reconstructive surgery (Taylor, 1997). In many surgical disciplines, topical administration of antibacterial drug is not possible or practicable, and achieving of a sufficient antibacterial dose by systemic delivery may lead to adverse reactions negatively influencing overall patient's c by conditions. Especially the use of specific antibiotics may be limited by their high cumulative cell and organ toxicity (Ruszczak & Friess, 2003). Moreover, insufficiency in local blood supply due to post-traumatic or post-operative tissue damage as well as inadequate tissue penetration or bacterial resistance increase the local ineffectiveness of systemic antibiotic therapy, both in terms of preventive or curative drug administration (Mehta et al, 1996). This dilemma can be resolved by local delivery of antibiotics.

The ideal local drug delivery system has been a pursuit of scientists and physicians for the past fifty years. The concept of delivering drugs locally to the area of disease rather than through the systemic circulation without the concomitant secondary systemic complications is appealing both physiologically and psychologically (Nelson, 2004). The ideal local antibiotic delivery system would produce high antibiotic levels at the site of infection and safe drug levels in the systemic circulation. Antibiotic levels would need to be controlled to allow the systemic to be either therapeutic, bellow the toxic level, or absent, and to allow these features to be controlled independently from each other. Furthermore, the antibiotic elution curves, the factors that influence elution, and the most suitable local delivery system for the environment into which the material is to be placed, would need to be known. These materials would need to be easily placed, easily removed or changed, patient friendly and inexpensive. According to Hanssen, the ideal local antibiotic delivery system "would provide a more efficient delivery of higher levels of antibiotics to the site of infection and yet minimize the risks of systemic toxicity associated with traditional methods of intravenous antibiotics" (Hanssen, 2005).

2.1 Carrier materials for local antibiotic delivery

The consequent need for local drug delivery has been recognized since many years. During the last decades, different forms of local antibiotic delivery have been used. The most common and simple way was to spread the drug in a powder form over the wound area after an extensive debridement and before wound closure (Rushton, 1997). Consequently, high local concentrations for a short period of time are achieved which potentially result in tissue damage. Another approach was to applied antibiotics in liquid form by injection or irrigation or, to extend the effectiveness by continuous perfusion. However, this method is labor intensive and requires experienced nursing staff to avoid leakage and drain blockage. Furthermore, the use of implantable pumps which can be refilled percutaneously is described (Perry & Pearson, 1991). An additional method used was to soak the cotton gauze or linen operative material with the antibiotic and leave it in the wound until the final closure. This procedure is still in use in many countries to minimize the post-operative risk of infection, e.g. in dirty abdominal wounds or in trauma patients.

Although the ideal local antibiotic delivery system has not been discovered, several promising materials are present in modern research. The most common carrier systems of antibiotics that successfully release the drug according to prescribed dosage are listed in Table 1.

Carrier System	Antibiotic Released	References
Non-biodegradable		
1. Bone cement	Gentamicin	Baker & Greenham, 1988; Buchholz et al, 1984
	Vancomycin	Kuechle et al, 1990
	Cefazolin	Marks et al, 1976
	Ciprofloxacin	Tsourvakas et al, 2009
2. Bone cement beads	Gentamicin	Buchholz et al, 1984; Mendel et al, 2005
	Tobramycin	Seligson et al, 1993
	Cefuroxime	Mohanty et al, 2003
	Vancomycin	Chohfi et al, 1998
Biodegradable		
1. Plaster of Paris pellets	Gentamicin Santschi & McGarvey, 2003	
	Teicoplanin	Dacquet et al, 1992
2. Collagen-Sponge	Gentamicin	Ruszczak & Friess, 2003
3. Fibrin-sealant	Cefazolin	Tredwell et al, 2006
	Ciprofloxacin	Tsourvakas et al, 1995
4. Hydroxyapatite blocks	Vancomycin	Shirtliff et al, 2002
5. Polylactide/polyglycolide implants	Gentamicin	Garvin et al, 1994b
	Ciprofloxacin	Koort et al, 2008
	Vancomycin	Calhoun & Mader, 1997
6. Dilactate polymers	Fluoroquinolones	Dounis et al, 1996; Kanellakopoulou et al, 1999
7. Cancellous bone	Vancomycin, Ciprofloxacin	Witso et al, 2000
8. Calcium Sulfate	Tobramycin	Nelson et al, 2000
9. Calcium phosphate cement	Teicoplanin	Lazarettos et al, 2004
Miscellaneous		
1. Fibres	Tetracycline	Tonetti et al, 1998
2. Chitosan	Vancomycin	Chevher et al, 2006
3. Biomedical polyourethanes	Gentamicin, Ciprofloxacin	Schierholz et al, 1997

Table 1. Carriers used for local delivery of antibacterial agents

Drug delivery carriers developed for local delivery of antibiotics can be divided into non-biodegradable and biodegradable carriers (Kanellakopoulou & Giamarellos-Bourboulis, 2000). Non-biodegradable delivery systems such as polymethylmethacrylate (PMMA)

beads containing gentamicin have been approved for use in treatment of osteomyelitis in Europe (Klemm, 2001; Seligson et al, 1993). Antibiotic-loaded bone cement represent the current gold standard for local antibiotic delivery in orthopedic surgery (Nelson, 2004). This product has been proven to be efficacious but suffers from the major drawback of requiring subsequent operation to remove the bone cement beads at the completion of antibiotics release.

In recent years, various biodegradable delivery systems have been developed and evaluated for local delivery of antibiotics in the treatment of bone and soft tissue infections (Garvin et al, 1994b; Gursel et al, 2000). One of the primary advantages of a biodegradable system is the avoidance of secondary surgical procedures to remove foreign materials, such as bone cement, once antibiotic elution has ceased. Biodegradable implants could provide high local bactericidal concentrations in tissue for the prolonged time needed to completely eradicate the infection and the possibility to match the rate of implant biodegradability according to the type of infection treated (Kanellakopoulou & Giamarellos-Bourboulis, 2000). Biodegradation also makes surgical removal of the implant unnecessary. The implant can also be used initially to obliterate the dead space and, eventually to guide its repair. Additional possibilities with the use of biodegradable systems include variation in the magnitude and duration of antibiotic delivery as well as the potential for purposely adjusting the wound environment with breakdown products of some biodegradable materials (Hanssen, 2005).

Additional methods have included adding antibiotics to bone graft and to bone substitutes (Li & Hu, 2001; Shinto et al, 1992; Witso et al, 2000) or other naturally occurring polymers (Kawanabe et al, 1998) whereby the antibiotic is adsorbed to the surface of these materials and is then released into the wound environment. These materials can be include to the biodegradable antibiotic carriers.

The major drawback associated with non-biodegradable systems is the need to remove from the application site upon completion of their task. This removal surgery is usually more difficult than the implantation because of local tissue scaring and adhesion and may lead to postoperative infection due to both the patient local and systemic condition. In addition, the second procedure poses the risk of additional pain, anesthetic complications, and inferring extra costs. Recently, a Dutch group of scientists has found that despite of antibiotic release, cement beads act as a biomaterial surface at which bacteria preferentially adhere, grow and potentially develop antibiotic resistant (Neu et al, 2001).

2.2 Antibiotic selection

In order to select the appropriate antibiotic, an understanding of the microbiology of bone and soft tissue infections is imperative. Normal bone is highly resistant to infection, which can only develop as a result of trauma, very large inocula, or due to the presence of foreign material. Irrespective of the advancement in making surgeries and prosthesis, available sterile, and achieving aseptic conditions in operation theatres , infection associated with major trauma or surgeries are still unavoidable. Due to their application for prophylaxis and therapeutic antibiotics need to be applied to bone in every case of trauma or surgery, in addition to cases of bone and soft tissues infections. When the microbial load has crossed a critical density, they form biofilms that are quite hard for antibiotics to penetrate, often resulting in relapse of infection (Fux et al, 2005). Very high concentrations of antibiotics are required to eradicate them, which could hardly be attained by conventional routes of delivery without serious side effects.

The most commonly described microbes to cause bone and soft tissue infections, especially chronic osteomyelitis, are staphylococcus aureus; Group A beta hemolytic streptococcus and gram-negative bacteria, particularly Enterobacteriaceae and Pseudomonas aeruginosa (Galanakis et al, 1997; Rissing et al, 1997).

Numerous of antibiotics are available for use in antibiotic impregnated carriers. Considering the above criteria and on bacteriological finding in bone and soft tissue infections, the most acceptable agents in local delivery systems are aminoglycosides and to a lesser extent various β-lactam agents and quinolones (Rushton, 1997). A combination therapy of antibiotics is useful to reduce the toxicity of individual agents, to prevent the emergence of resistance and to treat mixed infections involved in chronic osteomyelitis (Mader et al, 1993). However, specific characteristics should be considered before the antimicrobial agents selected for use in local delivery systems: the antibiotic should be stable at body temperature and water soluble to ensure diffusion from the carrier; be active against the most common bacterial pathogens involved in bone and soft tissue infections; be locally released at concentrations exceeding several times (usually 10 times) the minimum inhibitory concentration (MIC) for the concerned pathogens; be unable to enter in systemic circulation; have a low rate of allergic reaction; a low rate of primary resistance; not produce supra infection and be readily available in powder form (Kobayashi et al, 1992; Popham et al, 1991). The choice of different classes of antibiotics for clinical use must be made according to a microbiologic sensitivity test (Popham et al, 1991; Ueng et al, 1997).

Antibiotics in general are hydrophilic drugs, hardly exhibit stability problems (except a few as cephalosporins) making them suitable to load with any kind of composite. Release of antibiotics shall depend on various factors. Release of the antibacterial agent in such systems is governed by the rate of dissolution of the drug in its matrix allowing its penetration through the pores of the carrier. For highly soluble agents, e.g. β-lactams agents, the amount of released drug depends on the surface area of the carrier and on the initial concentration of the drug in the prepared system. For relatively insoluble agents, e.g. quinolones, the rate of drug release depends on the porosity of the matrix and on dissolution of the drug in the matrix (Allababidi & Shah, 1998). However, insufficient release of antibiotics on the basis of time and concentration could lead to development of resistant strains and growth of microorganisms on the surface of the scaffolds (Soundrapandian et al, 2009).

3. Non-biodegradable systems

Antibiotic-impregnated non-biodegradable beads mainly polymethylmethacrylate (PMMA) have been widely used for the local administration of antibiotics. Buchholz and Engelbrecht in 1970 proposed delivering antibiotics to an infected site via elution of antibiotics from antibiotic-impregnated cement placed adjacent to the site of infection. The use of antibiotic-impregnated polymethylmethacrylate (PMMA) cement bead for the treatment of bone and soft tissue infections has many theoretical advantages. The beads, which release antibiotics by passive diffusion, combine with high local concentrations with low systemic levels of the antibiotic (Henry & Galloway, 1995), leading to more effective killing of the organisms and less risk of systemic toxicity. In addition, the beads can fill the dead space that may be left after debridement of infected tissue (Patzakis et al, 1993).

3.1 Antibiotic-loaded bone cement (PMMA)

Antibiotic impregnated beads have been employed in the treatment of bone and soft tissue infections for nearly 30 years; their use is well established in many European centers (Jenny, 1988). For the first time, antibiotic-loaded bone cement was used as a prophylactic agent against deep bone infections in orthopedic endoprosthetic surgery in human patients (Buchholz et al, 1984). Since then antibiotic-loaded bone cement has been an effective method for providing sustained high concentrations of antibiotics locally when used in numerous types of bone and soft tissue infections (Calhoun & Mader, 1989; Josefsson et al, 1990). Polymethylmethacrylate (PMMA) exist in two forms: that of antibiotic-impregnated bone cement applied in arthroplasties and antibiotic-impregnated bead chains for musculoskeletal infections (Henry & Galloway, 1995). The success of these carriers depend on two factors: PMMA does not usually trigger any immune response from the host and the form of a bead confers a wide surface area, allowing rapid release of the antibiotic.

Several factors influence the elution of antibiotics from PMMA cement. In addition to the type of antibiotic used, the type of cement also influences elution (Marks et al, 1976). Factors that increase the porosity of the cement (such as the addition of dextran or higher concentrations of antibiotic) also increase elution (Patzakis & Wilkins, 1989). Walenkamp in 1989, showed that the size of the bead influenced the amount of antibiotic that can be eluted. Small or mini beads provide better elution than larger beads, probably because of a more favorable surface to volume ratio (Holtom et al, 1998). Finally, the turnover of the fluid surrounding the beads will influence the local concentration as well as the maximum amount of antibiotic eluted.

Polymethylmethacrylate cement is available in various commercial and non-commercial brands and in-vitro elution of antibiotics from these varies between brands (Greene et al, 1998). Commercially available beads have a consistent diameter of 7mm and are available in stands of 10 or 30 (Nelson et al, 1992). Noncommercial preparations are generally prepared by the surgeons themselves. The main disadvantages associated with beads are improper mixing of antibiotic into the beads and a lack of the uniform size of bead, resulting in lower antibiotic availability (Nelson et al, 1992). Selection of antibiotic in commercially prepared beads depends on its stability at the high temperatures (up to 100°C) at which polymerization of bone cement occurs. The aminoglycosides are heat stable and are thus extensively used in these preparations. It has been documented for human being and in-vitro studies that elution of antibiotics from PMMA is bimodal (Henry et al, 1991). Approximately 5% of the total amount of antibiotic is released within the first 24 hours from the surface of beads or rods, followed by a sustained elution of antibiotic that diminishes during subsequent weeks or months. Elution properties of polymethylmethacrylate bone cement depend on the type of PMMA, type and concentration of antibiotic and structural characteristics of the bead or rods (Henry et al, 1991). Gas sterilization does not affect the properties of antibiotics or elution properties of PMMA (Henry et al, 1993).

There have been many in-vitro studies on the diffusion or elution of antibiotics from polymethylmethacrylate bone cement. Several different antimicrobial agents have been studied, including the aminoglycosides, primarily gentamicin but also tobramycin, amikacin and streptomycin (Greene et al, 1998; Masri et al, 1995; Wahlig et al, 1978), cephalosporins including cefazoline, cefotaxime, ceftriaxone and ceftazidime (Alonge & Fashina, 2000; Tomczak et al, 1989; Wilson et al, 1988), vancomycin (Kuechle et al, 1991) and ciprofloxacin (Tsourvakas et al, 2009). All antimicrobial agents go through an initial phase during which the concentration of fluid surrounding the beads or cement spacers is very high, followed by a gradual decrease to sustained low levels for many weeks or months. Although there are differences in elution between each different antimicrobial agent, all seem to have adequate elution for the treatment of bone and soft tissue infection, but the length of time that the drug levels remain above the minimum inhibitory concentration for the target organism (usually Staphylococcus aureus) varies depending on the drug selected and the conditions of the experiment. Cumulative data on the in-vitro elution of antibiotics in polymethylmethacrylate bone cement are presented in table 2, where it is clearly shown that both aminoglycosides and quinolones are released at very high concentrations, but the peak of release occurs on the first day. As the viscosity of PMMA decreases, the amount of released antibiotic increases (Bunetel et al, 1990). The same first day peak was also documented for tobramycin and vancomycin (Brien et al, 1993); the release lasted for a total period of only one week.

Antibiotic-loaded	Duration of release	Peak of release (μg/ml)	Study
PMMA	(days)	/day of peak	
Gentamicin	56	318.6/1	Hoff et al, 1981
Tobramycin	220	>250/1	Mader et al, 1997
Clindamycin	220	>250/1	Mader et al, 1997
Vancomycin	12	>200/1	Mader et al, 1997
Cefazolin	28	250/1	Adams et al, 1992
Penicillin	91	199.5/1	Hoff et al, 1981
Ciprofloxacin	360	80.8/1	Tsourvakas et al, 2009
Amikacin	5	200/1	Kuechle et al, 1990

Table 2. Characteristics of the in-vitro elution of different antibiotics from PMMA bone cement

To achieve adequate killing of bacteria, beads should not be used in combination with an irrigation system, and moisture should be excluded by artificial skin. With these precautions the amount of gentamicin releasd by the bone cement beads does not exceed 25% of the total amount implanted (Rushton, 1997). In chronic osteomyelitis, healing of the wound expected within 10 days but PMMA beads may remain implanted for up to 4 weeks, after his surgical removal is necessary followed by osseous reconstructive surgery. The need for removal is the major disadvantage of the beads, although in some patients small chains of beads be removed in the ward via a small skin incision (Walenkamp, 1997).

Antibiotic-loaded bone cement can be applied either in infected arthroplasties or as surgical prophylaxis during joint arthroplasties. Cumulative results of clinical studies involving its application for both purposes are given in table 3.

Study	Purpose of application	Patients	Favorable outcome (%)	Follow-up (months)
Josefsson et al, 1990	Prophylaxis in total hip arthroplasty	1688	99.2	60
Garvin et al, 1994a	Periprosthetic hip infection	40	95	17
Hanssen et al, 1994	Infected knee prosthesis	183	84.2	93
Whiteside, 1994	Infected knee prosthesis	33	96.9	24
Raut et al, 1995	Infected knee prosthesis	86	89.6	52
Cho et al, 1997	Chronic osteomyelitis	31	87	36

Table 3. Cumulative data from clinical trials with antibiotic-loaded PMMA bone cement

The primary basis for use of antibiotic-loaded polymethylmethacrylate bone cement as a prophylactic method to reduce the prevalence of deep periprosthetic infection has been the clinical experience obtained over the past three decades combined with data from several experimental studies (Jiranek et al, 2006). Gentamicin, cefuroxime and tobramycin have been the antimicrobials most commonly admixed into PMMA in clinical studies worldwide (Chiu et al, 2002; Engesaeter et al, 2003; Malchau et al, 1993). In United States, tobramycin has been used most commonly, primarily because the product is available in powdered form. Of the three antibiotics, gentamicin has been used most frequently and studied most extensively overall (Hanssen, 2004).

In a large retrospective study, data on 22170 primary total hip replacements from the Norwegian Arthroplasty Register during the period of 1987 to 2001 were analyzed (Engesaeter et al, 2003). Patients who received only systemic antibiotic prophylaxis had a 1.8 times higher rate of infection than patients who received systemic antibiotic prophylaxis combined with gentamicin-loaded bone cement. Another retrospective study, of 92675 hip arthroplasties listed in the Swedish Joint Registry, presented similar conclusions, with the use of antibiotic-loaded bone cement favored for both primary and revision hip arthroplasties (Malchau et al, 1993).

Recently, prosthesis of antibiotics loaded acrylic bone cement consisting of an acetabular cup filled with antibiotic loaded polymethylmethacrylate bone cement was developed for the treatment of infections at the site of total hip arthroplasty accompanied by the extensive loss of the proximal part of the femur (Younger et al, 1998). The antibiotic usually impregnated is tobramycin or vancomycin with an elution of the former at intra-articular concentrations between 4.35 and 123.88 mg/L and remains undetected in the latter (Masri et al, 1998). This has resulted in a success rate of 94% in 61 patients after an average follow-up of 43 months. Polymethylmethacrylate bone cement beads impregnated with vancomycin were successfully used for the treatment of osteomyelitis of the pelvis and of the hip (Ozaki et al, 1998).

The primary concern regarding antibiotic-loaded acrylic bone cement include the potential for detrimental effects on the mechanical or structural characteristics of polymethylmethacrylate bone cement when antibiotic are admixed. The addition of >4.5g of gentamicin powder per 40g package of cement powder or the addition of liquid antibiotics causes a decrease in compressive strength to a level below American Society for Testing and Materials standards (Lautenschlager et al, 1976). The use of high-dose antibiotics in acrylic bone cement spacers (>2g of antibiotic powder per 40g of acrylic bone cement powder) implanted in staged revision procedures can lead to substantial cost savings to the hospital and improvement in patient care. However, the routine use of high-dose antibiotics in cement employed for fixation of prostheses is not supported by evidence (Jiranek et al, 2006).

Another basic concern regarding antibiotic-loaded polymethylmethacrylate bone cement include the potential for development of drug-resistant bacteria. Many of the bacterial pathogens involved in bone and soft tissue infections, particularly Staphylococcus epidermidis, produce a biofilm that limits the activity of antibiotics (Gracia et al, 1998). The biofilm, known as the extracellular slime of glycocalyx, is produced by strains of Staphylococcus aureus and Staphylococcus epidermidis, it also provides these strains with the capacity to adhere the foreign materials, such as the acrylic bone cement beads (Bayston & Rogers, 1990). Consequently, despite adequate killing of these micro-organisms by in-vitro elution of antibiotic in close proximity to the beads, the same micro-organisms survive on their surface (Kendall et al, 1996). This stable adherence might provide a mechanism of recurrence of the infection and of development of resistance, since small colony variants of Staphylococcus aureus resistant to gentamicin have been isolated from the wounds of patients with bone and soft tissue infections treated with gentamicin-impregnated acrylic bone cement beads (vonEiff et al, 1997). In a report from the Ohio State University Medical Center, the overall rate of infection decreased with the introduction and use of antibiotic-loaded acrylic bone cement; however, the prevalence of aminoglycoside-resistant bacteria, particularly in Staphylococcus aureus and coagulase-negative staphylococcal infections, increased (Wininger & Fass, 1996). Because of the considerable data suggesting the potential for the development of bacterial antibiotic resistance, antibiotic-loaded polymethylmethacrylate bone cement should not be used routinely for prophylaxis. Rather, it should be used for prophylaxis only when there are clear indications, such as a high-risk primary procedure or a high-risk revision arthroplasty. Vancomycin should not be used as a primary agent for prophylaxis because of the emergence of resistant organisms and the need to reserve this antibiotic for patients who require it for treatment (Hanssen & Osmon, 1999).

4. Biodegradable materials

A variety of bone cement alternatives have been used experimentally and clinically as local antibiotic delivery vehicles and there are many additional products in development. Currently, there are no FDA-approved biodegradable materials available for use to treat established musculoskeletal infection (Nelson, 2004).

Biodegradable implants could provide high local bacteridical concentrations in tissue for the prolonged time needed to completely eradicate the infection and the possibility to match the rate of implant biodegradability according to the type of infection and the possibility to match the rate of implant biodegradability according to the type of infection treated.

Biodegradation also makes surgical removal of the implant unnecessary. The implant can also be used initially to obliterate the dead space and, eventually, to guide its repair. Furthermore, secondary release of the antibiotic may occur during the degradation phase of the carrier, which could increase antibacterial efficacy compared to non-biodegradable carriers (Nandi et al, 2009).

The biodegradable antibiotic delivery materials have been classified into four broad categories: bone graft and bone substitutes, protein-based materials (natural polymers), synthetic polymers and miscellaneous biodegradable materials (McLaren, 2004). Within these four categories there are several mechanisms of antibiotic release such as the first order kinetics associated with antibiotics attached by surface adsorption and variable antibiotic release rates that are observed with products whereby antibiotics are admixed within the substance of the biomaterial (Hanssen, 2005). In vitro and in vivo elution of antibacterial agents from biodegradable materials are show in tables 4 and 5.

Study	Carrier	Antibiotic	Duration of release (days)
Witso et al, 2000	Bone-graft	Vancomycin	7
		Ciprofloxacin	7
Jia et al, 2010	Calcium Sulfate	Teicoplanin	29
Wachol-Drewek et al, 1996	Collagen Sponge	Gentamicin	4
		Vancomycin	2
Tsourvakas et al, 2009	Fibrin-clot	Ciprofloxacin	60
Garvin et al, 1994b	Synthetic Polymers	Clindamycin	38-50
		Tobramycin	36-75
		Vancomycin	38-51
Kanellakopoulou et al, 1999	Polylactate	Ciprofloxacin	51-350
		Pefloxacin	56-295
Dounis et al, 1996	Polylactate	Fleroxacin	56
Santschi & McGarey, 2003	Plaster of Paris	Gentamicin	14
Shinto et al, 1992	Hydroxyapatite	Gentamicin	90

Table 4. Cumulative data from in-vitro studies with antibiotic-loaded in biodegradable materials

Study	Carrier	Antibiotic	Animal Model	Duration of release (days)
Witso et al, 2000	Bone-graft	Vancomycin	Rat	7
		Ciprofloxacin		3
Shinto et al, 1992	Hydroxyapatite	Gentamicin	Rat	90
Stemberger et al, 1997	Collagen Sponge	Gentamicin	Rabbit	56
Tsourvakas et al, 1995	Fibrin-clot	Ciprofloxacin	Rabbit	15
Kanellakopoulou et al, 2000	Lactic-acid	Pefloxacin	Rabbit	33
Garvin et al, 1994b	Synthetic Polymers	Gentamicin	Canine	42
Koort et al, 2008	Synthetic Polymers	Ciprofloxacin	Rabbit	42

Table 5. Cumulative data from in-vivo studies with antibiotic-loaded in biodegradable materials

4.1 Bone grafts and bone substitutes

Bone graft, either as autograft or allograft, as a vehicle for local antibiotic delivery, has been used clinically for more than twenty years (McLaren, 2004).

Morselized cancellous bone has been used extensively as bone graft material. There are variations in the material that depend on the method of preparation. The use of morselized cancellous bone as a delivery carrier for antibiotics was developed in 1984 when there was limited choice in bone-grafting material and constraints related to biologic hazards were manageable (McLaren & Miniaci, 1986). Antibiotics can be added as a powered to morselized cancellous bone or by soaking the bone-graft in an antibiotic-loaded solution. The antibiotic is absorbed directly to the bone surfaces and subsequent release of antibiotics is based on first-order kinetics (McLaren, 2004). Although this clinical application protocols with a variety of different antibiotics, there are very little data regarding the actual concentration levels of the local antibiotics and the clinical effects that this practice has an eventual bone graft incorporation.

In vitro elution studies (McLaren & Miniaci, 1986) and in vivo studies in a rabbit model (McLaren, 1988) have shown first-order kinetics for release of tobramycin during a period of over three weeks. Tobramycin levels exceeded usual bactericidal concentrations for three weeks in the graft material implanted in a rabbit. In another study, the results showed that morselized bone graft can act as a carrier netilmicin, vancomycin, clindamycin and rifampicin in vitro and in vivo. Antibiotics levels exceeded usual bactericidal concentrations for seven days in the graft material implanted in a rat (Witso et al, 2000).

Application of antibiotic impregnated autogenic cancellous bone grafting has already been introduced in clinical practice. Chan et al, in 1998, reported results from 36 patients with infected fractures resulting from traffic accidents. After surgical debridement an iliac cancellous bone graft was taken and mixed by the surgeon with piperacillin and/or vancomycin, depending on the susceptibility of the isolated infective micro-organism. The graft was then implanted at the site of infection inside the osseous defect, which occurred principally in the proximal, middle or distal segment of the left or right tibia. Four to five months were necessary for bone union, and the only complications presented were skin rashes.

Impregnation of antimicrobial agents within osteoconductive biomaterials (calcium sulfate, calcium phosphate, hydroxyapatite or tricalcium phosphate) has been proposed for local treatment of osteomyelitis and to aid dead space management (Kawanabe et al, 1998; Makinen et al, 2005; Nelson et al, 2005). As a common feature, these implants show a rapid release of the antibiotic in a more or less controlled manner (McLaren, 2004). One of the benefits of this class of materials is that implantation provides the opportunity to deliver local antibiotics at high concentrations and simultaneously participate in the bone regeneration process during the time period of material degradation. These materials also avoid the risk of transmitting disease pathogens associated with the use of allograft bone.

Of these materials, commercial calcium sulfate has probably been used most commonly in the clinical setting of osteomyelitis treatment (Gitelis & Brebach, 2002). The most appropriate antibiotic dosage regimen not clear however, the most common formulation used clinically has been 3.64% vancomycin or 4.25% tobramycin per weight (Gitelis & Brebach, 2002). These percentages equate to 1g of vancomycin or 1.2g for tobramycin per 25g of calcium sulfate. Other antibiotic-loaded biomaterials being investigated in this category include calcium hydroxyapatites (Shirliff et al, 2002), calcium phosphates (Lazarettos et al, 2004), bioactive glasses (Kawanabe et al, 1998) and antibiotic loaded blood coated demineralized bone (Rhyu et al, 2003).

4.2 Natural polymers (protein-based materials)

This category includes antibiotic-loaded sponge collagen (Mehta et al, 1996; Ruszcak & Friess, 2003), fibrin (Tredwell et al, 2005; Tsourvakas et al, 1995), thrombin, and other commercially available systems that use clotted blood products. Although there are investigators actively involved in the use of these materials, their use as local antibiotic delivery vehicles is not as common as the use of antibiotic-loaded bone cement, antibiotic-loaded bone graft substitutes in the treatment of bone and soft tissue infections.

These materials function as delivery vehicles by providing a physical scaffold around the antibiotic mechanically limiting fluid flow, or by providing a protein to bind the antibiotic. Some data on release properties are published for all of these materials determined by either elution studies or by animal studies. Elution rates, tend to be rapid, leading to release of essentially all of the contained antibiotic in the range of hours to a few days. Antibiotic release in animal models is slower. Time to release the majority of contained antibiotic ranges from many days to several weeks. The investigations generating these data are limited, using a wide spectrum of methods, making a comparison of performance of these materials invalid. Clinical guidelines for the amount of the material to be used and for the dose of the contained antibiotic are not possible (McLaren, 2004).

Collagen sponge is the material in this group that was the best supporting data. It is a solid mesh of collagen-based spongy material, produced from sterile animal skin or tendo Achillis. Since collagen is a major component of connective tissue and the main structural protein of all organs, it has several desirable biological properties, including both biocompatibility and non-toxicity. Its ability to release drugs can be modified by changing the porosity of the matrix or by treating it with chemicals (Rao, 1995). It can also attract and stimulate the proliferation of osteoblasts, thereby promoting mineralization and the production of collagenous callus tissue, which aids the formation of new bone (Reddi, 1985).

Collagen sheets with impregnated gentamicin have been used to treat chronic osteomyelitis (Ipsen et al, 1991). It has been commercially available in Europe for ten years and is produced from sterilized bovine tendon in which gentamicin is suspended. In vitro studies of antibiotic release from collagen sponges showed four days to complete (Wachol-Drewek et al, 1996). When collagen sponge is combined with liposome encapsulated antibiotics, the duration of time for release of the antibiotics has been reported to be up to three times greater that that of collagen sponge alone (Trafny et al, 1996). Polymyxin-B and amikacin have been shown in other laboratory experiments to have significant sustained release action against Pseudomonas aeruginosa when attached to type I collagen (Trafny et al, 1995). Gentamicin impregnated collagen sponge shows up to 600 times MIC as compared to polymethylmethacrylate beads at 300 times MIC .It has also been observed that due to its release of large amounts of gentamicin the flexible gentamicin-contained collagen sponge proved to be superior to the rigid polymethylmethacrylate beads. Other authors conclude that it is an effective delivery vehicle for up to 28 days in a rabbit model (Humphrey et al, 1998) and that it is effective clinically (Kanellakopoulou & Giamarellos-Bourboulis, 2000). Further characterization and technique refinement are required before it can be recommended as a delivery vehicle for antibiotics. Commercially prepared antibiotic-laden collagen sponge is not available for use in the United States.

Fibrin sealants are topical hemostatic materials derived from plasma coagulation proteins that are being used increasingly in surgical procedures (Jackson, 2001). Fibrin sealants have great potential for the delivery of antibiotics, chemotherapy, and even growth factors at surgical sites (Jackson, 2001). They are biocompatible and degrade by normal fibrinolysis within days or weeks depending on the site. The main use of fibrin sealants has been in cardiovascular, thoracic, dental, plastic and reconstructive surgery. More recently, orthopedic procedures, such as total knee arthroplasty or hip replacement, have also been shown to benefit from the use of fibrin sealants (Jackson, 2001).

Clearly, the compatibility of these materials with surgical wound sites makes fibrin sealant logical candidates for use as controlled-release carriers for local antibiotic delivery. It has been shown that antibiotics with low water solubility, such as tetracycline base, are particularly suited to this system (Woolveron et al, 2001), presumably because the precipitated drug dissolves and diffuses slowly from the fibrin clot. Even more water-soluble antibiotics such as gentamicin and ciprofloxacin have been shown to release in vitro from fibrin over 5-7 days for gentamicin (Kram et al, 1991) and over 60 days for ciprofloxacin (Tsourvakas et al, 1995), although more than 66% was released in the first two days. In an animal model the maximum level of ciprofloxacin in bone and soft tissues, after the implantation of composite in the medullary canal of rabbit tibia, was obtained on the second day after implantation, and the drug was undetectable after ten days (Tsourvakas et al, 1995).

Zilch and Lambiris (1986) measured the cefotaxime concentrations in both blood and wound drainage from 46 patients with osteomyelitis who were treated with a fibrin clot cefotaxime mixture injected into the bone cavity. These authors reported serum levels that were low within 12 hours after fibrin clot placement, but wound drainage fluid maintained high concentrations for more than 3 days.

Fibrin clot antibiotic mixtures are a promising approach to providing a biocompatible tissue sealant with local antibiotic release that may decrease the incidence of postoperative infections. Further in vitro work is necessary to characterize the effect the addition of antibiotics has on the rate and strength of fibrin clotting. Additional in vivo data are necessary to determine what effect low systemic levels of antibiotics might have on antibiotic resistance patterns.

4.3 Synthetic polymers

Although collagen sponge is an established method of managing infection, there is great interest in developing a carrier with longer lasting effects and better penetration. Biodegradable synthetic polymers have been used in surgery since the 1950s as suture material. Advances in processing have generated stronger, more reliable synthetic polymers based implants for consideration as carriers (El-Husseiny et al, 2011).

The most active area of current research using biodegradable polymers from glycolide and lactide is in the controlled delivery of drugs especially in antibiotics such as ampicillin, gentamicin, polymyxin B and quinolones (Calhoun & Mader, 1997; Kanellakopoulou et al, 1994; Nie et al, 1995). Polylactide/polyglycolide was selected to act as a carrier because it undergoes a gradual degradation in a controlled manner and dissolves at physiological pH and removal is thus not necessary in patients who have bone and soft tissue infections (Nandi et al, 2009). A second advantage is that the kinetics of the release of the antibiotic can be modified by the selection of copolymers of varying monometric composition, polymer crystallinity and molecular weight as well as by alteration of the geometry of the implant. Finally, preliminary studies indicated that these materials is highly compatible with a wide variety of antibiotics and the in vivo release of antibiotics occurs for a definite time period with therapeutic concentrations, which may minimize slow residual release at suboptimal concentrations (Makinen et al, 2005).

Polymers are available in different patterns such as polylactides, copolymers of lactide and glycolide, polyanhydride and polycarpolactone. Copolymers of polylactides and polyglycolic acid have been produced with a ratio between the two composites varying between 90:10 and 50:50. It has been observed from in vitro studies that the 90:10 ratio provides better stability, delayed decomposition and superior elution concentrations of tobramycin, clindamycin and vancomycin than copolymers produced at other ratios (Bunetel et al, 1990). Copolymers (50:50)-gentamicin implant was significantly more successful than the use of the standard parenteral therapy in experimental osteomyelitis in canine model (Garvin et al, 1994).

The biocompatibility of polylactide/polyglycolide acid has been well established. The tissue reaction to implanted materials is minimum, with the inflammatory response limited to a narrow region, which gradually diminishes as the polymer is desorbed (Brady et al, 1973).

Although lactide/glycolide polymers were suggested as carriers for antibiotics thirty years ago (Thies, 1982), it was ten years before linked lactic acid chains were proposed as a drug delivery system for the treatment of bone and soft tissue infections. Wei et al in 1991 implanted molded rods, made by heating a mixture of lactic acid oligomer and dideoxykanamycin B, into rabbit models. They showed that the MIC of antibiotic for the common causative organisms of osteomyelitis was exceeded for six weeks in the cortex, the cancellous bone, and in the bone marrow. Furthermore, the majority of the implant material has been absorbed, and the bone marrow had returned to a nearly normal state within nine weeks of implantation.

Sampath et al in 1992 demonstrated an alternative method of delivering gentamicin locally using polymers. They prepared microcapsules composed of a polylactic acid shell containing gentamicin which was then compressed into the desired shape. It was noted that more 80% of antibiotic was released in the first three weeks in vitro. The efficacy of microcapsules in osteomyelitis has also been demonstrated in a study by Garvin et al, in 1994.

The polylactate polymers achieve prolonged in vivo quinolones release at higher levels than the other systems and produced their peal drug release after 15 days (Kanellakopoulou et al, 1994). On the basis of the adequacy of elution of quinolones from the polylactate carrier, pefloxacin impregnated of this carrier was used for therapy of an experimental osteomyelitis caused by the local application of MRSA in rabbits (Kanellakopoulou et al, 2000).

One of the primary drawbacks with synthetic polymers has been the difficulties associated with designing implants that also providing structural integrity. For this specific reason, the use of this category of biomaterials, like the other non-cement alternatives, has primarily been for the treatment of osteomyelitis. Although the structural requirements necessary for other applications can be accomplished for these implants initially, the process of polymer degradation often has led to severe loss of structural integrity during the course of treatment (Hanssen, 2005).

Synthetic polymers could function as a delivery vehicle for antibiotics with further evaluation and development. Manipulation of the material properties and combinations of one or more of these material can lead to any clinically desirable release rate. Investigations have been exploring these variables (Ambrose et al, 2003). However, no one material has shown dominance with confirmatory investigations and progression in development towards a usable clinical preparation. There are not available for clinical use as a depot antibiotic delivery vehicle. This may be related in part to the economics of bringing these products to market premixed with antibiotic. Currently, there is no polymer available that can be hand mixed with antibiotics in the operating room.

4.4 Miscellaneous

The range of different intended functions of these materials include different rates and timing of antibiotic release, provision of physicochemical characteristics necessary for osteoconduction, and provision of a scaffold that allows osteoconduction, osseous integration, and sufficient structural properties.

Antibiotic loaded plaster of Paris pellets is an effective ancillary treatment in the surgery of infected cavities in bone. It is well tolerated and spontaneous absorbed over a period of weeks to months, being replaced by bone if normal architecture (Mackey et al, 1982). Many antibiotics can be added to plaster of Paris, such as gentamicin, fucidic acid, and teicoplanin (Dacquet et al, 1992; Mackey et al, 1982).

Fibres locally releasing tetracycline hydrochloride have been successfully introduced for the therapy of persistent or recurrent periodontitis (Tonetti et al, 1998). Chitosan is an excellent biomaterial with biodegradable and immunologic activity, the gentamicin loaded chitosan bar seems to be a clinically useful method for the treatment of bone and soft tissue infections (Aimin et al, 1999). Different types of gel like hyalouronic acid (Matsuno et al, 2006), fibrin gel with bone marrow derived mesenchymal stem cells (Hou et al, 2008), and monoolein-water gels (Ouedraogo et al, 2008) have been used as an alternative treatment for bone and soft tissue infections.

Some unconventional marine biomaterials like sponge skeleton, coral, snail slime with varied intraglanular porosity are future promising options as bone grafts substitute. Most of the commonly used and under trial bone graft substitutes only have osteoconductive and osteogenic characters. Therefore, it is of paramount necessity to develop an ideal novel smart biomaterials with all three properties which cannot only provide sufficient concentration of antibiotic at the target site but also act as a bone strut to accelerate the goal. This may be achieved by combining conventional and some unconventional growth factors with the carrier materials including the incorporation of stem cells (Nandi et al, 2009).

The necessary data on the efficacy of these new biodegradable materials still are in early stages of development and assessment. Despite the vast potential to develop composite biomaterials that can provide multiple functions, the complexity of the cellular and molecular interactions within the wound environment exposes the potential for unforeseen adverse consequences. In fact, many of the clinical scenarios of treatment of musculoskeletal infection include the need for local antibiotics and stimulation of the process of bone regeneration. One of the most obvious adverse effects of high level of local antibiotics is an osteoblast function and subsequent bone regeneration. The concern is valid for specific clinical situations such as antibiotic bead pouches for treatment of open fractures (Henry et al, 1993b), bone grafting for nonunions, and implantation of devices into bone defects where bone regeneration is an intended outcome of the dead-space management strategy (Gitelis & Brebach, 2002).

5. Conclusion

The appropriate use of antimicrobial agents has decreased morbidity and mortality from orthopedic-related infections. Although systemic antibiotic use has been used for many years, new methods of local antibiotic delivery may result in increased antibiotic levels, decreased toxicity, and possibly greater efficacy. Antibiotic impregnated polymethylmethacrylate beads are currently being used in a variety of applications, but this method require a second procedure for removal of the antibiotic delivery system.

There is considerable interest in finding methods of delivering effective doses of antimicrobial drugs locally, not only in orthopedics, but across a range of specialists. While most of the antibacterial agent contained within a biodegradable system may be eluted, only 25% is actually released from polymethylmethacrylate beads. Biodegradable materials could mimic bone substances like calcium phosphate based carriers can be chosen for local drug delivery system in osteomyelitis with potential clinical application in orthopedic surgery. Widespread research is currently being conducted in the area of local drug delivery systems to treat osteomyelitis. Despite this fact, much work is still desired in the areas of biodegradable and biocompatible materials, the kinetics of antibiotic release, and further development of current systems before many of these formulations can be used. The seer diversity of available systems and the lack of suitable trials comparing them in-vivo makes their evaluation difficult. Nonetheless, it is apparent that while collagen fleece is currently the most widely used antimicrobial carrier system, the duration of its antibiotic delivery is the shortest. Other delivery systems have shown greater promise, and these that are able both to stimulate the formation of new bone and provide a scaffold, such as composite antibiotic carriers, are most likely to gain widespread acceptance in the future.

In future, researchers remain optimistic that many of these systems can be developed with ideal zero-order release kinetics profiles, in-vivo, over long periods of time, allowing for widespread use in chronic osteomyelitis patients. By utilizing newer forms of sustained-release antibiotic delivery systems, it will be possible to deliver such antibiotics at constant rates over a prolonged period of time and would eliminate the need for multiple dosing. It is hoped that in the future, development of new implantable systems would be helpful to reduce the cost of drug therapy, increase the efficacy of drugs, and could enhance the patient's compliance.

6. References

Adams K., Couch L., Cierny G., Calhoun J., & Mader JT. (1992). In vitro and in vivo evaluation of antibiotic diffusion from antibiotic-impregnated polymethylmethacrylates beads. *Clinical Orthopaedics Related Research,* Vol. 278, (May 1992), pp. 244-252, ISSN 0009-921X

Aimin C., Chunlin H., Juliang B., Tinyin Z., & Zhichao D. (1999). Antibiotic loaded chitosan bar. An in-vitro, in-vivo study of a possible treatment of osteomyelitis. *Clinical Orthopaedics Related Research,* Vol. 366, (September 1999), pp. 239-247, ISSN 0009-921X

Allababidi S., & Shah JC. (1998). Kinetics and mechanism of release from glyceryl monostearate-based implants: evaluation of release in a gel stimulating in vivo implantation. *Journal Pharmaceutical Sciences,* Vol. 87, No 6, (June 1998), pp. 738-744, ISSN 0022-3549

Alonge TO., & Fashing AN. (2000). Ceftriaxone-PMMA beads – a slow release preparation? *International Journal Clinical Practice,* Vol. 54, No 6, (July 2000), pp. 353-355, ISSN 1368-5031

Baker AS., & Greenham LW. (1988). Release of gentamicin from acrylic bone cement. Elution and diffusion studies. *Journal Bone Joint Surgery*, Vol. 70-A, No 10, (December 1988), pp. 1551-1557, ISSN 0021-9355

Bayston R., & Rodgers J. (1990). Production of extra-cellular slime by Staphylococcus epidermis during stationary phase of growth: its association with adherence to implantable devices. *Journal Clinical Pathology*, Vol. 43, No 10, (October 1990), pp. 866-870, ISSN 0021-9746

Brady IM., Cutright DE., Miller RA., & Barristance GC. (1973). Resorption rate, route, route of elimination, and ultrastructure of the implant site of polylactic acid in the abdominal wall of the rat. *Journal Biomedical Materials Research*, Vol. 7, No 2, (March 1973), pp. 155-166, ISSN 0021-9304

Brien WW., Salvati EA., Brause B., & Stern S. (1993). Antibiotic impregnated bone cement in total hip arthroplasty. An in-vivo comparison of the elution properties of tobramycin and vancomycin. *Clinical Orthopaedics Related Research*, Vol. 296, (November 1993), pp.242-248, ISSN 0009-921X

Buchholz HW., & Engelbrecht H. (1970). Uber die depotwirkung einiger antibiotica bei vermischung mit dem kunstharz Palacos. *Chirurg*, Vol. 41, No 11, (November 1970), pp. 511-515, ISSN 0009-4722

Buchholz HW., Elson RA., & Heinert K. (1984). Antibiotic-loaded acrylic cement: current concepts. *Clinical Orthopaedics Related Research*, Vol. 190, (November 1984), pp. 96-108, ISSN 0009-921X

Bunetel L., Sequi A., Cormier M., & Langlais F. (1990). Comparative study of gentamicin release from normal and low viscosity acrylic bone cement. *Clinical Pharmacokinetic*, Vol. 19, No 4, (October 1990), pp. 333-340, ISSN 0312-5963

Calhoun JH., & Mader JT. (1989). Antibiotic beads in the management of surgical infections. *American Journal Surgery*, Vol. 157, No 4, (April 1989), pp. 443-449, ISSN 0002-9610

Calhoun JH., & Mader JT. (1997). Treatment of osteomyelitis with a biodegradable antibiotic implant. *Clinical Orthopaedics Related Research*, Vol. 341, (August 1997), pp. 206-214, ISSN 0009-921X

Cevher E., Orhan Z., Mulazimoglu L., Sensoy D., Alper M., Yildiz A., & Ozsoy Y. (2006). Characterization of biodegradable chitosan microspheres containing vancomycin and treatment of experimental osteomyelitis caused by methicillin-resistant staphylococcus aureus with prepared microspheres. *International Journal Pharmaceutics*, Vol. 317, No 2, (July 2006), pp. 127-135, ISSN 0378-5173

Chan YS., Ueng SW., Wang CJ., Lee SS., Chao EK. ,& Shin CH. (1998). Management of small infected tibial defects with antibiotic-impregnated autogenous cancellous bone grafting. *Journal of Trauma*, Vol. a5, No 4, (October 1998), pp. 758-764, ISSN 0022-5282

Chiu FY., Chen CM., Lin CF., & Lo WH. (2002). Cefuroxime-impregnated cement in primary total knee arthroplasty: a prospective randomized study of three hundred and forty knees. *Journal Bone Joint Surgery*, Vol. 84-A, No 5, (May 2002), pp. 759-762, ISSN 0021-9355

Cho SH., Song HR., Koo KH., Jeong ST., & Park YJ. (1997). Antibiotic-impregnated cement beads in the treatment of chronic osteomyelitis. *Bulletin Hospital Joint Diseases*, Vol. 56, No 3, (March 1997), pp. 140-144, ISSN 0018-5647

Chohfi M., Langlais F., Fourastier J., Minet J., Thomazeau H., & Cormic M. (1998). Pharmacokinetics, uses, and limitations of vancomycin-load bone cement. *International Orthopaedics,* Vol. 22, No 3, (April 1998), pp. 171-177, ISSN 0341-2695

Cierny G., & Mader JT. (1987). Approach to adult osteomyelitis. *Orthopaedic Review,* Vol. 16, No 4, (April 1987), pp. 259-270, ISSN 0094-6591

Cierny III G. (1999). Infected tibial nonunions (1989-1995). The evolution of change. *Clinical Orthopaedics Related Research,* Vol. 360, (March 1999), pp. 97-105, ISSN 0009-921X

Dacquet V., Varlet A., Tandogan RN., Tation MM., Fournier L., Jehl F., Monteil H., & Bascoulergue G. (1992). Antibiotic-impregnated plaster of Paris beads. Trials with teicoplanin. *Clinical Orthopaedics Related Research,* Vol. 282, (September 1992), pp. 241-249, ISSN 0009-921X

Dombrowski ET., & Dunn AW. (1965). Treatment of osteomyelitis by debridement and closed wound irrigation-suction. *Clinical Orthopaedics Related Research,* Vol.43, (September 1965), pp. 215-231, ISSN 0009-921X

Dounis E., Korakis T., Anastasiadis A., Kanellakopoulou K., Andreopoulos A., & Giamarellou H. (1996). Sustained release of fleroxacin in vitro from lactic acid polymer. *Bulletin Hospital Joint Disease,* Vol. 55, No 1, (January 1996), pp. 16-19, ISSN 0018-5647

El-Husseini M., Patel S., MacFarlane RJ., & Haddad FS. (2011). Biodegradable antibiotic delivery systems. *Journal Bone Joint Surgery,* Vol. 93-B, No 2, (February 2011), pp. 151-157, ISSN 0301-620X

Engesaeter LB., Lie SA., Espehaug B., Furnes O., Vollset SE., & Havelin LI. (2003). Antibiotic prophylaxis in total hip arthroplasty: effects of antibiotic prophylaxis systemically and in bone cement on the revision rate of 22170 primary hip replacements followed 0-14 years in the Norwegian Arthroplasty Register. *Acta Orthopaedica Scandinavica,* Vol. 74, No 6, (December 2003), pp. 644-651, ISSN 0001-6470

Fleming A. (1920). The action of chemical and physiological antiseptics in a septic wound. *British Journal Surgery,* Vol. 7, pp. 99-129

Fux CA., Costerton JW., Stewart PS., & Stoodley P. (2005). Survival strategies of infections biofilm. *Trends Microbiology,* Vol. 13, No 1, (January 2005), pp. 34-40, ISSN 0966-842X

Galanakis N., Giamarellou H., Moussas T., & Dounis E. (1997). Chronic osteomyelitis caused by multi-resistant Gram-negative bacteria: evaluation of treatment with newer quinolones after prolonged follow-up. *Journal Antimicrobial Chemotherapy,* Vol. 39, No 2, (February 1997), pp. 241-246, ISSN 0305-7453

Carvin KL., Evans BG., Salvati EA., & Brause BD. (1994a). Palacos gentamicin for the treatment of deep periprosthetic hip infections. *Clinical Orthopaedics Related Research,* Vol. 298, (January 1994), pp. 97-105, ISSN 0009-921X

Garvin KL., Miyono JA., Robinson D., Giger D., Novak J., & Radio S. (1994b). Polylactide/polyglycolide antibiotic implants in the treatment of osteomyelitis. A canine model. *Journal Bone Joint Surgery,* Vol. 76-A, No 10, (October 1994), pp. 1500-1506, ISSN 0021-9355

Gitelis S., & Brebach GT. (2002). The treatment of chronic osteomyelitis with a biodegradable antibiotic-impregnated implant. *Journal Orthopaedic Surgery (Hong-Kong),* Vol. 10, No 1, (June 2002), pp. 53-60, ISSN 1022-5536

Gracia E., Lacteriga A., Monzon M., Leiva J., Oteiza C., & Amorena B. (1998). Application of a rat osteomyelitis model to compare in vivo and in vitro the antibiotic efficacy against bacteria with high capacity to form biofilms. *Journal Surgical Research,* Vol. 79, No 2, (October 1998), pp. 146-153, ISSN 0022-4804

Greene N., Holtom PD., Warren CA., Shepherd L., McPherson EJ., & Patzakis MJ. (1998). In vitro elution of tobramycin and vancomycin polymethylmethacrylate beads and spacers from Simplex and Palacos. *American Journal Orthopaedics,* Vol. 27, No 3, (March 1998), pp. 201-205, ISSN 1078-4519

Gursel I., Korkusuz F., Turesin F., Alaeddinoglu NG., & Hasirci V. (2001). In vivo application of biodegradable controlled antibiotic release system for the treatment of implant-related osteomyelitis. *Biomaterials,* Vol. 22, No 1, (January 2001), pp. 73-80, ISSN 0142-9612

Haddad FS., Muirhead-Allwood SK., Manktelow AR., & Bacarese-Hamilton I. (2000). Two stage uncemented revision hip arthroplasty for infection. *Journal Bone Joint Surgery,* Vol. 82-b, No 5, (July 2000), pp. 689-694, ISSN 0301-620X

Hanssen AD., Rand JA., & Osmon DR. (1994). Treatment of the infected total knee arthroplasty with insertion of another prosthesis. The effect of antibiotic-impregnated bone cement. *Clinical Orthopaedics Related Research,* Vol. 309, (December 1994), pp. 44-55, ISSN 0009-921X

Hanssen AD., & Osmon DR. (1999). The use of prophylactic antimicrobial agents during and after hip arthroplasty. *Clinical Orthopaedics Related Research,* Vol. 369, (December 19999), pp. 124-138, ISSN 0009-921X

Hanssen AD. (2004). Prophylactic use of antibiotic bone cement: an emerging standard-in opposition. *Journal of Arthroplasty,* Vol. 19, No 4, (June 2004), pp. 759-762, ISSN 0883-5403

Hanssen AD. (2005). Local antibiotic delivery vehicles in the treatment of musculoskeletal infection *Clinical Orthopaedics Related Research,* Vol. 437, (August 2005), pp. 91-96, ISSN 0009-921X

Hanssen AD., Osmon DR., & Patel R. (2005). Local antibiotic delivery systems: what are and where are we going? *Clinical Orthopaedics Related Research,* Vol. 437, (August 2005), pp. 111-114, ISSN 0009-921X

Henry SL., Seligson D., Mangino P., & Popham GJ. (1991). Antibiotic-impregnated beads. Part I: bead implantation versus systemic therapy. *Orthopaedic Review,* Vol. 20, No 3, (March 1991), pp. 242-247, ISSN 0094-6591

Henry SL., Hood GA., & Seligson D. (1993). Long term implantation of gentamicin-polymethylmethacrylate antibiotic beads. *Clinical Orthopaedics Related Research,* Vol. 295, (October 1993), pp. 47-53, ISSN 0009-921X

Henry SL., Ostermann PA., & Seligson D. (1993). The antibiotic bead pouch technique. The management of severe compound fractures. *Clinical Orthopaedics Related Research,* Vol. 295, (October 1993), pp. 54-62, ISSN 0009-921X

Henry SL., & Galloway KP. (1995) local antibiotic therapy for the management of orthopaedic infections. Pharmacokinetic considerations. *Clinical Pharmacokinetics,* Vol. 29, No 1, (July 1995), pp. 36-45, ISSN 0312-5963

Hoff SF., Fitzgerald RH Jr., & Kelly PJ. (1981). The depot administration of penicillin G and gentamicin in acrylic bone cement. *Journal Bone Joint Surgery,* Vol. 63-A, No 5, (June 1981), pp. 798-804, ISSN 0021-9355

Holtom PD., Warren CA., Greene NW., Bravos PD., Ressler RL., Shepherd L., McPherson EJ., & Patzakis MJ. (1998). Relation of surface area to in vitro elution characteristics of vancomycin-impregnated polymethylmethacrylate spacers. *American Journal Orthopaedics*, Vol. 27, No 3, (March 1998), pp. 207-210, ISSN 1078-4519

Hou T., Xu J., Li Q., Feng J., & Zen L. (2008). In vitro evaluation of a fibrin gel antibiotic delivery system containing mesenchymal stem cells and vancomycin alginate beads for treating bone infections and facilitating bone formation. *Tissue Engineering Part A*, Vol. 14, No 7, (July 2008), pp. 1173-1182, ISSN 2152-4947

Humphrey JS., Mehta S., Seober AV., & Vail TP. (1998). Pharmacokinetics of a degradable drug delivery system in bone. *Clinical Orthopaedics Related Research*, Vol. 349, (April 1998), pp. 218-224, ISSN 0009-921X

Ipsen T., Jorgensen PS., Damholt V., & Torholm C. (1991). Gentamicin-collagen sponge for local applications. 10 cases of chronic osteomyelitis followed for 1 year. *Acta Orthopaedica Scandinavica*, Vol. 62, No 6, (December 1991), pp. 592-594, ISSN 0001-6470

Izquierdo RJ., & Northmore-Ball MD. (1994). Long term results of revision hip arthroplasty. Survival analysis with special reference to the femoral component. *Journal Bone Joint Surgery*, Vol. 76-B, No 1 (January 1994), pp. 34-39, ISSN 0301-620X

Jackson MR. (2001). Fibrin sealants in surgical practice: An overview. *American Journal Surgery*, Vol. 182, No 2 Suppl., (August 2001), pp. 1-7, ISSN 0002-9610

Jenny G. (1988). Local antibiotic therapy using gentamicin-PMMA chains in post-traumatic bone infections. Sort and long-term results. *Reconstruction Surgery Traumatology*, Vol. 157, No 4, (March 1988), pp. 36-46, ISSN 0080-0260

Jensen NK., Johnsrud LW., & Nelson MC. (1939). The local implantation of sulfonamide in compound fractures. *Surgery*, Vol. 6, pp. 1-12

Jia WY., Luo SH., Zhang CQ., & Wang JQ. (2010). In vitro and in vivo efficacies of teicoplanin-loaded calcium sulfate of chronic methicillin-resistant Staphylococcus aureus osteomyelitis. *Antimicrobial Agents Chemotherapy*, Vol. 54, No 1, (January 2010), pp. 170-176, ISSN 0066-4804

Jiranek WA., Hanssen AD., & Greenwald AS. (2006). Antibiotic-loaded bone cement for infection prophylaxis in total joint replacement. *Journal Bone Joint Surgery*, Vol. 88-A, No 11, (November 2006), pp. 2487-2500, ISSN 0021-9355

Josafsson G., Gudmudsson G., Kolmert L., & Wijkstrom S. (1990). Prophylaxis with systemic antibiotics versus gentamicin bone cement in total hip arthroplasty. A five-year survey of 1688 hips. *Clinical Orthopaedics Related Research*, Vol. 253, (April 1990), pp. 173-178, ISSN 0009-921X

Kanellakopoulou K., Tsourvakas S., Korakis T., Andreopoulos A., Dounis E., & Giamarellou H. (1994). The release of pefloxacin from acrylic bone cement and lactic-acid polymer. A comparative in vitro study. *Proceeding of 5th International Symposium on New Quinolones*, Singapore, August 1994

Kanellakopoulou K., Kolia M., Anastasiadis A., Korakis T., Giamarellos-Bourboulis EJ., Andreopoulos A., Dounis E., & Giamarellou H. (1999). Lactic-acid polymers as biodegradable carriers of fluoroquinolones: an in vitro study. *Antimicrobial Agents Chemotherapy*, Vol. 43, No 3, (March 1999), pp. 714-716, ISSN 1532-0227

Kanellakopoulou K., & Giamarellos-Bourboulis EJ. (2000). Carrier systems for the local delivery of antibiotics in bone infections. *Drugs*, Vol. 59, No 6, (June 2000), pp. 1223-132, ISSN 0012-6667

Kanellakopoulou K., Galanakis N., Giamarellos-Bourboulis EJ., Rifiotis C., Papakostas K., Andreopoulos A., Dounis E., Karagiannakos P., & Giamarellou H. (2000). Treatment of experimental osteomyelitis caused by methicillin-resistant Staphylococcus aureus with a biodegradable system of lactic acid polymer releasing pefloxacin. *Journal Antimicrobial Chemotherapy*, Vol. 46, No 2, (August 2000), pp. 311-314, ISSN 0365-7453

Kawanabe K., Okada Y., Matsusue Y., Iida H., & Nakamura T. (1998). Treatment of osteomyelitis with antibiotic-soaked porous glass ceramic. *Journal Bone Joint Surgery*, Vol. 80-B, No 3, (May 1998), pp. 527-530, ISSN 0301-620X

Kendall RW., Duncan CP., Smith JA., & Nqui-Yen JH. (1996). Persistence of bacteria on antibiotic loaded acrylic depots. A reason of caution. *Clinical Orthopaedics Related Research*, Vol. 329, (August 1996), pp. 273-280, ISSN 0009-921X

Klemm K. (2001). The use of antibiotic-containing bead chains in the treatment of chronic bone infections. *Clinical Microbiology Infection*, Vol. 7, No 1, (January 2001), pp. 28-31, ISSN 1198-743X

Kobayasi H., Shiraki K., & Ikada Y. (1992). Toxicity test of biodegradable polymers by implantation in rabbit cornea. *Journal Biomedical Materials Research*, Vol. 26, No 11, (November 1992), pp. 1463-1476, ISSN 0021-9304

Koort JK., Makinen TJ., Suokas E., Veiranto M., Jalava J., Tormala P., & Aro HT. (2008). Sustained release of ciprofloxacin from an osteoconductive poly(DL)-lactide implant. *Acta Orthopaedica*, Vol. 79, No 2, (April 2008), pp. 295-301, ISSN 1745-3674

Kram HB., Bansal M., Timberlake O., & Shoemaker WC. (1991). Antibacterial effects of fibrin glue-antibiotic mixtures. *Journal Surgical Research*, Vol. 50, No 2, (February 1991), pp. 175-178, ISSN 0022-4804

Kuechle DK., Landon GC., Musher DM., & Noble PC. (1991). Elution of vancomycin, daptomycin, and amikacin from acrylic bone cement. *Clinical Orthopaedics Related Research*, Vol. 264, (March 1991), pp. 302-308, ISSN 0009-921X

Lautenschlager EP., Jacobs JJ., Marshal GW., & Meyer PRJr. (1976). Mechanical properties of bone cements containing large doses of antibiotic powders. *Journal Biomedical Materials Research*, Vol. 10, No 6, (November 1976), pp.929-938, ISSN 0021-9304

Lazarettos J., Efstathopoulos N., Papagelopoulos PJ., Savidou OD., Kanellakopoulou K., Giamarellou H., Giamarellos- Bourboulis EJ., Nikolaou V., Kapranou A., Papalois A., & Papachristou G. (2004). A bioresorbable calcium phosphate delivery system with teicoplanin for treating MRSA osteomyelitis. *Clinical Orthopaedics Related Research*, Vol. 423, (June 2004), pp. 253-258, ISSN 0009-921X

Lazzarini L., Mader TT., & Calhoun JH. (2004). Osteomyelitis in long bones. *Journal Bone Joint Surgery*, Vol. 86-A. No 10, (October 2004), pp. 2305-2318, ISSN 0021-9355

Li XD., & Hu YY. (2001). The treatment of osteomyelitis with gentamicin-reconstituted bone xenograft-composite. *Journal Bone Joint Surgery*, Vol. 83-B, No 7, (September 2001), pp. 1063-1068, ISSN 0301-620X

Mackey D., Varlet A., & Debeaumant D. (1982). Antibiotic loaded plaster of Paris pallet: an in vitro study of a possible treatment of osteomyelitis. *Clinical Orthopaedics Related Research*, Vol. 366, (July 1982), pp. 263-268, ISSN 0009-921X

Mader JT., Landon GC., & Calhoun J. (1993). Antimicrobial treatment of osteomyelitis. *Clinical Orthopaedics Related Research*, Vol. 295, (October 1993), pp87-95, ISSN 0009-921X

Mader JT., Calhoun J., & Cobos J. (1997). In vitro evaluation of antibiotic diffusion from antibiotic-impregnated biodegradable beads and polymethylmethacrylate beads. *Antimicrobial Agents Chemotherapy,* Vol. 41, No 2, (February 1997), pp. 415-418, ISSN 0066-4804

Makinen JT., Veiranto M., Lankinen P., Moritz N., Jalava J., Tormala P., & Aro HT. (2005). In vitro and in vivo release of ciprofloxacin from osteoconductive bone defect filler. *Journal Antimicrobial Chemotherapy,* Vol. 56, No 6, (December 2005), pp. 1063-1068, ISSN 0305-7453

Malchau H., Herberts P., & Ahnfelt L. (1993). Prognosis of total hip replacement in Sweden. Follow up of 92675 operations performed 1978-1990. *Acta Orthopaedica Scandinavica,* Vol. 64, No 5, (October 1993), pp. 497-506, ISSN 0001-6470

Marks KE., Nelson CL., & Lautenschlager EP. (1976). Antibiotic-impregnated acrylic bone cement. *Journal Bone Joint Surgery,* Vol. 58-A, No 3, (April 1976), pp., 358-364, ISSN 0021-9355

Masri BA., Duncan CP., Adams KR., Nqui-Yen J., & Smith J. (1995). Streptomycin-loaded bone cement in the treatment of tuberculous osteomyelitis: an adjunct to conventional therapy. *Canadian Journal Surgery,* Vol. 38, No 1, (February 1995), pp. 64-68, ISSN 0008-428X

Masri BA., Duncan CP., & Beauchamp CP. (1998). Long term elution of antibiotics from bone cement: an in vivo study using the prosthesis of antibiotic-loaded acrylic cement (PROSTALAC) system. *Journal Arthroplasty,* Vol.13, No 3, (April 1998), pp. 331-338, ISSN 0883-5403

Matsuno H., Yudoh K., Hashimoto M., Himeda Y., Miyoshi T., Yoshida K., & Kano S. (2006). A new antibacterial carrier of hyaluronic acid. *Journal Orthopaedic Science,* Vol. 11, No 5, (October 2006), pp. 497-504, ISSN 0949-2658

McLaren AC., & Miniaci A. (1986). In vivo study to determine the efficacy of cancellous bone graft as a delivery vehicle for antibiotics. *Proceeding of 12th Annual Meeting of the Society for Biomaterials,* Minneapolis-St Paul, Minnesota, USA, September 1986

McLaren AC. (1988). Antibiotic impregnated bone graft. Postop levels of vancomycin and tobramycin. *Proceeding of Orthopaedic Trauma Association Annual Meeting,* Boston-Mass, USA, September 1998

McLaren AC. (2004). Alternative materials to acrylic bone cement for delivery of depot antibiotics in orthopaedic infections. *Clinical Orthopaedics Related Research,* Vol. 427, (October 2004), pp. 101-106, ISSN 0009-921X

Mehta S., Humphrey JS., Dchenkmann DI., Seaber AV., & Vail TP. (1996). Gentamicin distribution from collagen carrier. *Journal Orthopaedic Research,* Vol. 14, No 5, (September 1996), pp. 749-754, ISSN 0736-0266

Mendel V., Simanowski HJ., Scholz HC., & Heymman H. (2005). Therapy with gentamicin-PMMA beads, gentamicin-collagen sponge, and cefazolin for experimental osteomyelitis due to Staphylococcus aureus in rats. *Archives Orthopaedic Trauma Surgery,* Vol. 125, No 6, (July 2005), pp. 363-368, ISSN 0936-8051

Mohanty SP., Kumar MN., & Murthy NS. (2003). Use of antibiotic-loaded polymethylmethacrylate beads in the management of musculoskeletal sepsis-a retrospective study. *Journal of Orthopaedics Surgery,* Vol. 11, No 1 (January 2003), pp. 73-79, ISSN 1022-5536

Nandi SK., Munkeherjee P., Ray S., Kundu B., De DK., & Basu D. (2009). Local antibiotic delivery systems for the treatment of osteomyelitis. – A review. *Materials Science and Engineering*, Vol. 29, No 8 (October 2009), pp. 2478-2485, ISSN 0928-4931

Nelson CL., Griffin FM., Harrison BH., & Cooper RE. (1992). In vitro elution characteristics of commercially and noncommercially prepared antibiotic PMMA beads. *Clinical Orthopaedics Related Research*, Vol. 284, (November 1992), pp. 303-309, ISSN 0009-921X

Nelson CL., McLaren SG., Skinner RA., Smeltzer MS., Thomes JR., & Olsen KM. (2002). The treatment of experimental osteomyelitis by surgical debridement and the implantation of calcium sulfate tobramycin pellets. *Journal Orthopaedic Research*, Vol. 20, No 4, (July 2002), pp. 643-647, ISSN 0737-0266

Nelson CL. (2004). The current status of material used for depot delivery of drugs. *Clinical Orthopaedics Related Research*, Vol. 427, (October 2004), pp. 72-78, ISSN 0009-921X

Neut D., van der Belt H., Stokroos L., van Hom JR, van der Mei HC., & Busscher HJ. (2001). Biomaterial-associated infection of gentamicin-loaded PMMA beads in orthopaedic revision surgery. *Journal Antimicrobial Chemotherapy*, Vol. 47, No 6, (July 2001), pp. 885-891, ISSN 0305-7453

Nie L., Nicolau DP., Nightingale CH., Browner BD., & Quintiliani R. (1995). In vitro elution of ofloxacin from a bioabsorbable polymer. *Acta Orthopaedica Scandinavica*, Vol. 66, No 4, (August 1995), pp. 365-368, ISSN 0001-6470

Noel SP., Courtney H., Bumgardner JD., & Haggard WO. (2008). Chitosan films: a potential local drug delivery system for antibiotics. *Clinical Orthopaedics Related Research*, Vol. 466, (June 2008), pp. 1377-1382, ISSN 0009-921X

Organ CH. (1971). The utilization of massive doses of antimicrobial agents with isolation perfusion in the treatment of chronic osteomyelitis. *Clinical Orthopaedics Related Research*, Vol. 76, (October 1971), pp. 185-193, ISSN 0009-921X

Ouedraogo M., Semde R., Some IT., Traore-Ouedraogo R., Guisson IP., Henschel V., Dubois J., Amighi K., & Ervard B. (2008). Monoolein-water liquid crystalline gels of gentamicin as bioresorbable implants for the local treatment of chronic osteomyelitis: in vitro characterization. *Drug development Industrial Pharmacy*, Vol. 34, No 7, (July 2008), pp. 753-760, ISSN 0363-9045

Ozaki T., Yoshitaka T., Kunisada T., Dan'ura T., Naito N., & Inoue H. (1998). Vancomycin-impregnated polymethylmethacrylate beads for methicillin-resistant Staphylococcus aureus (MRSA) infection: report of two cases. *Journal Orthopaedic Science*, Vol. 3, No 3, (June 1998), pp., 163-168, ISSN 0949-2658

Patzakis MJ., & Wilkins J. (1989). Factors influencing infection rate in open fracture wounds. *Clinical Orthopaedics Related Research*, Vol. 243, (June 1989), pp. 36-40, ISSN 0009-921X

Patzakis MJ., Mazur K., Wilkins J., Sherman R., & Holtom P. (1993). Septopal beads and autogenous bone grafting for bone defects in patients with chronic osteomyelitis. *Clinical Orthopaedics Related Research*, Vol. 295, (October 1993), pp. 112-118, ISSN 0009-921X

Perry CR., & Pearson RL. (1991). Local antibiotic delivery in the treatment of bone and joint infections. *Clinical Orthopaedics Related Research*, Vol. 263, (February 1991), pp. 215-226, ISSN 0009-921X

Popham GJ., Mangino P., Seligson D., & Henry SL. (1991). Antibiotic-impregnated beads. Part II: Factors in antibiotic selection. *Orthopaedic Review*, Vol. 20, No 4, (April 1991), pp. 331-337, ISSN 0094-6591

Rao KP. (1995). Recent developments of collagen-based materials for medical applications and drug delivery systems. *Journal Biomaterial Science*, Vol. 7, No 7, (July 1995), pp. 623-645, ISSN 0920-5063

Raut W., Siney PD., & Wroblewski BM. (1995). One-stage revision of total hip arthroplasty for deep infection. Long-term follow-up. *Clinical Orthopaedics Related Research*, Vol. 321, (December 1995). Pp. 202-207, ISSN 0009-921X

Reddi AH. (1985). Implant-stimulated interface reactions during collagenous bone matrix-induced bone formation. *Biomedical materials Research*, Vol. 19, No 3, (March 1985), pp. 233-239, ISSN 0021-9304

Rhyu KH., Jung MH., Yoo JJ., Seong SC., & Kim HJ. (2003). In vitro release of vancomycin from vancomycin-loaded blood coated demineralized bone. *International Orthopaedics*, Vol. 27, No 1, (January 2003), pp. 53-55, ISSN 0341-2695

Rissing JP. (1997). Antimicrobial therapy for chronic osteomyelitis. *Clinical Infectious Diseases*, Vol. 25, No 6, (December 1997), pp. 1327-1333, ISSN 1058-4838

Rushton N. (1997). Applications of local antibiotic therapy. *European Journal Surgery*, Vol.163, Suppl. 578, (September 1997), pp. 27-30, ISSN 1102-416X

Ruszcak Z., & Friess W. (2003). Collagen as a carrier for on-site delivery on antibacterial drugs. *Advanced Drug Delivery Reviews*, Vol. 55, No 12, (November 2003), pp. 1679-1698, ISSN 0169-409X

Sampath SS., Garvin KL., & Robinson DH. (1992). Preparation and characterization of biodegradable poly(L-lactic acid) gentamicin delivery systems. *International Journal of Pharmaceutics*, Vol. 78, No 1, (January 1992), pp. 165-174, ISSN 0378-5173

Santschi EM., & McGarvey L. (2003). In vitro elution of gentamicin from Plaster of Paris beads. *Veterinary Surgery*, Vol. 32, No 2, (March-April 2003), pp. 128-133, ISSN 0161-3499

Schierhoz JM., Steinhauser H., Rump AF., Berkels R., & Pulverer G. (1997). Controlled release of antibiotics from biomedical polyurethanes: morphological and structural features. *Biomaterials*, Vol. 18, No 12, (June 1997), pp. 839-844, ISSN 0142-9612

Seligson D., Popham GJ., Voos K., Henry SL., & Faghri M. (1993). Antibiotic-leaching from polymethylmethacrylate beads. *Journal Bone Joint Surgery*, Vol. 75-A, No 5, (May 1993), pp. 714-720, ISSN 0021-9355

Shinto Y., Uchida A., Korkusuz F., Araki N., & Ono K. (1992). Calcium Hydroxyapatite ceramic used as a delivery system for antibiotics. *Journal Bone Joint Surgery*, Vol. 74-B, No 4, (July 1992), pp. 600-604, ISSN 0301-620X

Shirtliff ME., Calhoun JH., & Mader JT. (2002). Experimental osteomyelitis treatment with antibiotic-impregnated Hydroxyapatite. *Clinical Orthopaedics Related Research*, Vol. 401, (August 2002), pp. 239-247, ISSN 0009-921X

Soundrapandian C., Sa B., & Datta S. (2009). Organic-inorganic composites for bone drug delivery. *AAPS PharmSciTech*, Vol. 10, No 4, (December 2009), pp. 1158-1171, ISSN 1530-9932

Stemberger A., Grimm H., Boder F., Rahn HD., & Ascherl R. (1997). Local treatment of bone and soft tissue infections with the collagen-gentamicin sponge. *European journal Surgery Supplement*, Vol. 578, (January 1997), pp. 17-26, ISSN 1102-416X

Taylor EW. (1997). Surgical infection: current concerns. *European Journal Surgery,* Vol. 163, Suppl. 578, (June 1997), pp. 5-9, ISSN 1102-416X

Thies C. (1982). Microcapsules as drug delivery devices. *Critical Reviews Biomedical Engineering,* Vol. 8, No 4, (April 1982), pp. 335-383, ISSN 0278-940X

Tomczak RL., Dowdy N., Storm T., Lane J., & Coldarella D. (1989). Use of ceftazidime-impregnated polymethylmethacrylate beads in the treatment of Pseudomonas osteomyelitis. *Journal Foot Surgery,* Vol. 28, No 6, (November-December 1989), pp. 542-546, ISSN 0449-2544

Tonetti MS., Cortellini P., Carnevale G., Cattabriga M., de Sanctis M., & Pini-Prato GP. (1998). A controlled multicenter study of adjunctive use of tetracycline periodontal fibers in mandibular class II furcations with persistent bleeding. *Journal Clinical Periodontology,* Vol. 25, No 9, (September 1998), pp. 728-736, ISSN 0303-6979

Trafny EA., Stepinska M., Antos M., & Grzybowski J. (1995). Effect of free and liposome encapsulated antibiotics on adherence to Pseudomonas aeruginosa to collagen type I. *Antimicrobial Agents Chemotherapy,* Vol. 39, No 12, (December 1995), pp. 2645-2649, ISSN 0066-4804

Trafny EA., Grzybowski J., Olszowska-Golec M., Antos M., & Struzyna J. (1996). Anti-pseudomonal activity of collagen sponge with liposomal polymyxin B. *Pharmacological Research,* Vol. 33, No 1, (January 1996), pp. 63-65, ISSN 1043-6618

Tredwell S., Jackson J., Hamilton D., Lee V., & Burt H. (2006). Use of fibrin sealants for the localized controlled release of cefazolin. *Canadian Journal Surgery,* Vol. 49, No 5, (October 2006), pp. 347-352, ISSN 0008-428X

Tsourvakas S., Hatzigrigoris P., Tsibinos A., Kanellakopoulou K., Giamarellou H., & Dounis E. (1995). Pharmacokinetic study of fibrin clot-ciprofloxacin complex: an in vitro and in vivo experimental investigation. *Archives Orthopaedic Trauma Surgery,* Vol. 114, No 5, (June 1995), pp. 295-297, ISSN 0936-8051

Tsourvakas S., Alexandropoulos C., Karatzios C., Egnatiadis N., & Kampagiannis N. (2009). Elution of ciprofloxacin from acrylic bone cement and fibrin clot: an in vitro study. *Acta Orthopaedica Belgica,* Vol. 75, No 4, (August 2009), pp. 537-542, ISSN 0001-6462

Ueng SW., Wei FC., & Shih CH. (1997). Management of large infected tibial defects with antibiotic beads local therapy and staged fibular osteoseptocutaneous free transfer. *Journal of Trauma,* Vol. 43, No 2, (August 1997), pp. 268-274, ISSN 0022-5282

von Eiff C., Bettin D., Proctor RA., Lindner N., Winkelmann W., & Peters G.(1997). Recovery of small colony variants of Staphylococcus aureus following gentamicin bead placement for osteomyelitis. *Clinical Infectious Diseases,* Vol. 25, No 5, (November 1997), pp. 1250-1251, ISSN 1058-4838

Wachol-Drewek Z., Pfeiffer M., & Scholl E. (1996). Comparative investigation of drug delivery of collagen implants saturated in antibiotics solutions and a sponge containing gentamicin. *Biomaterials,* Vol. 17, No 17, (September 1996), pp. 1733-1738, ISSN 0142-9612

Wahlig H., Dingeldein E., Bergmann R., & Reuss K. (1978). The release of gentamicin from polymethylmethacrylate beads. An experimental and pharmacokinetic study. *Journal Bone Joint Surgery,* Vol. 60-B, No 2, (May 1978), pp. 270-275, ISSN 0301-620X

Walenkamp GH. (1989). Small PMMA beads improve gentamicin release. *Acta Orthopaedica Scandinavica,* Vol. 69, No 6, (December 1989), pp. 668-669, ISSN 0001-6470

Walenkamp GH. (1997). Chronic osteomyelitis. *Acta Orthopaedica Scandinavica,* Vol. 68, No 5, (October 1997), pp.497-506, ISSN 0001-6470

Wei G., Kotoura Y., Oka M., Yamamuto T., Wada R., Hyon SH., & Ikada Y. (1991). A bioabsorbable delivery system for antibiotic treatment of osteomyelitis. The use of lactic acid oligomer as a carrier. *Journal bone joint Surgery,* Vol. 73-B, No 2, (March 1991), pp. 246-252, ISSN 0301-620X

Whiteside LA. (1994). Treatment of infected total knee arthroplasty. *Clinical Orthopaedic Related Research,* Vol. 299, (February 1994), pp. 169-172, ISSN 0009-921X

Wilson KJ., Cierny G., Adams KR., & Mader JT. (1988). Comparative evaluation of the diffusion of tobramycin and cefotaxime out of antibiotic-impregnated polymethylmethacrylate beads. *Journal Orthopaedic Research,* Vol. 6, No 2, (March 1988), pp. 279-286, ISSN 0736-0266

Wininger DA., & Fass RJ. (1996). Antibiotic-impregnated cement and beads for orthopedic infections. *Antimicrobial Agents Chemotherapy,* Vol. 40, No 12, (December 1996), pp. 2675-2679, ISSN 0066-4804

Witso E., Persen L., Loseth K., Benum P., & Bergh K. (2000). Cancellous bone as an antibiotic carrier. *Acta Orthopaedica Scandinavica,* Vol. 71, No 1, (February 2000), pp.80-84, ISSN 0001-6470

Woolverton CJ., Fulton JA., Salstrom SJ., Hayslip J., Haller NA., Wildroudt ML., & McPhee M. (2001). Tetracycline delivery from fibrin controls peritoneal infection without measurable systemic antibiotic. *Journal Antimicrobial Chemotherapy,* Vol. 48, No 6, (December 2001), pp. 861-867, ISSN 0305-7453

Younger AS., Duncan CP., & Masri BA. (1998). Treatment of infection associated with segmental bone loss in the proximal part of the femur in two stages with use of an antibiotic loaded interval prosthesis. *Journal Bone Joint Surgery,* Vol. 80-A, No 1, (January 1998), pp. 60-69, ISSN 0021-9355

Zilch H., & Lambiris E. (1986). The sustained release of cefotaxim from a fibrin-cefotaxim compound in treatment of osteitis. Pharmacokinetic study and clinical results. *Archives Orthopaedic Trauma Surgery,* Vol. 106, No 1, (January 1986), pp. 36-41, ISSN 0936-8051

Part 2

Topographic Reconstruction Strategies

4

Acellular Dermal Matrix for Optimizing Outcomes in Implant-Based Breast Reconstruction: Primary and Revisionary Procedures

Ron Israeli

Hofstra North Shore-LIJ School of Medicine
USA

1. Introduction

The benefits of using acellular dermal matrices (ADMs) in implant-based breast reconstruction have recently been reported both for primary reconstructions as well as revisionary procedures. Techniques using ADMs in these settings have been shown to assist in controlling implant position by defining the inframammary fold (IMF) and lateral mammary fold (LMF). In addition, they may provide a decreased risk of capsular contracture and may be used in the management of already developed contractures. The purpose of this chapter is to review the newest trends in the use of ADMs in implant-based breast reconstruction. A direct-to-implant approach to primary breast reconstruction following nipple-areola sparing mastectomy (NASM) is detailed and the revisionary procedures highlighted include the correction of implant malposition and the management of capsular contracture.

2. Primary reconstruction

Immediate direct-to-implant breast reconstruction after skin-sparing or NASM (Breuing & Warren, 2005; Breuing & Colwell, 2007; Cassileth et al., 2011; Salzberg, 2006; Salzberg et al., 2011; Topol et al., 2008; Wang et al., 2008; Zienowicz & Karacaoglu, 2007) is gaining popularity as a viable alternative to immediate expander/implant reconstruction which is the current standard of care for implant-based breast reconstruction postmastectomy (American Society of Plastic Surgeons [ASPS], 2009). While both approaches allow immediate creation of the breast mound offering pyschologic and aesthetic benefits, the direct-to-implant approach allows maximal use of the preserved mastectomy skin at the time of reconstruction. This eliminates the need for serial tissue expansions and potentially avoids a second surgery.

The use of ADMs has greatly facilitated direct-to-implant as well as expander/implant reconstruction. By extending the reach of the pectoralis major muscle, ADMs not only provide complete coverage of the subpectorally placed implant or expander but they also increase the volume of the subpectoral pocket. In expander/implant reconstructions, the increased subpectoral volume allows greater initial expansion of the expander, thus reducing the total number of expansions and time to full expansion (Collis et al., 2011; Hanna et al., 2011; Spear et al., 2008). In direct-to-implant reconstructions, the increased subpectoral volume allows a permanent implant to be placed in suitable patients. Several series have reported low complication rates and good aesthetic outcomes with ADM-assisted direct-to-implant reconstruction (Breuing & Warren, 2005; Breuing & Colwell, 2007; Cassileth et al., 2011; Salzberg, 2006; Salzberg et al., 2011; Topol et al., 2008; Zienowicz & Karacaoglu, 2007) that are comparable to those reported with ADM-assisted expander/implant reconstructions (S. Becker et al., 2009; Newman et al., 2011; Rawlani et al., 2011). In particular, in the largest series (260 patients representing 466 reconstructions) with the longest follow-up (mean 28.9 months; range 0.3-97.7 months), the overall complication rate was 3.9%. Complications included implant loss 1.3%, skin breakdown/necrosis 1.1%, hematoma 1.1%, ADM exposure 0.6%, capsular contracture 0.4%, and infection 0.2% (Salzberg et al., 2011).

2.1 Review of experience

The author's initial clinical experience with the use of ADM-assisted immediate direct-to-implant reconstruction following NASM consists of 47 reconstructions (24 therapeutic and 23 prophylactic) performed in 27 patients from January 2007 to June 2009 (Israeli et al., 2011). Patients were selected to undergo ADM-assisted immediate direct-to-implant reconstruction if they were not candidates for or did not desire an autologous procedure. Patients had an average age of 49 years (range 27-72 years). During the early postoperative period (<30 days) complications occurred in 21 breasts and included mild nipple-areola skin slough (13), moderate nipple-areola skin slough (2), full-thickness nipple loss (2), cellulitis (3), and capsular contracture (1). All cases of nipple-areola skin slough were resolved with local care and all cases of cellulitis were resolved with oral antibiotics. There were no cases of device loss or failed reconstruction during an average follow-up period of 17 months (range 2-28 months). There was one case of NA occult tumor that required NA removal. Two patients required revisionary surgery; one patient underwent implant exchange as she desired a larger implant and the other underwent nipple reconstruction to regain nipple projection after nipple flattening. Our results suggest that ADM-assisted direct-to-implant breast reconstruction can be reliably accomplished after NASM and are in concordance with other published series of ADM-assisted direct-to-implant reconstruction (Breuing & Warren, 2005; Breuing & Colwell, 2007; Cassileth et al., 2011; Salzberg, 2006; Salzberg et al., 2011; Topol et al., 2008; Zienowicz & Karacaoglu, 2007).

The success of direct-to-implant reconstruction after NASM is dependent on proper patient selection. Patients with evidence of direct nipple involvement of tumor, Paget's disease, inflammatory breast cancer, tumor size > 3 cm, or tumor < 2 cm from nipple center may not be suitable candidates for NASM because of an increased risk of local tumor recurrence (Brachtel et al., 2009; Cunnick & Mokbel, 2006). Following NASM, the quality of the preserved skin is an important consideration for direct-to-implant reconstruction because extremely thin skin or compromised skin increases the risk of ischemia and skin necrosis which can eventually lead to implant loss (Woerdeman et al., 2006). Moreover, patients with preoperative macromastia or breast ptosis who undergo direct-to-implant reconstruction are at increased risk of perioperative complications and revisionary surgery (Roostaeian et al.,

Acellular Dermal Matrix for Optimizing Outcomes in Implant-Based Breast Reconstruction:
Primary and Revisionary Procedures

63

2011). Further, age > 65 years and comorbid conditions such as smoking, obesity, and hypertension increase the risk of perioperative complications and the latter three also increase the risk of reconstructive failure (McCarthy et al., 2008). Thus, a careful evaluation of these risk factors needs to be taken into consideration when selecting patients for direct-to-implant reconstruction.

2.2 Operative details

The use of ADM to extend the pectoralis major muscle at the lower pole to provide complete soft tissue coverage of the implant (Figure 1) has been previously described (Breuing & Warren, 2005; Salzberg, 2006; Zienowicz & Karacaoglu, 2007). NASM is performed via a periareolar incision (Figures 2A & 2B). In some patients, a lateral extension to the periareolar incision may be required to facilitate mastectomy. Following

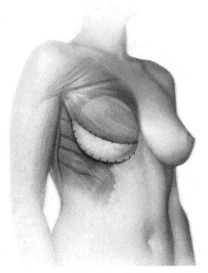

Fig. 1. ADM placement at the inferolateral border of the implant.

mastectomy, nipple coring is performed (Figure 2C) and specimens are taken and sent for permanent fixation and evaluation of tumor presence. Immediate reconstruction is then performed with subpectoral implant placement. The inferolateral origin of the pectoralis major muscle is elevated off the chest wall and a subpectoral pocket is created based on the dimensions of the previous breast perimeter and the desired implant size. The LMF is defined and marked on the chest wall in-continuity with the IMF. A prehydrated sheet of ADM (AlloDerm®, human acellular dermal matrix, LifeCell Corporation, Branchburg, NJ) is then sutured to the chest wall using running 2-0 Vicryl sutures (Ethicon, Inc., Somerville, NJ) along the marked fold. The deep dermal side of the ADM is placed facing the overlying lower breast skin. An implant is introduced into the subpectoral pocket under the muscle. The ADM is then brought over the implant, tapered as needed, and secured to the free border of the pectoralis muscle using running 2-0 Vicryl sutures, completely covering the implant (Figure 2D). Mastectomy flaps are then tailored as necessary and closed in layers over two closed suction drains brought out laterally. One drain is placed between the ADM and the overlying skin at the IMF and a second drain is placed deep to the superior mastectomy skin.

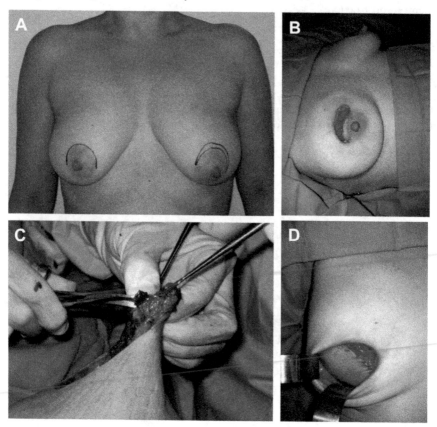

Fig. 2. Operative details. A: Preoperative markings. B: Periareolar incision. C: Nipple coring. D: ADM-assisted reconstruction.

2.3 Patient cases

Case 1

Patient is a 53-year-old with the BRCA 2 genetic mutation and a family history of breast cancer. She opted to undergo prophylactic mastectomy with immediate implant-based breast reconstruction. Physical examination revealed no contraindications for NASM. She had nearly symmetric B-cup breasts with grade 2 ptosis (Figure 3). Patient underwent NASM via the supra-areolar approach. Immediate ADM-assisted, direct-to-implant breast reconstruction was performed with 400 cc, smooth round gel implants. Her postoperative course was uneventful. At 11-month follow-up, she exhibited good symmetry, lower-pole projection, and volume match compared with preoperative size with well-camouflaged periareolar scars.

Acellular Dermal Matrix for Optimizing Outcomes in Implant-Based Breast Reconstruction:
Primary and Revisionary Procedures

65

Preoperative

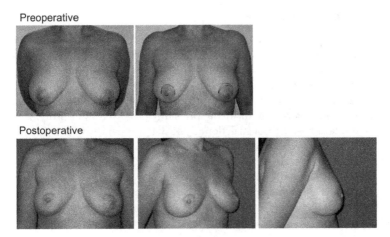

Postoperative

Fig. 3. A 53-year-old patient who underwent bilateral prophylactic mastectomy via the supra-areolar approach and received smooth round gel implants. Her postoperative course was uneventful. Postoperative: at 11 months follow-up.

Case 2

Patient is a 46-year-old diagnosed with right invasive ductal carcinoma. She elected to undergo right therapeutic mastectomy and left prophylactic mastectomy. There were no contraindications to proceeding with NASM. She had bilateral B-cup breasts with a slightly more ptotic right side. Patient underwent bilateral NASM via the supra-areolar approach with immediate ADM-assisted breast reconstruction using 325 cc smooth round gel implants. She had an uneventful postoperative course. At 4-month follow-up, she had good implant position, breast symmetry, and a well-healed periareolar scar.

Preoperative

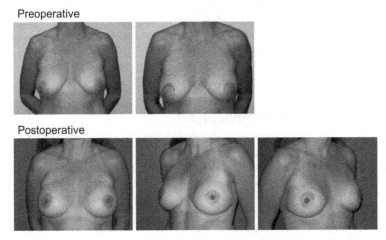

Postoperative

Fig. 4. A 46-year-old patient who underwent bilateral mastectomy, left prophylactic and right therapeutic for invasive ductal carcinoma, via the supra-areolar approach and received smooth round gel implants. Postoperative: at 4 months follow-up.

3. Revisionary procedures

Implant-based reconstruction is the most widely used approach to breast reconstruction postmastectomy because of its simplicity (ASPS, 2009). As opposed to autologous procedures, it is technically less demanding, has shorter operative times, results in brief hospital stays, has decreased short-term costs, and has no associated donor site morbidity (Ahmed et al., 2005). In addition, good to excellent aesthetic outcomes and high patient satisfaction have been reported with this approach (Cordeiro & McCarthy, 2006). Despite these benefits, implant-based reconstruction is not without concerns; it is associated with a high rate of implant-related complications notably capsular contracture, implant malposition, asymmetry, and rippling (Cunningham & McCue, 2009; Handel et al, 2006; Spear et al, 2007). Consequently, rates of revisionary surgery are also high; approximately 34%-52% of reconstruction patients undergo revision surgery within 3-6 years of their primary procedure and 36% of revision reconstruction patients undergo further revisionary surgery (Cunningham & McCue, 2009; Handel et al, 2006; Spear et al, 2007).

Corrective techniques for capsular contracture, implant malposition, and rippling have traditionally involved capsulotomy or capsulectomy, implant pocket change, implant replacement, use of capsular flaps, or a combination of these (Baxter, 2003; Maxwell & Gabriel, 2009). These techniques, however, have not always been reliable and recurrence is common (H. Becker et al, 2005; Chasan & Francis, 2008; Massiha, 2002; Spear et al., 2003). Given the safety, efficacy, and aesthetic results obtained with the use of ADM in primary breast reconstruction, there is an emerging trend to use ADM for the correction and prevention of implant-related complications in both reconstructive and aesthetic patients. The feasibility of using ADM for the correction of visible implant rippling and breast deformities due to implant malposition was initially reported almost a decade ago in breast reconstruction and aesthetic patients (Baxter, 2003; Duncan, 2001). Since then several studies have demonstrated a significant reduction in recurrence and improved cosmesis with the use of ADM for the correction of capsular contracture, implant malposition, and rippling (Breuing & Colwell, 2007; Maxwell & Gabriel, 2009; Grabov-Nardini et al., 2009; Hartzell et al., 2010; Spear et al., 2011). Overall, > 87% of implant-related complications were successfully managed using ADMs. Although promising, it should be noted that the follow-up period in most of these studies was relatively short averaging 9-12 months which may not be sufficiently long to evaluate recurrence rates.

3.1 Correction of implant malposition

Implant malposition manifesting as inferior, medial (symmastia), or lateral malposition is a commonly encountered complication of implant-based reconstructions. In primary reconstruction patients, a 20% reoperation rate due to implant malposition has been reported over a 6-year period (Spear et al., 2007). A number of factors may cause implant malposition including inadequate or excessive pocket dissection; overzealous release of the IMF, lateral and/or medial release of breast tissues, or lateral and/or medial release of the pectoralis major muscle; placement of excessively large implants; or attenuated capsular tissues (Baxter, 2003). Traditional approaches to surgical correction of implant malposition have included capsulorrhaphy with or without mirror-image capsulotomy (Chasan, 2005; Chasan & Francis, 2008; Spear & Little, 1988), implant site change from subglandular to subpectoral or subpectoral to neosubpectoral (Maxwell et al., 2009; Spear et al., 2009), and use of an adjustable implant (H. Becker et al., 2005). These approaches are often technically demanding and not always reliable (Spear et al., 2011). Capsulorrhaphy, the mainstay of corrective surgery, often does not sufficiently prevent the implant from falling against the suture line or moving across it (Voice & Carlsen, 2001). Consequently, reinforcement of the suture line with capsular flaps has been attempted (Voice & Carlsen, 2001) and a recent case study has noted success with this technique, albeit with a short follow-up period of 3-6 months (Yoo & Lee, 2010). However, capsular flaps have limited applicability in patients with attenuated capsules who are unlikely to have adequate tissue. As an alternative to capsular flaps, recent studies have advocated the use of ADM to reinforce the capsulorrhaphy suture line and maintain the implant within its pocket (Maxwell & Gabriel, 2009; Hartzell et al., 2010; Spear et al., 2011). In addition, the use of ADM also helps to redefine the IMF and LMF. Successful correction of implant malposition has been reported with the use of ADM with good aesthetic results, no recurrence, and minimal complications and failures.

3.1.1 Review of experience

The author's initial clinical experience with the correction of implant malposition with ADM assistance is derived from 12 patients who collectively had 21 inferior and lateral implant malpositions (Israeli & Cody, 2011). Patients were treated between December 2009 and March 2010. All patients underwent corrective surgery as described below with ADM reinforcement of the capsulorrhaphy suture line. Patients have been followed for a mean of 7 months (range 3-15 months) with no evidence of complications or recurrences. Proper implant position was reestablished in all patients with well-defined folds.

3.1.2 Operative details

The technique of using ADM to reinforce fold correction after capsulorrhaphy has been recently reported (Spear et al., 2011). The essential steps of corrective surgery include fold recreation by capsulorrhaphy, reinforcement of the fold with overlapping ADM secured to capsule, and pocket size correction, including mirror image capsulotomy when necessary (Figure 5).

Preoperatively, planned capsulorrhaphy fold correction and IMF position are marked with the patient in the upright standing position (Figure 6). The implant is accessed and removed via the previous mastectomy incision. If needed, the new IMF location can be remarked intraoperatively with the help of 25-gauge needles (Figures 7A & 7B). A capsulorrhaphy is then performed to create the new IMF and LMF with several rows of running 0-TiCron™ sutures (Covidien, Mansfield, MA) to the chest wall (Figure 7C). The desired fold location can be verified with the help of a sizer or implant. If needed, a superior capsular incision is made along the entire superior aspect of the breast to allow for improved implant positioning. The newly created IMF and lMF positions are then reinforced with a sheet of prehydrated ADM (AlloDerm) (Figure 7D). The ADM is placed over the fold suture line, with its deep dermal side facing the skin flaps, overlapping ~1.5 to 2 cm on either side of the repair. It is secured with multiple interrupted or with running 2-0 Vicryl sutures through the capsule to the chest wall posteriorly and to the capsule over the anterior surface along the entire length of the IMF and LMF. A new implant is introduced into the pocket and muscle, capsule, and skin closure are performed completing the corrective surgery (Figure 8).

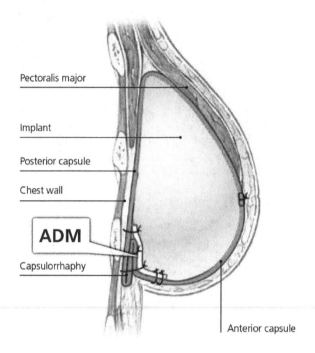

Fig. 5. Schematic representation of ADM reinforcement of recreated IMF and LMF. Illustration with permission from LifeCell Corporation (Branchburg, New Jersey).

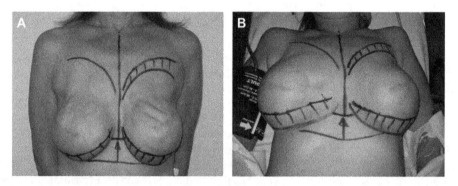

Fig. 6. Preoperative markings. A: Midline, planned capsulorrhaphy fold corrections, and planned IMF positions are marked with patient upright. The extent of inferior malposition is noted in this position. B: Examination of the patient in the supine position reveals the extent of lateral malposition.

Acellular Dermal Matrix for Optimizing Outcomes in Implant-Based Breast Reconstruction:
Primary and Revisionary Procedures

69

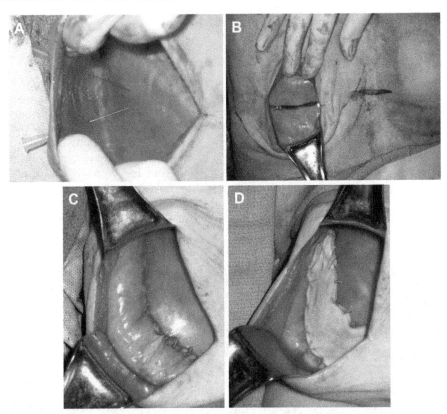

Fig. 7. Intraoperative view. A: The location of the new IMF is defined intraoperatively with the help of 25-gauge needles. B: The blue marking on the capsule indicates the new IMF position. C: Recreation of the new IMF and LMF by capsulorrhaphy. D: Reinforcement of the capsulorrhaphy suture line with ADM.

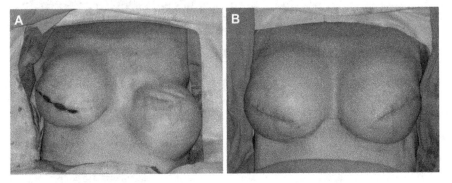

Fig. 8. Immediate postoperative stage. A: Revisionary surgery completed on right breast; implant is repositioned higher up on the chest wall compared with the unrevised left breast. B: Completion of revisionary surgery on the left breast establishes symmetry.

3.1.3 Patient cases

Case 3

A 48-year-old woman with a history of lobular carcinoma in situ presented with inferior implant malposition, breast asymmetry, and severe implant rippling at the superomedial aspect of her breasts after second stage bilateral tissue expander/implant reconstruction (Figure 9). Her implant-related problems were due to loss of IMFs and LMFs. To address these, she underwent bilateral recreation of the folds by capsulorrhaphy. Because she had thinned tissue, her native tissues were insufficient to reinforce the folds and ADM was used to reinforce the folds. An implant exchange was also performed and her silicone implants (450 cc) were replaced with slightly larger silicone implants (475 cc) to better fit the pocket size correction. The larger implants would also help toward reducing rippling. At 7 months post-revisionary surgery, the patient exhibited well-proportioned, symmetrical breasts with good contour as a result of well-defined IMFs and LMFs. Implant rippling was greatly reduced.

Preoperative

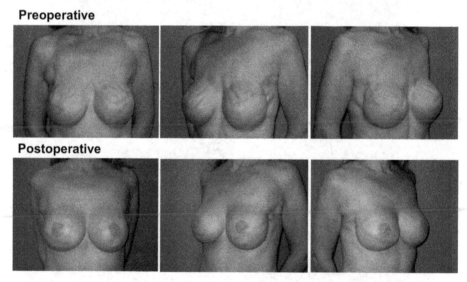

Postoperative

Fig. 9. Preoperative stage: patient presented with implant malposition, asymmetry, and significant implant rippling after second stage bilateral tissue expander/implant breast reconstruction. Postoperative stage: at 7 months of follow-up (with interim nipple-areola reconstruction) after correction of implant malposition using the technique described. The IMF and LMF are well-defined and rippling is improved.

Case 4

A 45-year-old woman with a history of left breast cancer presented with implant malposition and significant rippling after first stage bilateral tissue expander breast reconstruction. She was found to have inferior and lateral implant malposition as well as excess breast skin laxity with rippling. She underwent bilateral IMF and LMF correction with capsulorrhaphy. Each fold repair was reinforced with ADM and the breast skin

Acellular Dermal Matrix for Optimizing Outcomes in Implant-Based Breast Reconstruction:
Primary and Revisionary Procedures

71

envelope was tapered to accommodate 450 cc silicone gel implants. At 7 months after undergoing expander-implant exchange with revision reconstruction, the patient is found to have good breast contour and symmetry. Due to the improved balance between her breast skin, fold placement and implant position, her rippling is markedly reduced.

Preoperative

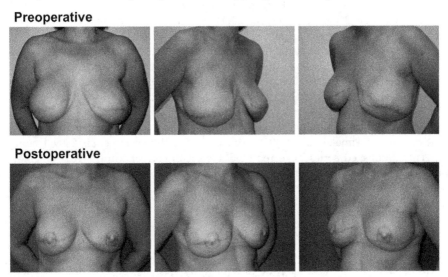

Postoperative

Fig. 10. Preoperative stage: patient presented with implant malposition and significant rippling after first stage bilateral tissue expander breast reconstruction. Postoperative stage: at 7 months of follow-up (with interim nipple-areola reconstruction) after correction of implant malposition using the technique described. The IMF and LMF are well-defined and rippling is improved.

3.2 Correction of capsular contracture

Capsular contracture is the most common complication associated with implant-based breast reconstruction (Adams, 2009). Core clinical studies from device manufacturers have reported a 6-year cumulative incidence of capsular contracture rate of 14%-16% in primary and 25% in revision reconstruction patients (Cunningham & McCue, 2009; Spear et al., 2007). Capsular contracture was also the most common reason for revisionary surgery in these studies.

The true cause of capsular contracture is unknown. Current evidence suggests that subclinical infection with biofilm-forming or nonbiofilm-forming bacteria may be a primary cause. A causal link between subclinical infection, biofilm formation, and capsular contracture has been demonstrated in a recent porcine study (Tamboto et al., 2010). Irrespective of the cause of capsular contracture, it is believed that inflammation at the cellular level eventually leads to pathologic capsular contracture (Adams, 2010). Support for this hypothesis comes from a clinical study where foreign body inflammatory response in capsular tissue was shown to be directly correlated to capsule thickness and Baker score (Prantl et al., 2007).

Traditionally, corrective surgery for capsular contracture has entailed open capsulotomy or partial/total capsulectomy, followed by implant site change, and implant exchange (Maxwell & Gabriel, 2009), although this does not always prevent recurrence. More recently, ADMs have been used at the inferolateral pole after capsulotomy or capsulectomy to help correct and prevent capsular contracture (Breuing & Colwell, 2007; Hartzell et al., 2010; Maxwell & Gabriel, 2009; Spear et al., 2011). In ADM-assisted implant-based primary reconstructions, a low rate of capsular contracture (0%-2%) has been observed (S. Becker et al., 2009; Bindingnavele et al., 2007; Breuing & Colwell, 2007; Namnoum, 2009; Salzberg, 2006; Salzberg et al., 2011; Spear et al., 2008; Zienowicz & Karacaoglu, 2007), suggesting that ADMs may help prevent or reduce the risk of capsular contracture; hence, the rationale for using ADMs for the correction and prevention of capsular contracture. Animal and clinical studies suggest that ADMs may prevent capsular contracture by minimizing the inflammatory response, thereby reducing capsule formation around implants (Basu et al., 2010; Komorowska-Timek et al., 2009; Orenstein et al., 2010; Stump et al., 2009; Uzunismail et al., 2008). Published series have reported successful correction of > 90% of grade 3/4 capsular contractures with the use of ADMs with no recurrences during a mean follow-up period of 9-21 months (Breuing & Colwell; 2007; Maxwell & Gabriel, 2009; Hartzell et al., 2010; Spear et al., 2011).

3.2.1 Review of experience

Between November 2005 and April 2010, the author used ADM for the correction of capsular contracture (grade 3 or 4) in 18 patients (21 breasts) (Israeli, 2011). All patients developed capsular contracture after tissue expander/implant reconstruction postmastectomy. Nine breasts had received prior radiotherapy. During a follow-up period of 3-43 months, initial successful correction of capsular contracture (ie, achievement of grade ≤ 2) was noted in 17 patients. There was 1 case of early post-operative cellulitis requiring oral antibiotics in a patient with a history of radiotherapy who later developed recurrent contracture. There were no cases of implant loss.

3.2.2 Operative details

We have previously described the technique of using ADM for the correction of capsular contracture (Israeli & Feingold, 2011) which is essentially the same as for a primary reconstruction (Figure 1). Key steps of corrective surgery include capsulectomy, expansion of implant pocket using a sheet of ADM, and redefining the IMF and LMF. Using the previous mastectomy incision, the implant or expander is accessed and removed. A circumferential capsulotomy is performed around the implant pocket at the level of the chest wall and the inferolateral border of the pectoralis major muscle is mobilized. A partial anterior capsulectomy is performed, the extent of which depends on capsule thickness, recreating the original inferolateral defect postmastectomy prior to primary reconstruction. Steps are then taken to correct this defect by recreating the IMF and LMF as in a primary reconstruction. A sheet of prehydrated ADM (AlloDerm) of standard thickness is utilized to recreate the inframammary and lateral mammary folds. The size of ADM used is dependent on the extent of capsulectomy performed. The ADM is placed at the inferolateral border of the breast and is secured laterally, inferiorly, and medially to the chest wall with 2-0 Vicryl sutures. The ADM is placed with the deep

Acellular Dermal Matrix for Optimizing Outcomes in Implant-Based Breast Reconstruction:
Primary and Revisionary Procedures

73

dermal side facing the inferior breast skin. A new implant is introduced into the pocket and with the patient in a sitting position proper implant and inframammary fold position are verified. The superior edge of the ADM is then sutured to the elevated lower border of the pectoralis major muscle or to the superior border of the capsulectomy defect. Through a separate lateral stab incision, one closed suction drain is placed along the inframammary fold between the ADM and the skin flap inferiorly where the capsulectomy was completed. Final incision closure is performed in standard fashion.

3.2.3 Patient cases

Case 5

A 44-year-old woman with a history of infiltrating ductal carcinoma and ductal carcinoma-in-situ on her right breast presented with right capsular contracture (grade 3) after first stage bilateral ADM-assisted expander reconstruction (Figure 11A). Capsular contracture developed secondary to radiotherapy. Corrective surgery for capsular contracture was performed in conjunction with second stage implant reconstruction and included capsulectomy (Figure 11B) followed by expansion of the implant pocket using a sheet of ADM (AlloDerm) and repositioning of the IMF (Figure 11C). On the left breast, excess skin was excised laterally to improve the breast contour during exchange. No complications occurred during a follow-up period of 10 months (Figures 11D & 11E). Capsular contracture was successfully treated and breast projection and ptosis on the irradiated side were well-matched to the contralateral nonirradiated side.

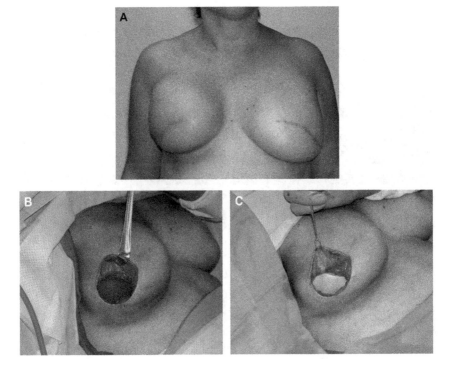

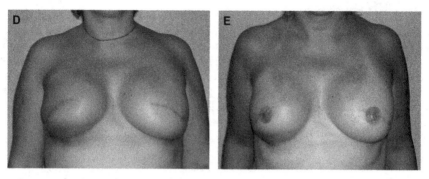

Fig. 11. Correction of capsular correction in the setting of radiation. A: Right breast capsular contracture after bilateral ADM-assisted expander reconstruction followed by postoperative radiation of the right breast. B: Expander exchange for implant after capsulectomy. C: ADM used in redefining the pocket. D: At 3 months postoperative. E: At 10 months postoperative with interim nipple areola reconstruction and tattooing.

Case 6

A 46-year-old woman presented with early right capsular contracture (grade 3) and left inferior implant malposition after ADM-assisted implant reconstruction (Figures 12A & 12B). On her right breast, she underwent partial capsulectomy at the IMF (Figure 12C) followed by reinforcement of the capsulectomy site with ADM (Figure 12D) as corrective

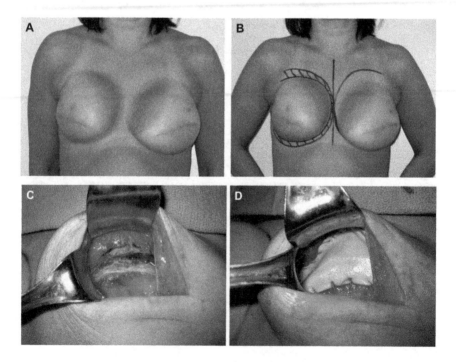

Acellular Dermal Matrix for Optimizing Outcomes in Implant-Based Breast Reconstruction:
Primary and Revisionary Procedures

75

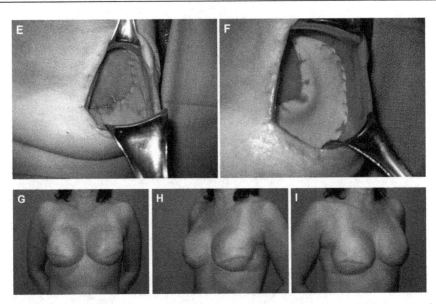

Fig. 12. Correction of right breast capsular contracture and correction of left breast inferior malposition. A: Early right capsular contracture and left malposition after bilateral ADM-assisted implant reconstruction. B: Planned corrective surgery included right capsulectomy with ADM reinforcement and left IMF/LMF capsulorrhaphy with ADM reinforcement. C: Right breast after IMF capsulectomy. D: Right breast, ADM secured in place overlapping IMF capsulectomy. E: Left breast after IMF and LMF capsulorrhaphy. F: Left breast, ADM secured in place reinforcing IMF and LMF capsulorrhaphy. G-I: At 4 months postoperative.

surgery for capsular contracture. On her left breast, she underwent capsulorrhaphy at the IMF and LMF (Figure 12E) with reinforcement of suture lines with ADM (Figure 12F) to address implant malposition. Both breasts were fitted with new implants. Four-month postoperative photographs showed correction of capsular contracture and inferior malposition (Figures 12G-I).

4. Conclusion

ADMs have become an integral part of implant-based breast reconstruction with the expectation that their use would result in low complication rates, improved aesthetic outcomes, and greater patient satisfaction. In the setting of immediate postmastectomy breast reconstruction, the ADM acts as an extension to the pectoralis muscle thereby allowing a direct-to-implant and potentially single-stage approach. This technique is particularly effective in patients that are candidates for NASM, where the entire breast skin envelope is preserved. Emerging evidence also indicates that ADMs may play a role in revisionary surgery assisting in reestablishing proper implant positioning and preventing capsular contracture. The ability of ADMs to fulfill these roles is attributed to their biomechanical properties of strength and pliability and biologic property of supporting tissue regeneration.

5. Acknowledgement

The author would like to thank LifeCell Corporation (Branchburg, NJ) for editorial assistance.

6. References

Adams, W. P., Jr. (2009). Capsular contracture: What is it? What causes it? How can it be prevented and managed? *Clinics in Plastic Surgery*, Vol.36, No.1, (January 2009), pp. 119–126, vii, ISSN 0094-1298

Adams, W. P., Jr. (2010). Discussion: Subclinical (biofilm) infection causes capsular contracture in a porcine model following augmentation mammaplasty. *Plastic and Reconstructive Surgery*, Vol.126, No.3, (September 2010), pp. 843-844, ISSN 0032-1052

Ahmed, S., Snelling, A., Bains, M., & Whitworth, I. H. Breast reconstruction. (2005). *British Medical Journal*, Vol.330, No.7497, (April 2005), pp. 943-948, ISSN 0959-8138

American Society of Plastic Surgeons. (2010). 2009 Reconstructive Breast Procedures, In: *American Society of Plastic Surgeons*, September 13, 2011, Available from http://www.plasticsurgery.org/Documents/news-resources/statistics/2009-statistics/2009breastreconsurgery.pdf

Basu, C. B., Leong, M., & Hicks, M. J. (2010). Acellular cadaveric dermis decreases the inflammatory response in capsule formation in reconstructive breast surgery. *Plastic and Reconstructive Surgery*, Vol.126, No.6, (December 2010), pp. 1842-1847, ISSN 0032-1052

Baxter, R. A. (2003). Intracapsular allogenic dermal grafts for breast implant-related problems. *Plastic and Reconstructive Surgery*, Vol.112, No.6, (November 2003), pp. 1692-1696, ISSN 0032-1052

Becker, H., Shaw, K. E., & Kara, M. (2005). Correction of symmastia using an adjustable implant. *Plastic and Reconstructive Surgery*, Vol.115, No.7, (June 2005), pp. 2124-2126, ISSN 0032-1052

Becker, S., Saint-Cyr, M., Wong, C., Dauwe, P., Nagarkar, P., Thornton, J. F., & Peng, Y. (2009). AlloDerm versus DermaMatrix in immediate expander-based breast reconstruction: a preliminary comparison of complication profiles and material compliance. *Plastic and Reconstructive Surgery*, Vol.123, No.1, (January 2009), pp. 1-6, ISSN 0032-1052

Bindingnavele, V., Gaon, M., Ota, K. S., Kulber, D.A., & Lee, D. J. (2007). Use of acellular cadaveric dermis and tissue expansion in postmastectomy breast reconstruction. *Journal of Plastic, Reconstructive and Aesthetic Surgery*, Vol.60, No.11, (n.d.), pp. 1214-1218, ISSN 1748-6815

Brachtel, E. F., Rusby, J. E., Michaelson, J. S., Chen, L. L., Muzikansky, A., Smith, B. L., & Koerner, F. C. (2009). Occult nipple involvement in breast cancer: clinicopathologic findings in 316 consecutive mastectomy specimens. *Journal of Clinical Oncology*, Vol.27, No.30, (October 2009), pp. 4948-4954, ISSN 0732-183X

Breuing, K. H., & Colwell, A.S. (2007). Inferolateral AlloDerm hammock for implant coverage in breast reconstruction. *Annals of Plastic Surgery*, Vol.59, No.3, (September 2007), pp. 250-255, ISSN 0148-7043

Acellular Dermal Matrix for Optimizing Outcomes in Implant-Based Breast Reconstruction:
Primary and Revisionary Procedures

77

Breuing, K. H., & Warren, S. M. (2005). Immediate bilateral breast reconstruction with implants and inferolateral AlloDerm slings. *Annals of Plastic Surgery*, Vol.55, No.3, (September 2005), pp. 232-239, ISSN 0148-7043

Cassileth, L., Kohanzadeh, S., & Amersi, F. (2011). One-Stage Immediate Breast Reconstruction With Implants: A New Option for Immediate Reconstruction. *Annals of Plastic Surgery*, (Jul 5 2011), [Epub ahead of print], ISSN 0148-7043

Chasan, P. E. (2005). Breast capsulorrhaphy revisited: A simple technique for complex problems. *Plastic and Reconstructive Surgery*, Vol.115, No.1, (Januar 2005), pp. 296–301, ISSN 0032-1052

Chasan, P. E., & Francis, C. S. (2008). Capsulorrhaphy for revisionary breast surgery. *Aesthetic Surgery Journal*, Vol.28, No.1, (January-February 2008), pp. 63-69, ISSN 1090-820X

Collis, G. N., Terkonda, S. P., Waldorf, J. C., & Perdikis, G. (2011). Acellular Dermal Matrix Slings in Tissue Expander Breast Reconstruction: Are There Substantial Benefits? *Annals of Plastic Surgery*, (Aug 5 2011), [Epub ahead of print], ISSN 0148-7043

Cordeiro, P. G., & McCarthy, C. M. (2006). A single surgeon's 12-year experience with tissue expander/implant breast reconstruction: part II. An analysis of long-term complications, aesthetic outcomes, and patient satisfaction. *Plastic and Reconstructive Surgery*, Vol.118, No.4, (September 2006), pp. 832-839, ISSN 0032-1052

Cunnick, G. H., & Mokbel, K. (2006). Oncological considerations of skin-sparing mastectomy. *International Seminars in Surgical Oncology*, Vo.3, (May 2006), pp. 14, ISSN 1477-7800

Cunningham, B., & McCue, J. (2009). Safety and effectiveness of Mentor's MemoryGel implants at 6 years. *Aesthetic Plastic Surgery*, Vol.33, No.3, (May 2009), pp. 440-444, ISSN 0364-216X

Duncan, D. I. (2001). Correction of implant rippling using allograft dermis. *Aesthetic Surgery Journal*, Vol.21, No.1, (January 2001), pp. 81-84, ISSN 1090-820X

Grabov-Nardini, G., Haik, J., Regev, E, & Winkler, E. (2009). AlloDerm sling for correction of synmastia after immediate, tissue expander, breast reconstruction in thin women. *Eplasty*, Vol.9, (November 2009), pp. e54, ISSN 1937-5719

Handel, N., Cordray, T., Gutierrez, J., & Jensen, J. A. (2006). A long-term study of outcomes, complications, and patient satisfaction with breast implants. *Plastic and Reconstructive Surgery*, Vol.117, No.3, (March 2006), pp. 757-767, ISSN 0032-1052

Hanna, K. R., Degeorge, B. R. Jr, Mericli, A. F., Lin, K. Y., & Drake, D. B. (2011). Comparison Study of Two Types of Expander-Based Breast Reconstruction: Acellular Dermal Matrix-Assisted Versus Total Submuscular Placement. *Annals of Plastic Surgery*, (Aug 22 2011), [Epub ahead of print], ISSN 0148-7043

Hartzell, T. L, Taghinia, A. H, Chang, J., Lin, S. J, & Slavin, S. A. (2010). The use of human acellular dermal matrix for the correction of secondary deformities after breast augmentation: results and costs. *Plastic and Reconstructive Surgery*, Vol.126, No.5, (November 2010), pp. 1711-1720, ISSN 0032-1052

Israeli, R. (2011). Correction of capsular contracture with acellular dermal matrix. Poster presented at Breast Cancer Coordinated Care Conference, Washington, DC, February 3-5, 2011.

Israeli, R., & Cody, D. G. (2011). Correction of implant malposition after breast reconstruction using acellular dermal matrix. Poster presented at Breast Cancer Coordinated Care Conference, Washington, DC, February 3-5, 2011.

Israeli, R., Cody, D. G., Busch-Devereaux, E., Mishkit, A., & Romanelli, J. N. (2011). Periareolar approach to nipple-areola sparing mastectomy and acellular dermal matrix-assisted direct-to-implant breast reconstruction. Poster presented at Breast Cancer Coordinated Care Conference, Washington, DC, February 3-5, 2011.

Israeli, R., & Feingold, R. S. (2011). Acellular dermal matrix in breast reconstruction in the setting of radiotherapy. *Aesthetic Surgery Journal*, Vol.31 (7 suppl), (September 2011), pp. 51S-64S, ISSN

Komorowska-Timek, E., Oberg, K. C., Timek, T. A., Gridley, D. S., & Miles, D. A. (2009). The effect of AlloDerm envelopes on periprosthetic capsule formation with and without radiation. *Plastic and Reconstructive Surgery*, Vol.123, No.3, (March 2009), pp. 807-816, ISSN 0032-1052

Massiha, H. (2002). Scar tissue flaps for the correction of postimplant breast rippling. *Annals of Plastic Surgery*, Vol.48, No.5, (May 2002), pp. 505–507, ISSN 0148-7043

Maxwell, G. P., Birchenough, S. A., & Gabriel, A. (2009). Efficacy of neopectoral pocket in revisionary breast surgery. *Aesthetic Surgery Journal*, Vol.29, No.5, (September-October 2009), pp. 379–385, ISSN 1090-820X

Maxwell, G. P. & Gabriel, A. (2009). Use of the acellular dermal matrix in revisionary aesthetic breast surgery. *Aesthetic Surgery Journal*, Vol.29, No.6, (November-December 2009), pp. 485-493, ISSN 1090-820X

McCarthy, C. M., Mehrara, B. J., Riedel, E., Davidge, K., Hinson, A., Disa, J. J., Cordeiro, P. G., & Pusic, A. L. (2008). Predicting complications following expander/implant breast reconstruction: an outcomes analysis based on preoperative clinical risk. *Plastic and Reconstructive Surgery*, Vol.121, No.6, (June 2008), pp. 1886-1892, ISSN 0032-1052

Namnoum, J. D. (2009). Expander/implant reconstruction with AlloDerm: recent experience. *Plastic and Reconstructive Surgery*, Vol.124, No.2, (August 2009), pp. 387-394, ISSN 0032-1052

Newman, M. I., Swartz, K. A., Samson, M. C., Mahoney, C. B., & Diab, K. (2011). The true incidence of near-term postoperative complications in prosthetic breast reconstruction utilizing human acellular dermal matrices: a meta-analysis. *Aesthetic Plastic Surgery*, Vol.35, No.1, (February 2011), pp. 100-106, ISSN 0364-216X

Orenstein, S. B., Qiao, Y., Kaur, M., Klueh, U., Kreutzer, D. L., & Novitsky, Y. W. (2010). Human monocyte activation by biologic and biodegradable meshes in vitro. *Surgical Endoscopy*, Vol.24, No.4, (April 2010), pp. 805-811, ISSN 0930-2794

Prantl, L., Schreml, S., Fichtner-Feigl, S, Pöppl, N., Eisenmann-Klein, M., Schwarze, H., & Füchtmeier, B. (2007). Clinical and morphological conditions in capsular contracture formed around silicone breast implants. *Plastic and Reconstructive Surgery*, Vol.120, No.1, (July 2007), pp. 275-284, ISSN 0032-1052

Rawlani, V., Buck, D. W. 2nd, Johnson, S. A., Heyer, K. S., & Kim, J. Y. (2011). Tissue expander breast reconstruction using prehydrated human acellular dermis. *Annals of Plastic Surgery*, Vol.66, No.6, (June 2011), pp. 593-597, ISSN 0148-7043

Roostaeian, J., Pavone, L., Da Lio, A., Lipa, J., Festekjian, J., & Crisera, C. (2011). Immediate placement of implants in breast reconstruction: patient selection and outcomes.

Acellular Dermal Matrix for Optimizing Outcomes in Implant-Based Breast Reconstruction:
Primary and Revisionary Procedures

79

    Plastic and Reconstructive Surgery, Vol.127, No.4, (April 201001), pp. 1407-1416, ISSN 0032-1052

Salzberg, C. A. (2006). Nonexpansive immediate breast reconstruction using human acellular tissue matrix graft (AlloDerm). *Annals of Plastic Surgery*, Vol.57, No.1, (July 2006), pp. 1-5, ISSN 0148-7043

Salzberg, C. A., Ashikari, A. Y., Koch, R. M., & Chabner-Thompson, E. (2011). An 8-year experience of direct-to-implant immediate breast reconstruction using human acellular dermal matrix (AlloDerm). *Plastic and Reconstructive Surgery*, Vol.127, No.2, (February 2011), pp. 514-524, ISSN 0032-1052

Spear, S. L., Carter, M. E., & Ganz, J. C. (2003). The correction of capsular contracture by conversion to "dual-plane" positioning: Technique and outcomes. *Plastic and Reconstructive Surgery*, Vol.112, No.2, (August 2003), pp. 456–466, ISSN 0032-1052

Spear, S. L, Dayan, J. H., Bogue, D., Clemens, M. W., Newman, M., Teitelbaum, S., & Maxwell, G. P. (2009). The "neosubpectoral" pocket for the correction of symmastia. *Plastic and Reconstructive Surgery*, Vol.124, No.3, (September 2009), pp. 695–703, ISSN 0032-1052

Spear, S. L., & Little, J. W. III. (1988). Breast capsulorrhaphy. *Plastic and Reconstructive Surgery*, Vol.81, No.2, (February 1988), pp. 274-279, ISSN 0032-1052

Spear, S. L., Murphy, D. K., Slicton, A., & Walker PS; Inamed Silicone Breast Implant U.S. Study Group. (2007). Inamed silicone breast implant core study results at 6 years. *Plastic and Reconstructive Surgery*, Vol.120(7 Suppl 1), (December 2007), pp. 8S-16S, ISSN 0032-1052

Spear, S. L., Parikh, P. M., Reisin, E., & Menon, N. G. (2008). Acellular dermis-assisted breast reconstruction. *Aesthetic Plastic Surgery*, Vol.32, No.3, (May 2008), pp. 418-425, ISSN 0364-216X

Spear, S. L., Seruya, M., Clemens, M. W., Teitelbaum, S., & Nahabedian, M. Y. (2011). Acellular dermal matrix for the treatment and prevention of implant-associated breast deformities. *Plastic and Reconstructive Surgery*, Vol.127, No.3, (March 2011), pp. 1047-1058, ISSN 0032-1052

Stump, A., Holton, L. H. 3rd, Connor, J., Harper, J. R., Slezak, S., & Silverman, R. P. (2009). The use of acellular dermal matrix to prevent capsule formation around implants in a primate model. *Plastic and Reconstructive Surgery*, Vol.124, No.1, (July 2009), pp. 82-91, ISSN 0032-1052

Tamboto, H., Vickery, K., & Deva, A. K. (2010). Subclinical (biofilm) infection causes capsular contracture in a porcine model following augmentation mammaplasty. *Plastic and Reconstructive Surgery*, Vol.126, No.3, (September 2010), pp. 835-842, ISSN 0032-1052

Topol, B. M., Dalton, E. F., Ponn, T., & Campbell, C. J. (2008). Immediate single-stage breast reconstruction using implants and human acellular dermal tissue matrix with adjustment of the lower pole of the breast to reduce unwanted lift. *Annals of Plastic Surgery*, Vol.61, No.5, (November 2008), pp. 494–499, ISSN 0148-7043

Uzunismail, A., Duman, A., Perk, C., Findik, H., & Beyhan, G. (2008). The effects of acellular dermal allograft (AlloDerm®) interface on silicone-related capsule formation – experimental study. *European Journal of Plastic Surgery*, Vol.31, No.4, (n.d.), pp. 179-185

Voice, S. D., & Carlsen, L. N. (2001). Using a capsular flap to correct breast implant malposition. *Aesthetic Surgery Journal*, Vol.21, No.5, (September 2001), pp. 441–444, ISSN 1090-820X

Wang, H. Y., Ali, R. S., Chen, S. C., Chao, T. C., & Cheng, M. H. (2008). One-stage immediate breast reconstruction with implant following skin-sparing mastectomy in Asian patients. *Annals of Plastic Surgery*, Vol.60, No.4, (April 2008), pp. 362-366, ISSN 0148-7043

Woerdeman, L. A., Hage, J. J., Smeulders, M.J., Rutgers, E. J., & van der Horst, C. M. (2006). Skin-sparing mastectomy and immediate breast reconstruction by use of implants: An assessment of risk factors for complications and cancer control in 120 patients. *Plastic and Reconstructive Surgery*, Vol.118, No.2, (August 2006), pp. 321–330, ISSN 0032-1052

Yoo, G., & Lee, P. K. (2010). Capsular flaps for the management of malpositioned implants after augmentation mammoplasty. *Aesthetic Plastic Surgery*, Vol.34, No.1, (February 2010), pp. 111-1115, ISSN 0364-216X

Zienowicz, R. J., & Karacaoglu, E. (2007). Implant-based breast reconstruction with allograft. *Plastic and Reconstructive Surgery*, Vol.120, No.2, (August 2007), pp. 373-381, ISSN 0032-1052

5

Head and Neck
Reconstructive Surgery

J.J. Vranckx and P. Delaere
KU Leuven University Hospitals, Department of Plastic & Reconstructive Surgery
Department of Otorhinolaryngology, Head and Neck Surgery
Belgium

1. Introduction

1.1 Floor-of-the-mouth defects

The oral cavity is the most common location in the head and neck region for primary malignant tumors. In the Western world, primary squamous cell carcinomas of the oral cavity most frequently involve the tongue and the floor of the mouth. In countries in which betel nut and tobacco chewing are common, the buccal mucosa and retromolar trigone are the most frequently encountered primary tumor sites. Initial treatment depends on parameters of the primary tumor, patient factors and factors related to the treatment team (Shah & Patel, 2003; Ariyan, 1997).

Reconstruction of defects in the oral cavity after tumor extirpation and anticipated radiotherapy requires well-vascularized pliable tissues with limited tissue bulk (Gurtner & Evans, 2000). The radial forearm flap has been used conventionally for decades to repair defects of the floor of the mouth and oral sidewalls. Its major disadvantage is significant donor site morbidity when the flap is harvested as a conventional fasciocutaneous flap. Webster described a suprafascial dissection that permits leaving the fascia on top of the forearm tendons and musculature (Webster & Robinson, 1995). The harvest requires meticulous cleavage of the anterior sleeve of the conjoint tendon that stretches between the flexor carpi radialis and the brachioradialis tendons and envelops the radial vascular pedicle (Fig 1). The suprafascial harvest, in combination with a full-sheet skin graft, strongly reduces adhesions, neurotrophic pain and loss in range of motion, and its superiority over the conventional "subfascial" technique has been clearly demonstrated (Chang et al.,1996).

The anterolateral thigh flap (ALT) has been popular for decades in Asia for head and neck reconstructions and offers reliable, pliable tissues for intraoral lining. When a thin flap is needed in more obese patients, a suprafascial dissection towards the perforators allows immediate thinning down to 4 mm. The ALT flap provides a large skin paddle and can be combined with anterolateral thigh fascia and the thick tensor fascia lata. If more bulk is required, a segment of the vastus lateralis can also be incorporated as a monobloc, or each segment based on its perforator can be used as a chimera flap that allows for optimal positioning in the defect (Fig 2).

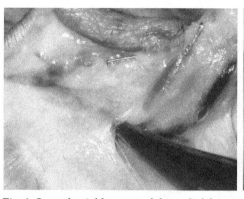
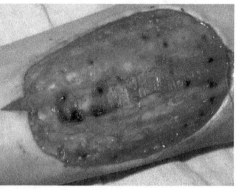

Fig. 1. Suprafascial harvest of the radial forearm flap. Left: The conjoint tendon of the anterior and posterior fascia wraps the radial vascular pedicle. The anterior sleeve is sectioned at the position of the scissors, leaving the conjoint tendon intact. Right: The donor bed after harvesting a suprafascial radial forearm flap. No tendons are exposed. A fatty layer covers the superficial nerves. There is no tenting between the flexor carpi radialis and brachioradialis tendons.

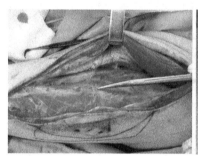
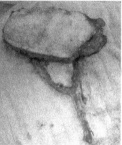
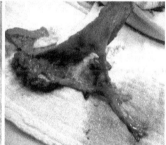

Fig. 2. The anterolateral thigh flap. Left: A septocutaneous perforator is visible between the vastus lateralis and rectus femoris muscles. Middle: The anterolateral thigh flap harvested on 2 perforators. Right: A multi-unit ALT flap is harvested with a large fascia segment on one perforator, and a small muscle cuff on a second perforator and a small skin island are used as monitor.

The vascular pedicle is the descending branch of the lateral circumflex femoral artery (LCFA) system. This pedicle is long and of good caliber. The ALT flap is notorious for its anatomic variations. The skin perforators of the anterolateral thigh can be either musculocutaneous (87%) or septocutaneous (13%), whereas the pedicle of the flap can be either the descending or the oblique branch of the LCFA (Wong et al., 2009).The absence of significant perforators is rare (1%).

The SCIAP flap (superficial circumflex iliac artery perforator-based free groin flap) provides a thin and flexible lining for the reconstruction of the floor of the mouth and an inconspicuous donor site (Fig 3). A disadvantage, however, is the variable vasculature both of the artery and the veins, which often renders the harvest unpredictable in terms of pedicle length.

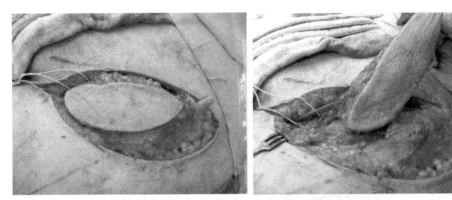

Fig. 3. A superficial circumflex artery perforator-based flap from the left groin. This flap offers thin pliable tissues ideal for the reconstruction of the floor of the mouth.

Full-thickness cheek-and-floor-of-the-mouth defects in combination require a double skin paddle and a long vascular pedicle that allows for optimal set-in and satisfactory volume to provide adequate lining of the cheek. A folded radial forearm flap is an option; however, its use requires either two skin paddles with one perforator each in the suprafascial dissection technique or use of the traditional harvesting technique with a de-epithelialized zone in between to permit plication and suturing to the sidewalls of the cheek. A folded anterolateral thigh flap can be used with the intervening folded portion de-epithelialized (Fig 4). These full-thickness defects often have a significant volume deficit, which may result in a long-term sunken appearance of the cheek.

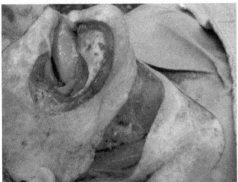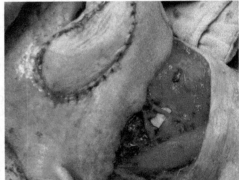

Fig. 4. Left: Full-thickness defect of the floor of the mouth and cheek. Right: A defect restored with an anterolateral thigh flap with 2 skin paddles. Venous anastomosis end-to-side on the IJV and artery end-to-end on the superior thyroid artery.

The anterolateral thigh flap provides more tissue volume than a radial forearm flap; in addition, vascularized fascia or a vastus lateralis muscle segment can be included to provide more tissue volume. If two suitable perforators are present, the skin paddle can be split as a chimeric flap, which allows for a more elegant reconstruction; if the oral commissure is involved in the defect, the fascia lata can be split and sutured into the upper and lower orbicularis oris muscle as a static sling (Huang, 2002).

1.2 Defects of the tongue

Hemitongue defects are preferably reconstructed using a thin sensate flap (Kimata et al., 1999, 2003). The suprafascial dissected radial forearm flap is particularly useful if a pliable, flexible, well-vascularized flap is required for lining of the tongue in cases where there is also a significant defect in the floor of the mouth or on the cheek (Fig 5). The anterolateral thigh flap with the lateral femoral cutaneous nerve delivers the required tissues. If the donor thigh is too bulky, a suprafascial dissection allows for immediate thinning of the flap. Also, partial tongue defects that include the floor of the mouth can be restored with an ALT flap; if required, a fascia extension or de-epithelialized segment can be used to drape the floor of the mouth or to fill the dead space in the submandibular zone.

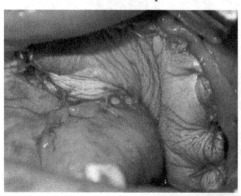 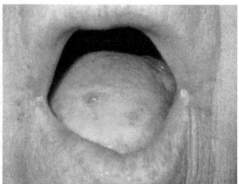

Fig. 5. Left: segmental tongue, floor of the mouth and internal defect of the cheek. Defect restored with a suprafascial radial forearm flap that drapes well over the U-shaped defect. Right: a total tongue reconstruction with an anterolateral thigh flap and small central segment of vastus lateralis muscle.

Total glossectomy defects require significant bulk to restore height and volume to the reconstructed tongue, and a myocutaneous flap is therefore required. Previously, the rectus abdominis myocutaneous flap was popular for the reconstruction of the tongue. However, donor site morbidity may be significant (Lyos et al., 1999 ; Hurvitz et al., 2006). The anterolateral thigh flap can provide as much volume as a rectus abdominis myocutaneous flap with a similar long vascular pedicle but with minimal donor site morbidity. The myocutaneous gracilis flap also allows access to the required tissues with minimal donor site morbidity (Yousif et al., 1999). However, pedicle length is limited, and in obese patients, it is difficult to align the skin portion on top of the gracilis muscle, which may result in shear stress or omission of a skin perforator and subsequent loss of the skin paddle.

2. Reconstruction of the mandible

When a primary tumor of the oral cavity extends to the alveolar ridge or infiltrates the mandible, surgical excision becomes mandatory. A marginal mandibulectomy is indicated when a primary tumor of the oral cavity approximates the alveolar process or the lingual site of the mandible. A marginal mandibulectomy preserves the mandibular arch and can be performed on the symphysis, at the body of the mandible or at the coronoid process and retromolar trigone. Mandibular reconstruction is not required following a marginal resection of the mandible. The defect is restored by primary suture of the mucosa of the floor of the mouth anteriorly to the lower lip or laterally to the cheek mucosa or with a split-thickness skin graft. For suitable patients, osteointegrated implants recreate denture.

When a primary malignant tumor infiltrates the gingiva over the alveolar process or infiltrates the mandible, a segmental mandibulectomy and stabilization or reconstruction are required. A commando composite operation consists of the resection of the intraoral primary tumor with a mandibular segment and ipsilateral neck dissection 'en bloc' (Shah & Patel, 2005).

Proper flap selection and operative planning is based on the extent and location of the resection, the quality of surrounding tissues, the status of the recipient vessels (ipsilateral versus contralateral) and the availability of donor sites. These variables are often related to the general condition of the patient and the patient's history of previous surgery or irradiation therapy.

Reconstruction of the mandible is accomplished either with the use of soft-tissue free flaps and a reconstruction plate or with the use of osseous free flaps. Despite early enthusiasm for soft-tissue free flaps (radial forearm and rectus abdominis) in conjunction with a reconstruction plate, there is a higher incidence of long-term failure, such as plate fracture and extrusion, of such flaps than with the use of osseous free flaps (Schusterman et al., 1991; Foster et al., 1999; Head C et al., 2003). Although the use of osseous free flaps in mandible reconstruction is more complex, their advantages far outweigh any disadvantages. Vascularized bone allows authentic bone healing, resulting in a stable union between the flap and graft within 2–3 months in the majority of patients, in spite of preoperative or postoperative radiation therapy (Cordeiro & Hidalgo, 1994). Moreover, vascularized bone serves as an excellent recipient substrate for the placement of osteointegrated dental implants. The four osteocutaneous donor sites most commonly used for mandible reconstruction are the fibula, the iliac crest, the radial forearm, and the scapula. Each donor site has its own intrinsic parameters with respect to the quality and quantity of available bone and soft tissue, the quality of the vascular pedicle, the feasibility of a two-team approach, and the potential for osseointegrated dental implants (Disa & Cordeiro, 2000).

The fibula has become the flap of choice for reconstruction of most segmental mandibular defects. The bony flap based on the peroneal artery and associated veins can deliver up to 27 cm of triangular- shaped bone, an amount that is ideal for lateral, anterior, or combination defects. Donor site morbidity is minimized by preserving 7 cm of distal fibula at the ankle and 6 cm at the knee. Blood supply to the fibula is both intraosseous and segmental; therefore, multiple osteotomies can be performed without risk of devascularizing the bone (Wei , 1994, 2003). The flap can be harvested as an osteocutaneous or osteomyocutaneous flap with a skin island based on perforators that travel within the posterolateral crural septum (Fig 6). Musculocutaneous perforators to the skin are often encountered proximally, while more septocutaneous perforators are present in the middle and distal third of the lower leg. The flexor hallucis longus muscle or segments of the soleus muscle can be integrated in the harvest to provide extra soft-tissue bulk.

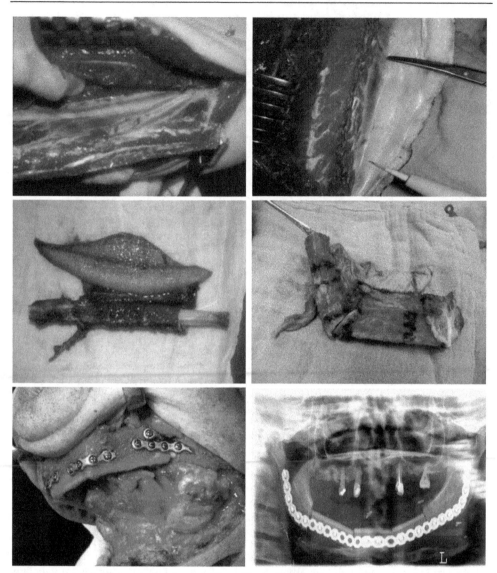

Fig. 6. Upper left: Harvest of osteocutaneous fibula (OCF). The transition zone between the peroneal and tibial pedicle in between the tibial nerve. Upper right: Two septocutaneous perforators in the posterolateral septum. Middle left: Harvest of the OCF with a minimal muscle cuff. Middle right: Restoration of the lateral ramus of the mandible with the OCF. One osteotomy required. Skin island covers the floor of the mouth and cheek. Lower left and right: Anterior ramus reconstructed with OCF. Four osteotomies required.

One advantage of the use of a fibular flap is the possibility of carrying out a simultaneous unimpeded dissection in a 2-team approach while the ablative procedure is being performed. After harvest, the flap can be left perfused on its vascular pedicle while the osteotomies are performed in order to minimize ischemia time. A disadvantage of the fibula is the straightness of the bone; this makes the fibula particularly suitable for anterior defects, but osteotomies are required for curvature. The fibula also has a low profile relative to the height of the native mandible in dentulous patients. In patients in whom osseointegrated implants are planned as either a primary or a secondary procedure, the fibula should be placed about 0.5 to 1 cm above the inferior border of the native mandible, closer to the superior alveolar edge, to facilitate the placement of implants; alternatively, a double-barrel fibula can be used (Chang et al., 1998; Urken ML et al., 1989 ; Sclaroff A, 1994). However, this requires an adequate skin paddle because more soft tissue is often needed to accommodate the extra bony volume. Another disadvantage of the fibula osteocutaneous flap is the unreliability of the skin island, which has been reported to be not useful in up to 10% of cases. The incorporation of flexor hallucis longus muscle or segments of soleus muscle with the skin paddle may result in a greater reliability of the skin island.

The iliac crest was the main method of mandible reconstruction in the 1980s. Its major advantages are its natural curvature, which is anatomically contoured for ipsilateral reconstruction, and the abundance of vertical and horizontal height of the bone for mandibular contour and osseointegration (Jewer et al., 1989). The flap has a large overlying skin island. It has a good cosmetic appearance of the donor site compared with the other free flaps that are used for mandibular reconstruction. The disadvantages of this flap include a short vascular pedicle and a lack of segmental perforating vessels, which limit the ability to perform osteotomies for graft shaping. In obese patients, the skin paddle can be thick and relatively nonmobile. In obese patients there may also be excess adipose tissue, and the harvest of the flap may become unreliable. This limits its utility for intraoral reconstruction. An additional limitation of the iliac crest flap is the donor site morbidity associated with its use. This includes numbness in the hip region and, especially, bulging as well as hernia formation due to the fact that all attaching muscles must be dissected from their origins. A modification of this flap leaves the superior anterior iliac spine intact with its muscle insertions. Also, only the inner table of the iliac crest can be used; this reduces donor site morbidity but also reduces the quantity of bone available for osseointegration. The versatility of the fibula has superseded the iliac crest in most situations.

The radial forearm flap has long and large donor site vessels. The skin paddle is thin, pliable and long and can perfectly drape over intraoral defects. The major disadvantage of the forearm osteocutaneous flap is the quality of the available bone, which is thin and not reliably osteotomized. Additional bulk can be added by harvesting a segment of the brachioradialis muscle. However, this adds to the already notorious donor site morbidity. Harvest of a unicortical segment of radius may destabilize the bone, resulting in fracture. The forearm osteocutaneous free flap is best suited to ramus defects requiring minimal bone but needing a large amount of skin. The available bone stock of the radius is usually unsuitable for osseointegration.

The scapula flap is versatile because the long circumflex scapular artery and vein can supply a large quantity of soft tissue with the bone. An axial parascapular and/or transverse scapular flap skin island can be based on this vascular pedicle in combination with a segment of the serratus anterior or latissimus dorsi muscles. The major drawback of the scapula flap is the marginal quality of the bone, which is not reliable for osteotomies or osseointegration. The location of the donor site prohibits simultaneous harvest of the flap and tumor ablation, thus drastically lengthening the time required for the procedure. The major indication for the use of the scapula flap in mandibular reconstruction is a posterior defect that does not require osteotomy of the bone but does require a large amount of external skin and soft-tissue reconstruction.

3. Reconstruction of the maxilla

If a primary tumor involves the hard palate, upper gum, or the upper gingivobuccal sulcus, or if the tumor is in direct continuity with the maxilla, maxillar resection is mandatory. The resection may consist of an alveolectomy, palatal fenestration or partial maxillectomy. Multiple classifications describe the maxillectomy and midface defects in terms of the vertical and horizontal aspect of the maxillary loss (Brown JS et al., Cordeiro P et al., Santamaria et al.). Classes I–IV describe the increasing extent of the maxillary defect in the vertical dimension as follows: class I—maxillectomy without oronasal fistula; class II—maxillectomy not involving the orbit; class III—involving the orbital adnexae with orbital retention; class IV—with orbital enucleation or exenteration; class V—orbitomaxillary defect; class VI—nasomaxillary defect (Fig 7). Horizontal classification is based on the increasing complexity of the dentoalveolar and palatal defect and describes the vertical

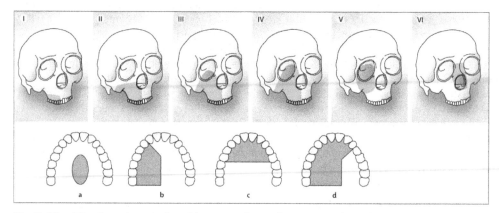

Fig. 7. Classification of vertical and horizontal maxillectomy and midface defects. Vertical classification: I—maxillectomy not causing an oronasal fistula; II—not involving the orbit; III—involving the orbital adnexae with orbital retention; IV—with orbital enucleation or exenteration; V—orbitomaxillary defect; VI—nasomaxillary defect. Horizontal classification: a—palatal defect only, not involving the dental alveolus; b—less than or equal to 1/2 unilateral; c—less than or equal to 1/2 bilateral or transverse anterior; d—greater than 1/2 maxillectomy. Letters refer to the increasing complexity of the dentoalveolar and palatal defect and qualify the vertical dimension. From Brown JS and Shaw RJ., The Lancet Oncol. 2010: 1001-08.

dimension: a—palatal defect only, not involving the dental alveolus; b—less than or equal to 1/2 unilateral; c—less than or equal to 1/2 bilateral or transverse anterior; d—greater than 1/2 maxillectomy. This classification provides a framework to explain the complexity of each defect and describes the rationale for the reconstructive options. Traditionally, the majority of midfacial defects were lined with split-thickness skin grafts, and obturators were used to fill the defect. Obturation is simple and provides the patient with immediate new dentition. However, the cavity behind the obturator may contract during the healing process, and the obturator should be repetitively adapted to the changing contour. In addition, radiotherapy may cause severe problems. Soiling from the oral and nasal cavity may occur, and the interface between a rigid non-flexible obturator and soft tissues may cause problems of skin irritation, maceration and poor hygiene.

For some defects, obturation may offer a simple non-invasive solution preventing oronasal communication and improving speech. For larger defects, however, there may be problems with stabilization of the obturator (McCarthy et al. 2010). Reconstruction with tissues obliterates the defect using vascularized tissues that are more resilient to irradiation and provide preservation of volume, flexibility and shape, allowing for more easy integration of dentures in the second stage. Moreno et al. reported on the largest comparative series between obturation and reconstruction of the maxillary defects. They found that reconstruction gave the better outcome for swallowing and speech, especially in larger defects in the horizontal component (class IId). In general, one could conclude that for larger alveolar class IId and class III-VI defects, a reconstruction with a composite free flap is preferred.

Brown et al. analyzed the literature from 1998-2009 and summarized the reconstructive options selected for each of the classes. For class I and class IIa midline hard palate defects, most authors report the use of the radial forearm free flap. For class IIb defects that consist of less than half of the lateral alveolus and palate, zygomatic implants have been reported to give good results. The temporoparietalis fascia flap can close the oroantral and nasal fistulae but provides no bulk. The most frequently reported soft tissue flap used for reconstruction of class II defects is a radial forearm fascia flap. However, the anterolateral thigh flap provides well-vascularized tissues and can be easily modified in terms of bulk and lining with fascia in addition to the skin paddle. A segment of bone can also be included based on the ascending branch of the lateral circumflex vascular pedicle.The most frequently reported composite flap is the fibula osteocutaneous flap, which provides easily maniable bone segments rooted on a large vascular pedicle and a skin paddle on fine septocutaneous perforators. The fibula also provides good bone stock for osteointegrated implants.

In class III defects, support of the orbital, cheek and dental arch must be provided in addition to a facial skin paddle and closure of the oral and nasal defects. The rectus abdominis myocutaneous flap provides a voluminous, well-vascularized paddle. The dissection is straightforward, and the vascular pedicle is predictable and long. However, long-term donor site morbidity may be cumbersome (Browne et al., 1999). Moreover, the rectus flap only provides soft tissue bulk without bone for support of the bony walls. Because postoperative irradiation is inevitable, the combination of a rectus abdominis flap with non-vascularized bone to restore the orbital rim and floor may result in wound breakdown and collapse due to bone loss (Cordeiro & Santamaria, 2000). For class IIIb defects, the most recent literature supports the use of a DCIA iliac crest flap with a segment of internal oblique muscle. The bony segment can be shaped into the defect with the curvature required for the orbital rim and the piriform aperture, and it provides sufficient bone for the restoration of the alveolar rim even for dental implants (Fig 8). The internal oblique muscle provides the lining of the nasal wall and the separation between the nasal and oral cavities (Brown et al.,2002).

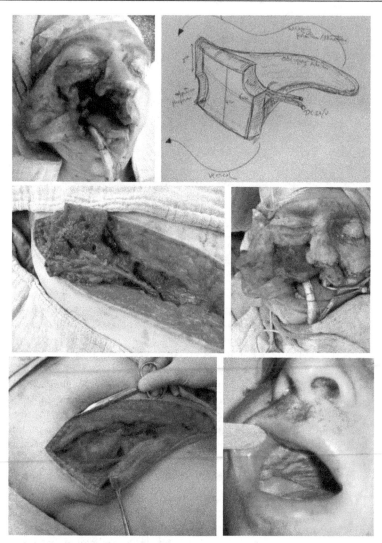

Fig. 8. Upper left: class IIIb defect involving maxilla and orbita at right side.Upper right: pre-op sketch of required iliac crest flap with internal obliquus muscle.Middle left: harvest of the iliac crest flap based on the DCIA. Middle right: flap fixed into the defect with mini plate and screws.Lower left: donor site carefully closed with a mesh graft and muscular approximation of abdominal wall and gluteal thigh layers.Lower right: the internal vestibular lining with obliquus internus muscle reepithelialises spontaneously.

The scapular angle osteomyocutaneous flap, a scapula flap with a latissimus dorsi segment, was proposed for class II and IV defects (Uglesic, 2000; Bidros, 2005). This chimera flap, which is based on the thoracodorsal angular artery, provides all required tissues for class II and IV defects. The advantage in comparison to the DCIA flap is the long thoracodorsal vascular pedicle, which facilitates flap set in. The angular scapula segment has also been described in combination with the serratus anterior or teres major muscle (Ugurlu et al., 2007; Clark et al., 2008). The osteocutaneous fibula flap can also be used for these defects. However, the challenge lies in aligning the skin paddles and the required bony osteotomies for the perfect fit (Futran et al., 2002; Peng et al., 2005). The advantage of using either of these composite vascularized bone flaps is that the intrinsic height of the bone allows good bony adaptation, which promotes union at the alveolus and zygomatic remnant, although the scapular bone is significantly thinner than the iliac crest. In addition, both flaps provide adequate muscle to obturate the oral, nasal, and orbital defects. The subsequent epithelialization produces a natural result. Harvest of the iliac crest flap with internal oblique muscle is more difficult than the scapular angle osteocutaneous flap. However, the patient does not need turning or tilting, and a two-team approach is possible, which significantly reduces operation time (Brown & Shaw, 2010).

Class V orbitomaxillary defects are usually restored with soft-tissue flaps because exenteration of the orbit is required, but the palate remains intact. No bone is required. The orbit should be lined to receive an orbital prosthesis. The pedicled temporoparietal fascia flap delivers excellent lining in unilateral cases. When the defect is larger, a suprafascial harvested anterolateral thigh flap or suprafascial radial forearm flap are appropriate options. The suprafascial dissection of the ALT facilitates flap thinning. The suprafascial dissection of the radial forearm flap significantly reduces donor site morbidity at the forearm and should be performed for all forearm flaps that require a skin paddle.

Class VI nasomaxillary defects that involve the nasal bone require a reconstruction with thin vascularized tissues such as a radial forearm flap. A split radius can be included to provide structural support of the flap. A rib cartilage or bone strut can support a suprafascial radial forearm flap as well. However, after radiotherapy there is a significant risk of graft loss.

4. Reconstruction of the hemilarynx after hemilaryngectomy

The accepted treatment modalities for laryngeal cancer are radio(chemo)therapy and surgery. A unilateral advanced tumor on one vocal fold can only be treated surgically by total laryngectomy because the reconstruction of a hemilarynx for sparing one vocal cord is so complex (Pearson et al., 1990). However, every attempt must be made to avoid total laryngectomy because the loss of speech and the need for a permanent tracheostome dramatically change the quality of life of these patients.

The technique for extended hemilaryngectomy is designed to allow for functional treatment of lateralized glottic cancer with subglottic extension (T2, T3) and of lateralized chondrosarcomas of the cricoid cartilage (Fig 9). The aim of the reconstruction is to restore the extended hemilaryngectomy defect and to obtain a morphology after reconstruction that is comparable to the vocal fold paralysis in the paramedial position.

In order to restore the cartilaginous framework after extended hemilaryngectomy, donor tissues should be used that mimic the resected tissues. The trachea represents good donor tissue: it has a similar cartilaginous structure and is internally lined with respiratory mucosa. When opened at the posterior membrane, a 4-ring horseshoe-shaped configuration can be obtained that mimics the hemilaryngeal convex shape. Because of the proximity of the cervical trachea to the larynx, a possible one-stage reconstruction of the hemilarynx would consist of a simple advancement of 4 cm of trachea with preservation of the tracheal continuity. To allow this upward mobilization, the trachea must be dissected from the surrounding tissues over

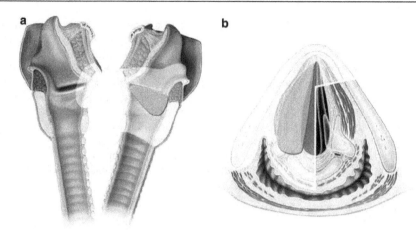

Fig. 9. Extended hemilaryngectomy defect. a: Internal view of the larynx after midline sagittal section. b: Axial section at the glottic level. The tumor (gray) is visible on one vocal fold. The bright area shows the amount of larynx resection necessary to remove the tumor. The resection includes one side of the thyroid cartilage and the full amount of the arytenoid and the cricoid cartilage at the tumor side. From Delaere P., *Vander Poorten V, Vranckx J, Hierner R. Eur. Arch. Otorhinolaryngol.* 2005 Nov; 262(11):910-6

about 8 cm, which means that this segment will have its extrinsic blood supply interrupted. Vascularity will further diminish after modification of the upper 4 cm of membranous trachea to create the convex patch and placement of a temporary tracheostomy at the anterior wall. Even in non-irradiated cases, advancement of a tracheal patch would inevitably lead to patch necrosis. Zur and Urken (2003) transferred the trachea pedicled on the thyroid artery and vein with the adjacent thyroid gland in a single stage. However, the thyrotracheal flap is not well suited for primary reconstruction of defects caused by epithelial-based neoplasms. There is an inherent risk of occult metastases to the thyroid gland and the paratracheal lymph nodes, and such metastases are commonly seen when there is significant subglottic extension. Therefore, a 2-stage prefabrication procedure is required to generate a revascularized autologous trachea segment. Delaere et al. reported a modification of the operative sequence compared to their initial procedure. In the first series of patients, the prefabrication of a 4-ring trachea segment was carried out by wrapping it with a radial forearm fascia flap, and a microvascular anastomosis was performed to head and neck blood vessels. The prefabrication step took 2 weeks. In a second stage, the tumor was resected and the hemilarynx restored with the prefabricated trachea construct. However, the prefabrication step used in the 1st stage before tumor resection in the second stage could manipulate tumor cells and elicit spreading. The conversion of sequence proved to be difficult; when the tumor is resected primarily, a hemilaryngeal defect exists at the time prefabrication of the trachea must begin. The hemilaryngeal defect must therefore be temporarily closed to permit breathing and swallowing during the time that the prefabrication step takes place. Experience after reconstruction of 50 cases allowed the authors to modify the sequence and to define an 'optimal reconstructive design' for extended hemilaryngectomy repair leading to optimal functional results without diminishing oncologic safety.

In the first stage of this design, an extended hemilaryngectomy is performed. For T3 glottic cancer, the tumor is resected with inclusion of the anterior commissure and with inclusion of half of the cricoid cartilage. The ipsilateral thyroid lobe and tracheoesophageal lymph nodes are removed, as well as the lymph nodes at levels II, III, and IV. Only tumors without extension to the supraglottic area are included2. Subsequently, a radial forearm flap comprising a proximal fasciocutaneous segment and a distal fascial component is harvested from the non-dominant arm (Fig 10). The fascial paddle is wrapped around the upper 4 cm of the cervical trachea. The fasciocutaneous paddle is used to temporarily close the extended

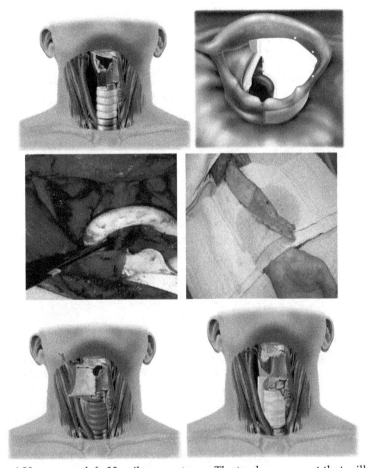

Fig. 10. Stage 1.Upper row, left: Hemilaryngectomy. The trachea segment that will be prefabricated by wrapping it with a radial forearm flap is shown in white. Upper row, right: tumor resection indicated in white. White dots locate the sutures used to close the aryepiglottic area to recreate the sphincter. Middle row, left: Hemilaryngeal defect to be restored with the free flap. Middle row, right: A radial forearm flap is harvested with a fascia (F) segment distally and fasciocutaneous (FC) segment proximally. Lower row, left: The FC segment restores temporarily the hemilaryngeal defect. The F segment wraps 4 trachea rings. After microsurgical anastomosis, this revascularised fascia flap will prefabricate the trachea segment introducing an intrinsic axial blood supply.

hemilaryngectomy defect. After microsurgical anastomosis of the radial vascular pedicle to the neck vessels, the flap and the pedicle are covered with an ePTFE membrane to prevent adhesion formation. An inferolateral corner of the fasciocutaneous segment is sutured in the skin of the neck as a monitor flap to control vascularization of the buried tissues after microsurgical anastomosis. It also serves as the roofing for the temporary tracheostome and can be used in the second stage to close the skin defect after removal of the tracheostome.

After 4 months, a second look at the section margins is performed. If histology confirms the absence of tumor recurrence, the definitive reconstruction is initiated (fig 11). The ePTFE membrane is removed, and the skin paddle of the radial forearm flap is dislodged from the laryngeal defect. The skin paddle is de-epithelialized to serve as posterior bulk at the end of reconstruction. The fascia-enwrapped segment of revascularized trachea is isolated, remodeled and transferred upward into the laryngeal defect. The mediastinal tracheal stump is mobilized and sutured to the reconstructed larynx. During the second stage, the microvascular pedicle of the radial forearm flap in which the trachea segment was wrapped remains unharmed. A tracheostomy is maintained in the suture line between the reconstructed larynx and the mediastinal trachea. That tracheostomy is closed after restoration of all laryngeal functions, usually 1 to 2 months after the second operation. The tracheostomy is closed by inverting the skin around the tracheostomy, a small procedure performed under local anesthesia.

Tracheal autotransplantation leads to optimal reconstruction of extended hemilaryngectomy defects. Swallowing function recovers within a week after the first and second interventions, and laryngeal respiratory function is fully regained after closure of the tracheostomy.

After the first operation, the radial fasciocutaneous forearm flap restores the sphincter function of the larynx[1]. Swallowing of solids and liquids is possible after 1 week, and speaking is possible during finger occlusion of the temporary tracheostomy. After the second operation, the tracheal patch and the vascularized forearm flap produce successful restoration of sphincteric and respiratory function.

Hand-free speech is possible after closure of the tracheostome 6 weeks after the definitive reconstruction. The voice sounds natural and moderately hoarse. Some aspiration of saliva can be seen during the first days after operation, and most patients resume oral feeding after 1 week. When the patient does not succeed in swallowing without aspiration, a conversion towards total laryngectomy is performed. The tracheostomy closure may be delayed because of swallowing problems caused by postirradiation pharyngeal hypocontractility.

At the subglottic level, the luminal concavity should be restored to preserve function. The revascularized tracheal patch graft meets these subglottic reconstructive requirements (Pearson, 1990 ; Delaere , 2007). At the glottic level, the reconstructive tissue should follow the midline posteriorly, and a luminal concavity should be preserved anteriorly (Fig 12). Two sutures placed at the lateral site of the defect between the epiglottis and the aryepiglottic fold bring the aryepiglottic fold into a midline position posteriorly. Such a configuration leads to optimal sphincter and respiratory function.

Complete posterior closure is important for obtaining a good voice and swallowing function; therefore, the reconstruction must be placed in the posterior midline. Complete glottic closure is less critical anteriorly; therefore, a paramedian position of the graft will allow good respiratory function.

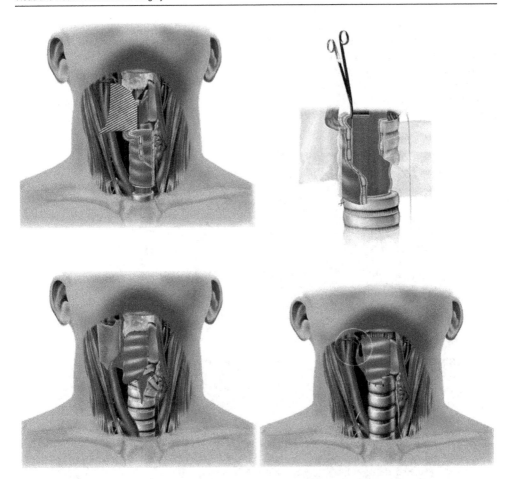

Fig. 11. Stage 2. Upper left: The FC segment is de-epithelialized while the vascular anastomosis remains intact. Right: The opened prefabricated trachea. Lower left: The hemilarynx defect is restored with a horseshoe-shaped prefabricated trachea segment. Lower right: The final state.

The most challenging part of the reconstruction is repair of the airway lumen at the subglottic level. Experimental research has shown that only revascularized tracheal autografts succeed in creating a luminal convexity (Delaere et al., 1998, 2005, 2007). Tracheal autografts have the combined characteristics of a respiratory mucosal lining, a cartilage support and a vascular supply, which are tissue characteristics that are necessary for restoration of a luminal convexity. The normal larynx was studied morphologically by Hirano et al. (1987), who concluded that, in the normal larynx, the anterior glottis plays the most important role in phonation while the posterior glottis plays an equally important role in respiration. Diseases of the anterior glottis usually cause voice problems. They disturb respiration only when they present a large obstruction to the airway. Diseases of the posterior glottis result in respiratory distress. They do not affect phonation until they become extensive and inhibit vocal fold closure. In the normal situation, the posterior glottis is a respiratory glottis, while the anterior glottis is a phonatory glottis. Closure of the posterior larynx is important for swallowing without aspiration. After extended hemilaryngectomy, the posterior larynx becomes a sphincteric larynx. After reconstruction, the phonatory glottis is moved from anterior to posterior while the respiratory glottis is moved from posterior to anterior. With the tracheal patch in a paramedial position, the amount of airway lumen that is lost in the posterior larynx will be gained anteriorly.

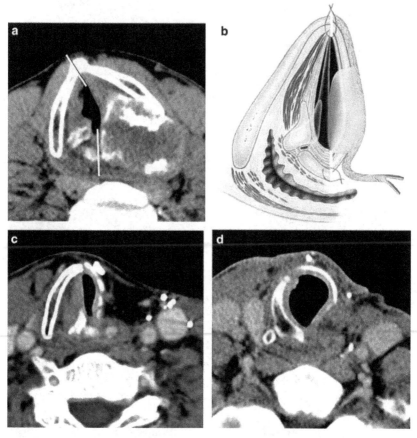

Fig. 12. Upper left: A preoperative CT scan at the glottic level showing a lateralized chondrosarcoma of the subglottic area at the left side with involvement of the vocal fold. The tumor was resected by performing an extended hemilaryngectomy (white lines indicate resection). Upper right: Schematic presentation of reconstruction at the glottic level. A combination of radial forearm skin and tracheal autotransplant gives a reconstruction against the midline posteriorly at the level of the vocal fold, while a small convexity is provided anteriorly by the tracheal autotransplant. Lower left: A postoperative CT scan, glottic level; the same situation as in b. Lower right: A postoperative CT scan, subglottic level. A tracheal autotransplant restores the airway lumen. From Delaere P.,*Vander Poorten V, Vranckx J, Hierner R., Eur. Arch. Otorhinolaryngol.* 2005 Nov; 262(11):910-6

The extended hemilaryngectomy allows for complete removal of a suitable tumor, for neck dissection, for hemithyroidectomy and for removal of the ipsilateral tracheoesophageal lymph nodes. The reconstruction is a combination of immediate reconstruction with a fasciocutaneous free flap and flap prefabrication with the help of the fascial part of the same fasciocutaneous free flap. The 4-month prefabrication period allows laryngeal repair with a well-vascularized tracheal patch in combination with a strip of forearm skin. During the second operation, the small piece of forearm skin is detached from the radial vascular pedicle, but it shows a sufficient marginal perfusion from the laryngeal remnant. The delay between tumor resection and definitive reconstruction permits a second look with control of the resection margins. In cases of local recurrence, a total laryngectomy can be performed during the second procedure.

5. Reconstruction of the trachea

5.1 Reconstruction of short-segment stenosis of the trachea

Segmental tracheal resection with end-to-end anastomosis is the treatment of choice for a stenosis encompassing less than 50% of the tracheal length. The advantage of a tracheal resection is that no graft is necessary, and there is no need for prolonged endotracheal intubation (Grillo, 1990). A requirement is that a direct end-to-end suture does not exert traction on the suture line, which may lead to local necrosis, leakage and fistulization. Scarring due to previous interventions may limit a tensionless suture (Delorimier, 1990; Idriss, 1984).

5.2 Reconstruction of recurrent short-segment stenosis of the trachea

Augmentation of the tracheal lumen by inserting local, regional, or distant tissue is necessary when a tracheal resection is not possible as, for example, in long-segment stenosis or in cases of restenosis after tracheal resection (Eliachar et al., 1989). Tracheal reconstruction using repair tissue is a second-choice solution because autologous donor tissues that resemble the mucosa-lined elastic cartilaginous framework of the trachea are not available. The most frequently used reconstructive tissues consist of cartilage grafts, pericardium, and muscle flaps, which are used as a carrier for skin, periosteum, or bone (Wright et al., 2004). Because these donor tissues all lack one or more features for optimal tracheal repair, the outcome is not constant. Experimental evaluation showed that for optimal laryngotracheal repair, the donor tissue should resemble the native tracheal tissue as closely as possible and be composed of a cartilaginous support, an internal lining consisting of respiratory mucosa, and a reliable blood supply (Fig 13).

Composite tissue consisting of vascularized fascia for blood supply, buccal mucosa for internal lining, and elastic cartilage for support are generally suitable as vascularized tracheal transplants.[5] However, bare cartilage undergoes necrosis when directly exposed to the airway lumen [6] and therefore should be vascularized. This can be done using a 'prefabrication' procedure [6,7]. The cartilage is sutured on a vascularized fascia layer, such as the radial forearm fascia and its intrinsic blood supply, which consists of the radial artery and comitant veins. After 2 weeks, the orthotopic transfer can be performed (Fig 14).

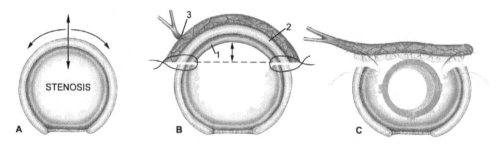

Fig. 13. Optimal reconstruction of anterior airway defect. (A) Axial section through tracheal stenosis. The stenotic airway is incised longitudinally (double arrow) and expanded (arrows). (B) Optimal reconstruction. The anterior tracheal defect is reconstructed with a revascularized tracheal allotransplant. The optimal tissue consists of a respiratory mucosal lining (1) and an elastic type of cartilage support (2). Vascularized fascia wrapped around the allotransplant will keep the reconstruction viable (3). The elastic nature of the cartilage component allows augmentation of the airway lumen (double arrow). (C) Reconstruction with vascularized mucosa. The airway defect is reconstructed with vascularized fascia and buccal mucosa. A laryngeal stent will prevent recollapse during the healing phase.

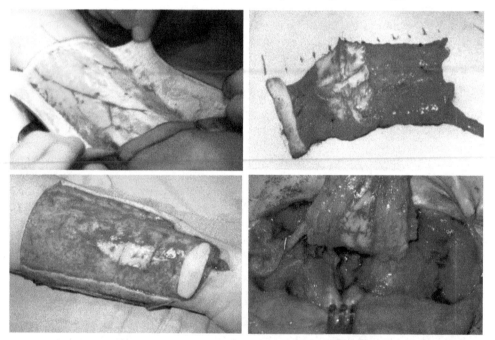

Fig. 14. Upper row. Left: Radial forearm fascia flap used as a vascular carrier. The skin is opened in an H-shaped pattern. After suturing the cartilage grafts on the fascia, the skin is closed until the 2nd stage 2 weeks later. Right: Auricular cartilage sutured on the radial forearm fascia flap. After the prefabrication step to vascularize the cartilage grafts, the transfer to the trachea defect is performed in a 2nd stage after 2 weeks.

Lower row. Left: The buccal mucosa is sutured on the radial forearm fascia flap, which serves as vascular carrier. A skin patch will serve as a monitor flap and will be sutured to the skin of the neck. Right: The prelaminated flap sutured into the defect on the trachea, mucosa patch downwards.

Because buccal mucosa is thinner than cartilage, composite tissue consisting of vascularized fascia and mucosa could be used in a one-stage procedure without a prefabrication step. Vascularized mucosa can repair airway defects with primary healing of the reconstructed site (Fig 14). A disadvantage of the mucosa-lined fascia is the absence of supportive tissue. The convexity of the airway lumen will be less because the cartilaginous supportive component is not available. When using a mucosa-lined fascia flap to repair an airway defect, it is essential that the mucosal patch and the defect be of similar size. Simultaneous use of the Dumon silicone stent will prevent prolapse of the mucosa-lined fascia and will prevent collapse of the incised and expanded airway. A short-term stenting period of 4 to 6 weeks is sufficient to anticipate collapse of the reconstructed airway during healing. This reconstruction technique is indicated for restenoses after segmental tracheal resection (Fig 15). Anastomotic stricture is usually related to excessive tension at the suture line and occurs in approximately 10% of patients undergoing tracheal resection (Delaere et al., 2005). Mucosa-lined fascia is currently the preferred tissue combination for the treatment of an airway stenosis in which segmental resection is difficult or impossible. The mucosa-lined reconstruction shows primary healing with a complete take of the oral mucosa on the fascial vascular carrier. The vascular supply and the epithelial lining guarantee a primary healing. No re-epithelialization is necessary during healing; this may be advantageous in the clinical situation of a restenosis where a scarred wound bed is encountered. Wound healing with mucosa-lined fascia is comparable to the wound healing seen when using skin-lined flaps.

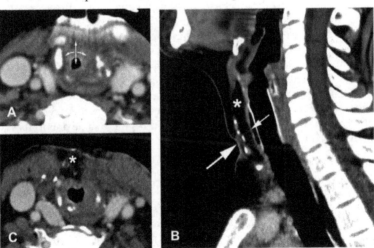

Fig. 15. Computed tomography (CT) scan of restenosis and tracheoplasty. (A) An axial CT scan at the stenotic site. The stenosis is incised longitudinally (double arrow) and expanded (arrows). (B) A sagittal reformatted CT scan. The silicone stent is visible. The buccal mucosa graft is visible as an internal lining (small arrow). Forearm fascia flap (asterisk); monitor skin flap (thick arrow). (C) An axial CT scan after reconstruction (same level as in A). Fascia flap (asterisk). The surface area after reconstruction is expanded by a factor of 2.

A mucosal lining is preferable, however, for airway lining to prevent the crusting and desquamation seen when using skin grafts. Another advantage of the mucosa-lined fascia is that the donor defect at the forearm site can be closed primarily, resulting in a less visible scar compared with the defect after dissection of a fasciocutaneous flap.

5.3 Reconstruction of long-segment stenosis of the trachea

For long airway defects, there are no autologous donor tissues available to use in restoring the mucosa-lined elastic cartilaginous framework. One option is a tissue engineering protocol in which a 3-dimensional vascularized tubular trachea is cultivated. Recently, successful restoration of a main-stem bronchus was reported in which a tissue-engineered transplant colonized by the recipient's epithelial and chondrogenic mesenchymal cells was used without the use of immunosuppressive therapy. The main drawback of this procedure was the lack of an intrinsic blood supply. An avascular tissue-engineered trachea would be unsuitable for use inside a major tracheal defect where the graft would be exposed to the airway lumen and to continuous movements during respiration, swallowing, and coughing. Without intrinsic vascularization techniques, scar tissue will be generated and healing becomes unpredictable. Ad hoc tissue engineering protocols do not allow us to generate a vascularized hollow tubular trachea that remains stable over time (Ott et al. 2011). The only other option is an allogenic trachea transplant. An allogenic trachea from a tissue bank could be used to bridge the gap in a manner similar to stored bone grafts. However, although the vascular requirements of the cartilaginous framework are limited and cartilage elicits limited immunologic rejection, the inner mucosal lining requires a significant vascular supply and, like regular skin, its immunologic response is strong. Because the blood supply to the trachea makes it unsuitable for direct revascularization, most previous attempts at tracheal transplantation have been performed after indirect revascularization. Rose et al. reported the first allogeneic tracheal transplantation in a human (Rose et al., 1979). The donor trachea was implanted heterotopically in the sternocleidomastoid muscle of the recipient and was transferred to the orthotopic position 3 weeks later. The recipient was not given immunosuppressive therapy; the report did not document the viability of the allograft or the long-term outcome. Klepetko et al. reported preserved viability of a heterotopically revascularized allograft by wrapping it in the omentum of a patient who received a lung transplant from the same donor. Its viability was documented after 60 days (Klepetko et al., 2004).

As with other composite-tissue allografts, restoration of arterial inflow and venous outflow is essential for the survival of the tracheal allograft. Indirect revascularization of a donor trachea is perfectly feasible, as demonstrated by the successful outcome of tracheal allografts and of autografts using vascularized fascia flaps in laboratory animals and humans (Buckwalter, 1998, Delaere et al., 1995). When this recipient tissue is perfused by an identifiable vascular pedicle, a microvascular transfer can be performed after the prefabrication step (Delaere et al. 2007).

Experiments in immunosuppressed rabbits showed complete revascularization and restoration of the mucosal lining in tracheal allografts after 2 to 4 weeks of heterotopic revascularization in the lateral thoracic area. Delaere et al. (2010) reconstructed a long-segment tracheal defect in a patient using an allograft that was revascularized in the first stage by heterotopic wrapping in vascularized radial forearm fascia. Immunosuppressive therapy during the prefabrication step was necessary for establishing connections between the donor's capillary network around the trachea and the recipient's fascial blood vessels.

This occurred quickly enough to maintain viability of the cartilaginous trachea. Nonetheless, unlike in the animal model, the posterior membranous trachea underwent avascular necrosis, and the necrotic segments were debrided and replaced with buccal mucosa (Fig 16).

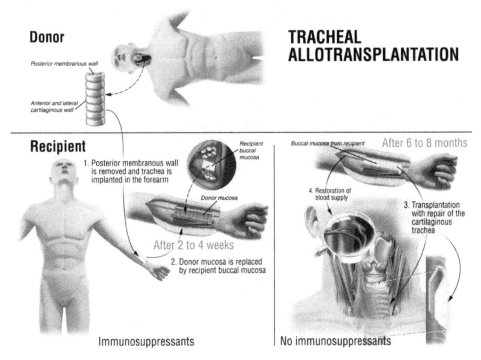

Fig. 16. Overview of trachea allotransplantation. A donor trachea is wrapped by radial forearm fascia in the forearm in a heterotopic position. The buccal recipient mucosa is sutured at the posterior membrane. After prefabrication, the vascularized trachea is transferred orthotopically to the neck. Immunosuppression is stopped when the trachea is in place. From Delaere P., Vranckx JJ., Verleden G.,De Leyn P,Van Raemdonck D. N.Engl.J.Med. 2010; 14, 362: 138-145.

The recipient buccal mucosa grew progressively over the lumen of the cartilaginous tracheal transplant, creating a chimeric patchwork of donor epithelium and recipient buccal mucosa; when this had occurred, immunosuppressive therapy was tapered and stopped. The authors report that FISH analysis of biopsies showed that endothelial and respiratory cells originating from the donor disappeared shortly after the withdrawal of immunosuppressive therapy. They presumed that the immunologic rejection occurred silently because of repopulation by the recipient's surrounding vascular network and buccal mucosal cells, and they speculated that the cartilaginous framework was not recognized by the immune system because adult cartilage lacks blood vessels. The viability of the tracheal cartilage was maintained after all immunosuppressive drugs had been discontinued. There is a meticulous balance between the speed of formation of neovascular connections and the oxygen requirements of the allogenic trachea. The metabolic demands of the cartilaginous framework may be low, while the oxygen requirements for the mucosal lining are rather high. The stealth activity of the highly differentiated chondrocytes may be based on their encasement in a dense matrix. This procedure confirmed the hypothesis that intact cartilage allografts are resistant to rejection and that the cartilaginous framework preserves its features when surrounded by well-vascularized recipient tissues. So far, 5 patients have been treated with allogenic trachea transplants with variable outcomes. The limiting factor remains the speed of the revascularization process of the inner mucosal lining of the trachea transplant. Further studies should indicate which strategies are useful in enhancing the neovascularization process in a clinical setting.

6. Reconstruction of the hypopharynx

The hypopharynx is an elementary component of the upper aerodigestive tract. Its boundaries consist of the pyriform sinuses bilaterally, the posterior pharyngeal wall and the post-cricoid zone. The hypopharynx ends at the lower border of the cricoid cartilage where the aerodigestive tract continues into the cervical esophagus. Surgical resection of any tumor in the hypopharynx results in disturbance of swallowing with aspiration in the respiratory tract due to the contiguity of the hypopharynx with the supraglottic larynx. Cancer of the cervical esophagus may result in resection of the larynx, post cricoid and proximal trachea. The most frequently encountered malignancies in this zone are squamous cell carcinomas. Adenocarcinomas of minor salivary glands and melanomas occur infrequently.

Cancer control is the primary goal of treatment of tumors of the hypopharynx. However, preservation of speech, avoidance of a tracheostome and preservation of normal swallowing are important aims if they are feasible. In cases where the larynx is uninvolved but the pharyngeal resection is extensive, careful judgment in the treatment plan is essential because postoperative aspiration is a major problem due to loss of sensation and muscular activity on the pharyngeal wall.

When the resection leaves a full-thickness defect of the pharyngeal wall, an immediate reconstruction is required. This can be performed with a pedicled flap such as the pectoralis major myocutaneous flap. However, this flap is bulky and may lessen the patient's ability to swallow. Microvascular free flaps with refined lining, such as a radial forearm flap, are better options for reconstructions of the posterior pharyngeal wall.

Advanced cancer of the pyriform sinus or the pharyngeal wall and primary post-cricoid tumors require a pharyngectomy with a total laryngectomy. If the cervical esophagus is involved, a pharyngolaryngoesophagectomy must be performed with immediate reconstruction. Immediate one-stage procedures that include reconstruction after the cancer extirpation are mandatory.

6.1 Reconstruction after tumor removal without laryngectomy

The funnel-shaped configuration of the hypopharynx is important for resection and reconstruction. The gradual transition in shape is maintained by the u-shaped hyoid bone and the spreading wings of the thyroid lamina. The posterior pharyngeal wall can be resected and reconstructed in selected tumors. The postcricoid area is a functionally important subunit that is not reparable with the larynx in situ. The main postoperative risk is from aspiration because of loss of sensation and muscular activity on the posterior pharyngeal wall.

6.2 Partial pharyngectomy

A partial laryngopharyngectomy can be performed only when the primary tumor is confined to the anatomical boundaries within the hypopharynx, signifying the ipsilateral pharyngeal wall and pyriform sinus, and the tumor may not extend up to the apex of the pyriform sinus nor to the base of the tongue. In addition, the ipsilateral hemilarynx must be mobile, and the tumor may not involve the larynx in a transglottic plane. Reconstructive options include the use of a vascularized skin island such as the anterolateral thigh perforator flap or the rectus abdominis flap. The ALT flap has the advantage of minimal donor site morbidity (Fig 17). A free jejunal flap can also be used as a jejunal patch sutured to the semicircular defect.

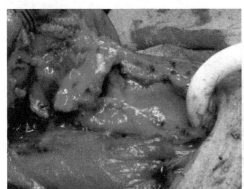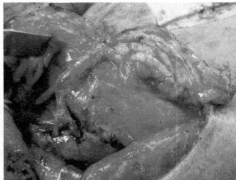

Fig. 17. Left: Semicircular defect of the pharynx. Right: Reconstruction with an anterolateral thigh flap. Two end-to-side anastomoses on the IJV and end-to-end to the facial artery.

6.3 Total pharyngectomy and circumferential pharyngeal defects

After pharyngolaryngectomy in advanced cancer, restoration of the continuity of the alimentary tract and the ability to swallow by mouth are important. If the resection is circular, restoration of the continuity is an integral part of the initial treatment strategy.

A total laryngo-pharyngectomy may be necessary in lower piriform fossa lesions and in lesions with extension to the posterior pharyngeal wall. The resultant defect is typically a circumferential defect and must be restored with gastric transposition (pharyngogastrostomy) or microvascular tubed flaps such as the radial forearm flap, anterolateral thigh flap, vertical rectus abdominis flap or jejunum free flap.

The choice of reconstructive technique for restoration of the continuity of the alimentary tract following pharyngeal resection must take into consideration the time required for restoration of the patient's ability to eat by mouth. Multi-staged operations that require long hospitalization and parenteral feeding until the last stage are not desired. Immediate reconstruction in a single-stage procedure is the goal (Shah & Patel, 2005). The time required to achieve normal swallowing after reconstruction of circular defects is the shortest after a free jejunum transfer (Fig 18) and gastric transposition. The jejunum is ideal for end-to-end anastomosis with the esophagus. It should be beveled at its proximal anastomosis with the oropharynx. A gastric transposition is employed for circumferential pharyngeal defects when a free jejunum vascularized transfer is not available.

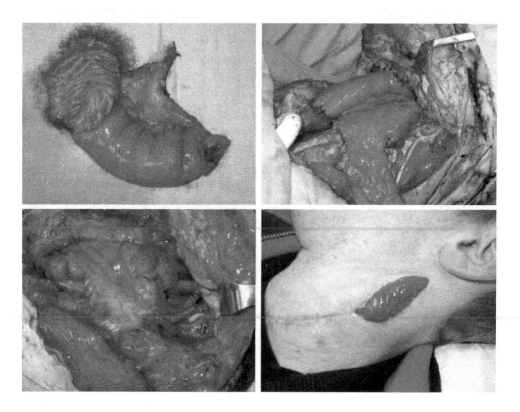

Fig. 18. Upper left: Harvest of a free jejunum flap. Upper right: Reconstruction of the circular hypopharynx defect with a free jejunum flap. Lower left: venous anastomosis end-to-side on the internal jugular vein and arterial anastomosis end-to-end to the facial artery. Lower right: a segment of the jejunum flap is isolated on a mesenterial vascular pedicle and sutured to the neck to serve as a monitor flap. After a few weeks, this monitor island is removed under local anesthesia.

Postcricoid hypopharyngeal stenosis

Although tremendous progress has been made in curing head and neck cancer with chemoradiation therapy, the toxicity of therapy may limit the number of patients who can achieve the ultimate goal of organ preservation, that is, normal speech and swallowing function, in hypopharynx cancer treatment. Postcricoid hypopharyngeal stenosis is a devastating complication of organ-sparing chemoradiation therapy for head and neck cancer. The radiosensitization effect of chemotherapy may lead to chemoradiation-induced mucositis, which may result in ulceration of opposing surfaces of redundant postcricoid mucosa. This may lead to circumferential scar formation and subsequent postcricoid stenosis (Lawrence et al., 2003), a rare complication that may occur short-or long-term after the termination of radiation therapy. A possible cause is progressive obliterative endarteritis and ischemia (Nguyen et al., 2000).

Postchemoradiation hypopharyngeal stenosis is a rare complication, but it is expected that it will become more frequent because the addition of chemotherapy, hyperfractionated, and concomitant boost radiation will result in higher toxicity and higher risk of stenosis (Silvain et al., 2003). Partial or complete stenosis of the postcricoid hypopharynx leads to an inability to swallow, resulting in aspiration and gastrostomy tube dependence. Patients with partial stenosis can be managed successfully with anterograde dilatation (Sullivan et al., 2004,). Patients with complete postcricoid hypopharyngeal stenosis have previously remained gastric tube dependent. Complete postcricoid hypopharyngeal stenosis requires reconstruction with preservation of the larynx whenever possible. Bypassing of the postcricoid area using reconstructive tissue with the larynx in situ is technically challenging.

To bypass the short stenosis, a tubed fasciocutaneous free flap, a free gastro-omental flap, or a free jejunum flap could be considered. A tubed fasciocutaneous free flap has a high prevalence of stenosis of the skin mucosa at the circular anastomosis. The majority of authors using fasciocutaneous flaps after total laryngopharyngectomy have described higher rates of distal anastomotic stricture than after enteric reconstructions (Genden et al. 2001, Varvares et al., 2000). The free gastro-omental flap delivers a large vascularized tissue bulk that protects the entire wound. While this may be advantageous for the total laryngopharyngectomy defect, the volume provided by the omentum cannot be accommodated in cases of larynx preservation; hence, it is less well indicated for the correction of post-chemoradiation hypopharyngeal stenosis. The free jejunal tube transfer is currently the most popular flap for reconstruction of the alimentary tract after total laryngopharyngectomy. A tube of about 12 cm is sutured between the base of the tongue and the distal cervical esophagus. The major shortcoming of this approach is that the transplanted jejunal segment maintains an intrinsic motor activity (Reese et al., 1994, 1995). This activity is autonomous and continues long after surgery. In addition, the transplanted segment remains temporally independent of the normal swallow reflex (Delaere et al., 2006, McConnel et al., 1988) and may create a functional obstruction of the jejunal conduit when the jejunum is contracting at the time of bolus delivery. Another shortcoming is that strictures may develop at the distal suture line resulting from kinking due to redundancy of the flap; this will be more pronounced when a short segment of 6 cm is used with the larynx in situ, as in hypopharyngeal stenosis. Delaere et al. (2006) used the jejunum as a patch with reorientation of the tube to avoid these complications. The jejunal tube was transformed into a short mucosal conduit with a large diameter and longitudinally oriented mucosal plicae, thus providing a tube without autonomous muscular activity (Fig 19 and 20).

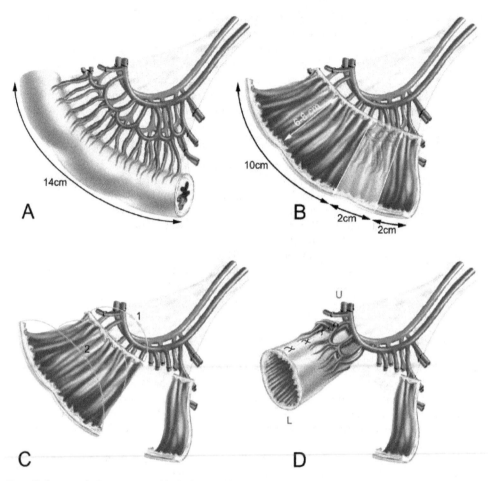

From Delaere et al., *Laryngoscope*, 2006 Mar; 116(3):502-4.

Fig. 19. Free jejunum used to bypass the postcricoid stenosis. (A) A 14-cm tube of jejunum is harvested on its vascular pedicle. (B) Patch of jejunum. The jejunum is divided longitudinally along its antimesenteric border. Circular mucosal folds are visible. The patch is divided (white double arrows) into a segment of 10 cm and two segments of 2 cm. The width of the patch measures 6 to 8 cm. (C) Formation of tube (arrows) with longitudinally oriented mucosal folds. First, the upper side of the patch is tabulated, and this side is sutured to the pharyngeal opening (1). The patch is progressively sutured into a tube; the reconstruction is completed by suturing the lower end (2) to the stump of the cervical esophagus. The circumference of the newly formed tube measures 10 cm, and its length is between 6 and 8 cm (the width of the jejunum patch). A 2-cm segment of jejunal mucosa is removed; the distal 2 cm of the jejunal patch will serve as the monitor flap. (D) Jejunum after tubulation (U, upper end of tube; L, lower end of tube). The vascularized jejunal patch monitor flap will be placed in the neck incision to allow direct observation.It is removed under local anesthesia at a later stage.

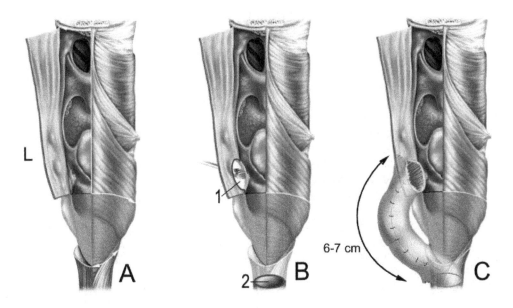

From Delaere et al., *Laryngoscope*, 2006 Mar; 116(3):502-4

Fig. 20. Postchemoradiation hypopharyngeal stenosis. (A) Schematic presentation of postcricoid stenosis from the posterior. The left side (L) of the pharynx is shown after opening; the postcricoid area shows a complete stenosis. (B) During the operation, an opening is made in the left lateral hypopharynx at the upper site of the stenosis. At the site of the hypopharyngeal opening (1), the lamina of the thyroid cartilage is removed with a burr. The cervical esophagus is incised at the lower site of the stenosis (2). (C) A loop is constructed between the upper pharyngeal opening and the lower esophageal stump. To bypass the postcricoid stenosis, the loop must be 6 to 7 cm in length. The width (6–7 cm) of an incised segment of jejunum is used to bridge the length of the stenosis.

After microvascular anastomosis of the jejunal tube with the local vasculature, a monitor flap is essential because the location of the tube within the hypopharynx buries the flap and essentially eliminates direct observation as a method of flap monitoring. Conventional hand-held Doppler ultrasonography is unreliable because it is difficult to discern whether the Doppler signal is emanating from the flap or from a surrounding vessel. More involved methods of monitoring include leaving a window over the jejunum for direct monitoring. However, the resulting skin defect may be a port of entry for infection or may create a chronic wound due to the fact that these tissues often become rigid for a longer period due to edema and inflammation. Based on one of the blood vessels of the mesenterial arcade, a vascularized jejunal monitoring patch can be sutured externally for direct observation.

Before operation, it is important to confirm that only the hypopharynx is involved. Jejunal reconstruction is no longer indicated when dealing with multiples sites of stenosis. A pedicled colon transfer may be considered for constructing the bridge between the hypopharynx and the stomach if the cervical esophagus is also involved (Maish et al., 2005).

7. References

Ariyan S, Ross DA, Sasaki CT. *Reconstruction of the head and neck.* Surg Oncol Clin N Am; 6:1–15,1997

Bidros RS, Metzinger SE, Guerra AB. *The thoracodorsal artery perforator-scapular osteocutaneous (TDAP-SOC) flap for reconstruction of palatal and maxillary defects.* Ann Plast Surg; 54:59–65,2005

Brown JS, Rogers SN, McNally DN, Boyle M. *A modified classification for the maxillectomy defect. Head Neck;* 22:17–26,2000

Browne JD, Burke AJ. *Benefits of routine maxillectomy and orbital reconstruction with the rectus abdominis free flap. Otolaryngol Head Neck Surg.;*121:203–209,1999

Buckwalter JA, Mankin HJ.Articular cartilage. *Part II: degeneration and osteoarthritis, repair, regeneration and transplantation.* J.Bone Joint Surg Am. 79: 612-32,1997

Chana JS, Wei F-C. *A review of the advantages of the anterolateral thigh flap in head and neck reconstruction.* Br J Plast Surg 2004

Chang SC-N, Miller G, Halbert CF, Yang KH, Chao WC, Wei F-C. *Limiting donor site morbidity by suprafascial dissection of the radial forearm flap.* Microsurgery ; 17:136–140,1996

Chang YM, Santamaria E, Wei F-C, et al. *Primary insertion of osseointegrated dental implants into fibula osteoseptocutaneous free flap for mandible reconstruction.* Plast Reconstr Surg;102:680–688,1998

Clark JR, Vesely M, Gilbert R. *Scapular angle osteomyogenous flap in postmaxillectomy reconstruction: defect, reconstruction, shoulder function, and harvest technique. Head Nec;* 30: 10–20,2008

Cordeiro PG, Hidalgo DA: *Soft tissue coverage of mandibular reconstruction plates.* Head Neck; 16:112–115,1994

Cordeiro PG, Santamaria E. *A classification system and algorithm for reconstruction of maxillectomy and midfacial defects. Plast Reconstr Surg.;*105:2331–2346; discussion 2347–2348,2000

Davison SP, Sherris DA, Meland NB. *An algorithm for maxillectomy defect reconstruction. Laryngoscope;*108:215–219,1998

Delaere P, goeleven A.,Vander Poorten V, Hermans R., Hierner R.,Vranckx JJ. *Organ Preservation Surgery for Advanced Unilateral Glottic and Subglottic Cancer* Laryngoscope, 117:1764–1769,2007

Delaere P, Hierner R, Vranckx J, Hermans R. *Tracheal stenosis treated with vascularized mucosa and short-term stenting.* Laryngoscope. Jun;115(6):1132-4,2005

Delaere P, Vander Poorten V, Goeleven A, Feron M, Hermans R. *Tracheal autotransplantation: a reliable reconstructive technique for extended hemilaryngectomy defects.* Laryngoscope 108:929–34,1998

Delaere P, Vander Poorten V, Vranckx J, Hierner R. *Laryngeal repair after resection of advanced cancer: an optimal reconstructive protocol.* Eur Arch Otorhinolaryngol. Nov;262(11):910-6,2005

Delaere P., Goeleven A.,Vander Poorten V.,Hermans R., Hierner R.,Vranckx JJ. *Organ preservation surgery for advanced unilateral glottic and subglottic cancer.* Laryngoscope 117: 1764-9,2007

Delaere P., Hierner R., Goeleven A., D'Hoore A. *Reconstruction for postcricoid pharyngeal stenosis after organ preservation protocols.* Laryngoscope., 116(3):502-4,2006

Delaere P., Liu ZY., Hermans R., Sciot R., Feenstra L. *Experimental tracheal allograft revascularization and transplantation.* J.Thorac Cardiovasc Surg 110:728-37,1995

Delaere P., Vranckx JJ., Verleden G.,De Leyn P., Van Raemdonck D. *Tracheal autotransplantation after withdrawal of immunosuppressive therapy.* N.Engl J Med 362: 138-45,2010

DeLorimier AA, Harrison MR, Hardy K, et al. *Tracheobronchial obstructions in infants and children.* Experience with 45 cases. *Ann Surg;* 212:277–285,1990

Disa JJ., Cordeiro P. *Mandible Reconstruction With Microvascular Surgery.* Seminars in Surg. Oncol.; 19:226–234,2000

Eliachar I, Roberts JJ, Welker KB, Tucker HM. *Advantages of the rotary door flap in laryngotracheal reconstruction: is skeletal support necessary? Ann Otol Rhinol Laryngol;* 98:37–40,1989

Foster RD, Anthony JP, Sharma A, Pogrel MA. *Vascularized bone flaps versus nonvascularized bone grafts for* mandibular *reconstruction: an outcome analysis of primary bony union and endosseous implant success.* Head Neck;21:66–71,1999

Futran ND, Mendez E. *Developments in reconstruction of midface and maxilla. Lancet Oncol.;*7:249–258,2006

Genden EM, Kaufman MR, Katz B, et al. *Tubed gastroomental free flap for pharyngoesophageal reconstruction. Arch Otolaryngol Head Neck Surg;*127:847–853,2001

Grillo HC. *Tracheal replacement. Ann Thorac Surg;* 49:864–865,1990

Gurtner GC, Evans GR. *Advances in head and neck reconstruction.* Plast Reconstr Surg;106 :672–682,2000

Head C, Alam D, Sercarz JA, et al. *Microvascular flap reconstruction of the mandible: a comparison of bone grafts and bridging plates for restoration of mandibular continuity.* Otolaryngol Head Neck Surg;129:48–54,2003

Hirano M, Kurita S, Kiyokawa K, Sato K Posterior glottis. *Morphological study in excised human larynges.* Ann Otol Rhinol Laryngol 95:576–581,1986

Huang WC , H.C. Chen HC , V. Jain *et al., Reconstruction of through-and-through cheek defects involving the oral commissure, using chimeric flaps from the thigh lateral femoral circumflex system. Plast Reconstr Surg* 109 2 , pp. 433–441 discussion 442–3,2002

Hurvitz KA, Kobayashi M, Evans GR. *Current options in head and neck reconstruction.* Plast Reconstr Surg;118:122e–133e,2006

Idriss FS, DeLeon SY, Ilbawi MN. *Tracheoplasty with pericardial patch for extensive tracheal stenosis in infants and children. J Thorac Cardiovasc Surg* 4; 88:527–536,1988

Jewer DD, Boyd JB, Manktelow RT, et al: *Orofacial and mandibular reconstruction with the iliac crest free flap: A review of 60 cases and a new method of classification.* Plast Reconstr Surg 84:391,1989

Kimata Y, Sakuraba M, Hishinuma S, et al. *Analysis of the relations between the shape of the reconstructed tongue and postoperative functions after subtotal or Total glossectomy.* Laryngoscope;113:905–909,2003

Kimata Y, Uchiyama K, Ebihara S, et al. *Comparison of innervated and noninnervated free flaps in oral reconstruction.* Plast Reconstr Surg;104:1307–1313, 1999

Klepetko W., Marta GM., Wisser W. *Heterotopic trachea transplantation with omentum wrapping in the abdominal position preserves functional and structural integrity of a human tracheal allograft.* J.Thorac Cardiovasc Surg 127: 862-7,2004

Lawrence TS, Blackstock AW, McGinn C. *The mechanism of action of radiosensitization of conventional chemotherapeutic agents.* Semin Radiat Oncol;13:13–21,2003

Lyos AT, Evans GR, Perez D, Schusterman MA. *Tongue reconstruction: outcomes with the rectus abdominis flap.* Plast Reconstr Surg;103:442–449,1999

Maish MS, DeMeester SR. *Indications and technique of colon and jejunal interpositions for esophageal disease.* Surg Clin North Am;85:505–514,2005

Mc Carthy C., Cordeiro P. *Microvascular reconstruction of oncologic defects of the midface.* Plast.Reconstr.Surg. 126,1947-1959,2010

McConnel FMS, Hester TR, Mendelsohn MS, et al. *Manofluorography of deglutition after total laryngopharyngectomy.* Plast Reconstr Surg;81:346–350,1988

Nguyen NP, Sallah S. *Combined chemotherapy and radiationin the treatment of locally advanced head and neck cancers.* In Vivo;14:35–39,2000

Ott LM., Weatherly RA., Detamore MS. *Overview of tracheal tissue engineering: clinical need drives the laboratory approach.* Ann.Biomed.Eng. (Epub ahead of print) 2011

Pearson BW, Keith RL. *Near-total laryngectomy.* In: JohnsonJT, Blitzer A, Ossoff RM, Thomas IR, eds. *American Academy of Otology-Head Neck Surgery*,vol 2. St Louis: Mosby,:309–330,1990

Peng X, Mao C, Yu GY, Guo CB, Huang MX, Zhang Y. *Maxillary reconstruction with the free fibula flap.* Plast Reconstr Surg; 115: 1562–69,2005

Reece GP, Bengtson BP, Schusterman MA. *Reconstruction of the pharynx and cervical esophagus using free jejunal transfer.* Clin Plast Surg;21:125–136,1994

Reece GP, Schusterman MA, Miller MJ, et al. *Morbidity and functional outcome of free jejunal transfer reconstruction for circumferential defects of the pharynx and cervical esophagus.* Plast Reconstr Surg;96:1307–1316,1995

Rose KG, Sesterhenn K., Wustrow F. *Tracheal allotransplantation in man.* Lancet 1: 433,1979

Santamaria E, Granados M, Barrera-Franco JL. *Radial forearm free tissue transfer for head and neck* reconstruction: *versatility and reliability of a single donor site.* Microsurgery; 20: 195–201,2000

Schusterman MA, Reece GP, Kroll SS, Weldon ME. *Use of the AO plate for immediate mandibular reconstruction in cancer patients.* Plast Reconstr Surg;88: 588–593,1991

Sclaroff A, Haughey B, Gay WD, Paniello R. *Immediate mandibular reconstruction and placement of dental implants at the time of ablative surgery.* Oral Surg Oral Med Oral Pathol;78:711–717,1994

Shah JP and Patel SG. *Head and Neck. Surgery and Oncology* (3rd Ed), *Oral cavity and oropharynx.* Mosby, *ISBN*02723432236, Edinburgh,2003

Silvain C, Barrioz T, Besson I, et al. *Treatment and long-term outcome of chronic radiation esophagitis after radiation therapy for head and neck tumors.* Dig Dis Sci;38: 927–31,1993

Sullivan CH, Jaklitsch M, Haddad R, et al. *Endoscopic management of hypopharyngeal stenosis after organ sparing therapy for head and neck cancer.* Laryngoscope;114: 1924–31,2004

Uglesic V, Virag M, Varga S, Knezevic P, Milenovic A. *Reconstruction following radical maxillectomy with flaps supplied by the subscapular artery.* J Craniomaxillofac Surg; 28: 153–60,2000

Ugurlu K, Sacak B, Huthut I, Karsidag S, Sakiz D, Bas L. *Reconstructing wide palatomaxillary defects using free flaps combining bare serratus anterior muscle fascia and scapular bone.* J Oral Maxillofac Surg; 65: 621–29,2007

Urken ML, Buchbinder D, Weinberg H, Vickery C, Sheiner A, Biller HF. *Primary placement of osseointegrated implants in microvascular mandibular reconstruction.* Otolaryngol Head Neck Surg;101:56–73,1989

Varvares MA, Cheney ML, Glicklich RE, et al. *Use of the radial forearm fasciocutaneous free flap and Montgomery salivary bypass tube for pharyngoesophageal reconstruction.* Head Neck;22:463–468,2000

Vranckx JJ, Delaere P, Vanderpoorten V, Segers K, Nanhekhan LL. Prefabrication of trachea for the reconstruction of hemilaryngectomy defects in unilateral laryngx cancer. Proc. WSRM 2011, ISBN 978-88-7587-612-8, pp41-45.

Vranckx JJ, Delaere P, Vanderpoorten V,Segers K, Nanhekhan LL. Trachea allotransplantation after withdrawal of immunosuppression. Proc. WSRM 2011, ISBN 978-88-7587-612-8, pp 37-41.

Webster HR, Robinson DW. *The radial forearm flap without fascia and other refinements.* Eur J Plast Surg;18:11–16,1995

Wei F-C, Celik N, Yang W-G, Chen I-H, Chang Y-M, Chen H-C. *Complications after reconstruction by plate and soft-tissue free flap in composite mandibular defects and secondary salvage reconstruction with osteocutaneous flap.* Plast Reconstr Surg;112:37–42,2003

Wei F-C, Seah CS, Tsai YC, Liu SJ, Tsai MS. *Fibula osteoseptocutaneous flap for reconstruction of composite mandibular defects.* Plast Reconstr Surg;93:294–304,1994

Wong CH, Wei FC, Fu B, Chen YA, Lin JY. *Alternative vascular pedicle of the anterolateral thigh flap: theoblique branch of the lateral circumflex femoral artery.*Plast.Reconstr.Surg., 123: 571-577,2009

Wright CD, Grillo HC, Wain JC, et al. *Anastomotic complications after tracheal resection: prognostic factors and management.* J Thorac Cardiovasc Surg; 128:731–739,2004

Yousif NJ, Dzwierzynski WW, Sanger JR, Matloub HS,Campbell BH. *The innervated gracilis musculocutaneous flap for total tongue reconstruction.* Plast Reconstr Surg;104:916–921, 1999

Zur KB, Urken ML *Vascularized hemitracheal autograft for laryngotracheal reconstruction: a new surgical technique based on the thyroid gland as a vascular carrier.* Laryngoscope 113:1494–1498,2003

6

Reconstruction of Perineum and Abdominal Wall

J.J. Vranckx[1] and A. D'Hoore[2]
[1]Dept. of Plastic & Reconstructive Surgery
[2]Dept. Abdominal Surgery
KUL Leuven University Hospitals, Leuven
Belgium

1. Introduction

Deep defects at the perineum most frequently result from colorectal or vaginal tumor resection. More superficial but often extensive defects may be caused by radiotherapy, burns or aggressive infections such as necrotizing fasciitis. Resection of colorectal tumors is the main reason for perineal defects that require reconstruction. Abdominoperineal excision of the rectum is largely reserved for larger T2-3 tumors of the distal rectum and poorly differentiated tumors when a safe anastomosis after an anterior resection is not practicable. With the patient in the supine position, the rectum is mobilized down to the pelvic floor via a subumbilical midline incision. After division of the colon, the distal sigmoid is removed as a left iliac fossa colostomy. The distal colon is sutured and folded down into the pelvis. The perineal resection is subsequently performed with the patient in a prone or left lateral position, where utmost care is taken not to allow any tumor spillage by dissecting too close to the rectum. The dissection is therefore performed well into the ischiorectal fossa. The pudendal vessels that supply the anorectal area need to be ligated. For posterior cancers, the coccyx also needs to be resected to provide efficient clearance. In males, damage to the urethra and urethral bulb needs to be avoided. In females, the posterior vaginal wall is resected along with the rectum. These parameters specific to an abdominoperineal rectum amputation determine the difficulty and requirement for reconstruction (Lefevre et al., 2009, Park et al., 2007).

Necrotizing fasciitis of the genito-perineal area (gangrene of Fournier) is a rather frequent cause of extensive tissue loss in the abdominal wall and genitoperineal areas. It is a rapidly progressive mixed infection by hemolytic streptococci or staphylococci and peptostreptococci that is associated with an excessive secretion of toxic metabolites and collagenases that results in the dissolution of connective tissues. These mechanisms make the infection spread rapidly in a suprafascial tissue plane. The infection may be immediately fulminant or initially dormant for some days before evolving rapidly. Typically, no specific port of entry is noted. Because of the suprafacial spreading, the wounds may be extensive but are usually not deep. However, the infection may penetrate through lacerations into muscle compartments or cause a compartment syndrome because of inflammation and edema formation. These events may cause secondary destruction of the muscles. Rapid aggressive debridement is the only strategy to halt the necrotizing fasciitis, and repetitive debridements are necessary to stop the progression. Reconstructive options after serial debridement focus on the restoration of the fascioadipocutaneous layers while avoiding tissue contraction.

1.1 Superficial and extensive defects of the perineal wall

Superficial extensive defects most often occur after necrotizing fasciitis and seldom occur after burns because this region is well protected by clothing. Serial debridements are required to eradicate the tissue infection. Coverage of the exposed fascia layers and muscle compartments is most commonly performed by split-thickness skin grafts because of the extent of the lesions. To avoid graft contractions, a 1:1 mesh graft pattern is often preferred. Artificial dermal sheets may restore the deep dermal layer and create a more flexible and elastic floor of the wound after skin grafting to prevent tissue contraction in the perineum. Especially in burn treatment, these dermal or skin equivalents have proven their value. The take and integration of these skin equivalents significantly decreases in contaminated areas, and they have no use in infected milieu. Therefore, their use after necrotizing fasciitis is limited. In several countries, there is a partial or total reimbursement for these expensive dermal templates or skin equivalents when the recipient sites are located in the face or over mobile joints. Otherwise, the steep costs may prevent widespread use of these skin equivalents despite their impact on tissue elasticity. In the genitoperineal area, tissue flexibility is important because tissue contraction in the lower abdomen, groin and genitoperineal zones could lead to chronic pain and tissue breakdown as well as loss of function during stance and mobilization. Ideally, a restoration with like-with-like elastic tissues is preferred for deeper defects. Local or locoregional flaps can provide all required donor tissues in this area. The rectus femoris flap has been widely reported to restore groin defects, but this flap can also reach the perianal and perineal areas. It may be estimated that donor site morbidity after prelevation of the rectus femoris muscle is more significant than occurs after harvest of the anterolateral thigh flap in conjunction with a vastus lateralis segment because the rectus femoris is considered the most significant quadriceps muscle. The scar after the prelevation of the rectus femoris flap is located on the anterior thigh and may flatten the natural aesthetic curvature. Depending on the BMI of the patient and skin elasticity, a skin paddle of approximately 7-10 cm can be harvested from the anterior thigh. To maintain the leverage of the quadriceps tendons for knee extension, it is important not to harvest the flap too distally on the thigh. The tendinous extensions of the vastus medialis, intermedius and lateralis should be reinforced after a rectus flap is harvested distally to preserve the strength of the quadriceps muscles (fig. 1).

The anterolateral thigh flap also offers ample tissues and is an excellent option for defects in the groin and perineum (Friji et al., 2010, Lannon et al., 2011). Its wide arc of rotation, with a pivot point medial to the sartorius muscle, allows an efficient transfer to the perineal floor. Because it is harvested as a fasciocutaneous or adipocutaneous perforator flap, the donor site is minimal in size. Care must be taken not to harm femoral nerve branches to the rectus femoris when the ALT is tunnelled medially under the rectus femoris and sartorius. However, without this maneuver, the flap will not be long enough to reach the perineal area.

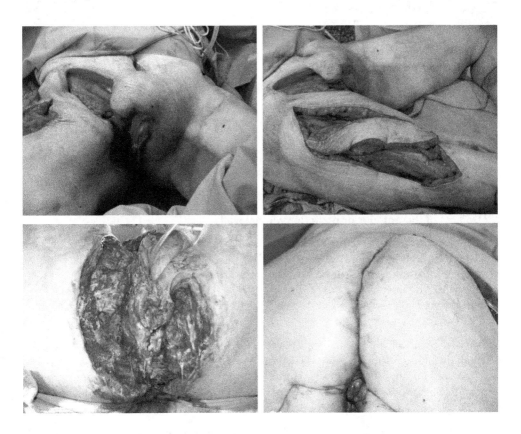

Fig. 1. Necrotizing fasciitis involving the groin and perianal region, sacral and gluteal zones. Upper row: rectus femoris myocutaneous flap harvested for closure of the deep inguinal defect. Lower row: A unilateral inferior gluteal artery perforator flap (IGAP) is dissected to close the sacral and perianal defects. A contralateral SGAP-based flap closes the transition zone between the perianal area and the groin.

For perianal defects and more posteriorly located defects in the gluteal crease and sacral areas, the gluteus maximus myocutaneous transposition flap has been the procedure of choice for decades (fig. 1). This flap can be rotated into the defect as a wide rotation flap or as a V-Y transposition flap. When considering donor site morbidity after harvesting the gluteus maximus muscle, muscle-sparing techniques are the procedure of choice. Flaps in the gluteal area can be harvested based on perforators of the superior (S-GAP) or inferior (I-GAP) gluteal vascular pedicle (Wagstaff et al., 2009). Because of an advantageous arc of rotation, the inferior gluteal artery perforator-based flap can be used to address large sacral and perineal defects (Fig. 2).

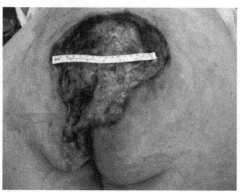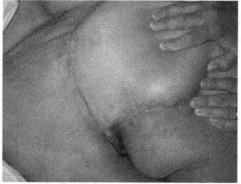

Fig. 2. Necrotizing fasciitis in the perianal area and sacral zones, reconstructed with a unilateral IGAP-based gluteal flap.

1.2 Defects of the anterior or posterior vaginal wall

For congenital vaginal aplasia with an intact vaginal canal, the Abbe-McIndoe procedure represents the easiest and most successful method for vaginal reconstruction because it does not require laparotomy. Split-thickness skin grafts are sutured around a vaginal stent with the epithelial side inward (Lesavoy & Carter , 1996). Patients should wear a conformer for 6 months to avoid contraction off the vaginal vault. Lubricants should prevent the grafts from drying, blistering, and eroding.

Primary sarcomas of the vaginal wall may result in deep vaginal defects of any size and orientation. Skin-grafting techniques using fine 1:1 meshed split-thickness skin grafts function well for superficial defects. However, to prevent tissue contraction and provide appropriate sensitivity in this sensitive area, local and locoregional fasciocutaneous flaps are preferred.

A traditional algorithm for vulvovaginal reconstruction distinguishes between partial IA and IB versus circumferential type II defects (Pusic & Mehrara , 2006). For partial type IA anterior or lateral defects, pudendal thigh flaps are the first choice for treatment because they provide well-vascularized innervated flaps based on the posterior labial vascular pedicle and the posterior labial branches of the pudendal nerve. The axis of these flaps lies within the groin creases and therefore leaves no donor site morbidity. During the harvesting, it is necessary to incise at both sides into the subcutis at the entrée of the pedicle and in a superficial plane above the pedicle. This maneuver facilitates rotation and donor-site closure. Flap inset is performed by tunneling under the labia majora to avoid creating dog ears in the skin at the pivot points.

Partial type IB posterior defects can also be reconstructed with a pudendal thigh flap. A perforator-based gluteal crease flap can also be harvested in a unilateral or bilateral fashion to allow restoration of the posterior or lateral wall with well-vascularized fasciocutaneous tissues with minimal donor site morbidity. For the reconstruction of an entire posterior vaginal wall, bilateral pudendal thigh flaps or bilateral gluteal crease flaps are required.

Type II defects are circumferential and are divided to type IIA upper $2/3^{rd}$ defects and type IIB total defects of the vagina. Most often, such defects are the result of advanced colorectal cancer, advanced cancer of the urinary bladder, primary sarcomas of the vaginal wall or extensive uterine or cervical neoplasms. A resection to negative oncologic borders may result in a cavity. Aside from restoration of the vaginal wall, tissue bulk is required to fill the cavity and avoid herniation of tissues within the cavity, infection, tissue breakdown and fistulization. In such situations, bilateral myocutaneous gracilis flaps are a good option. Segmental or total vaginal defects can be restored with the skin paddle whereas the muscle provides limited tissue bulk to fill a medium-sized cavity (Whetzel & Lechtman, 1997). The skin island overlaying the gracilis muscle at the medial thigh is not always distally reliable, which may lead to segmental skin necrosis of the distal tip. Incorporation of more fascia at the sides may prevent skin perforators from being harmed during flap harvest (Fig. 3). As a bilateral flap, the gracilis is efficient in restoring defects along the labia majora of the outer vaginal wall. The length from the medial circumflex femoral pedicle to the gracilis determines the arc of rotation. This pedicle should be dissected to the origin at the deep femoral pedicle to allow maximal mobilization of the flaps.

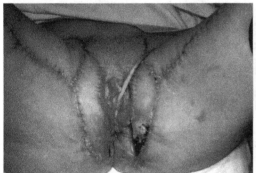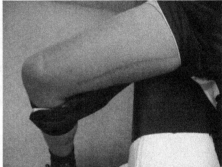

Fig. 3. Left: Bilateral gracilis musculocutaneous flaps restored the perineal wall and labia majora. The left distal skin island of the gracilis flap underwent necrosis. Right: limited donor site morbidity of a gracilis flap.

Often, however, the resection of advanced colorectal cancer leaves a deep cavity with a large risk of herniation of the bowels into the defect. After postoperative radiotherapy, there is a high incidence of fistulization if the cavity is not filled with bulky, well-vascularized tissues. These donor tissues also need to restore the posterior vaginal wall defect. An inferior gluteal artery perforator flap (IGAP) has a broad arc of rotation. A unilateral IGAP flap can be rotated medially, segmentally deepithelialized and set into the defect (Fig. 4). The most medially located segment can be left as a fasciocutaneous unit and used to close a segmental vaginal wall defect.

The primary choice for deep defects including those of the posterior vaginal wall is the vertical rectus abdominis musculocutaneous flap (VRAM), even when a colostomy and urostomy need to be placed in the abdominal wall. (Tobin & Day, 1988). The VRAM flap is harvested in an anterior fascia-sparing technique that facilitates donor-site closure. A transabdominal-transperineal approach transfers the VRAM flap through the perineal introitus and fills the perianal cavity after colorectal resection with bulky, well-vascularized

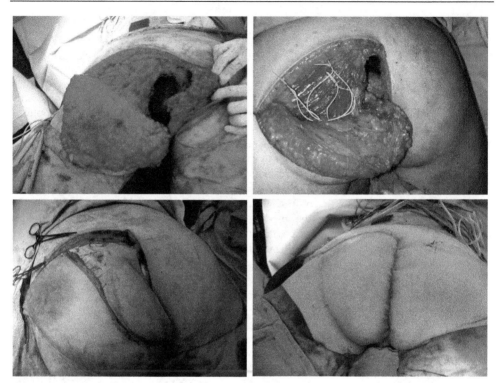

Fig. 4. Upper row: IGAP harvest for perineal reconstruction. Perforators marked with blue vessel loops. Lower row: The medial segment is deepithelialized and introduced into the defect. The contralateral buttock is sutured end-to-side to the IGAP flap at the lateral border of the deepithelialized area.

tissues (Fig. 5). The skin paddle can be located vertically on the mesogastrium over the proximal rectus abdominis muscle. Oblique and extended VRAM flaps based on perforators at the costal margin or at the distal mammary artery are reported. These modifications in the design of the skin island allow the physician to raise the skin paddle more proximally to reach defects located far up in the gluteal crease after transpelvic transfer (Taylor et al., 1993;Abbott et al., 2008 ;Villa et al., 2011). When the rectus abdominis muscle is harvested with a transverse skin island (TRAM-flap), a tubular circular neovagina can be created. After harvest, the flap is formed into a cone and transferred through the peritoneum at the origin of the deep inferior epigastric vessels in a transpelvic approach and sutured to a perineal introital incision (Lesavoy & Carter E, 1996). A pedicled rectus femoris and anterolateral thigh flap can also be used to create a tubular-shaped neovagina. The length of the neovagina depends on tissue elasticity and flap length and bulk. However, it should be marked that the vector of a unilateral anterolateral thigh or rectus femoris flap may distort tissues after inset and does not yield results that are as aesthetically pleasing as those achieved with a rectus abdominis flap. Fig. 6 represents our current algorithm.

For similar reasons, a myocutaneous gracilis flap should be harvested bilaterally, with each flap recreating one half of the neovaginal cone to prevent the distortion of tissues, as when a unilateral flap is used.

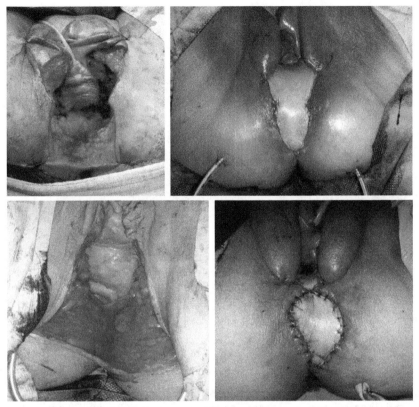

Fig. 5. Posterior vaginal wall defect restored with a vertical rectus abdominis flap by the intraperitoneal transpelvic approach. There is abundant remaining tissue close to the perineal defect. The base of the labia majora is sutured to a deepithelialized segment of the VRAM flap.

Complications

Infection has an incidence of approximately 10 %. Perioperative antibiotics, careful rinsing and meticulous wound-care are mandatory for postoperative care. Irradiation, smoking and obesity are the risk factors most strongly associated with delayed wound healing and infection. A VRAM flap has the most secure blood supply to the skin paddle. However, torsion should be avoided at the pedicle after full release of the rectus abdominis muscle at its origin at the pubic bone. Therefore, if length permits, which it usually does, it is advisable to leave the distal muscular attachment intact, especially when the patient is placed in a prone or lateral position during an abdominoperineal rectum amputation (Glatt et al, 2006). The musculocutaneous gracilis flaps carry a substantial risk of distal skin necrosis. This area is the deepest point of the newly shaped vaginal cone and difficult to treat with non-conservative measures after insertion into the pelvis. Side-wall restoration with an IGAP flap often collapses because of the intrinsic bulk of the flap in some patients. Several long-term complications have been described. Vaginal dryness is the most frequent complication because of inadequate secretion. Hypertrophy or dysesthesia at the scars may be significant. The neovagina is often too small after collapse and contraction.

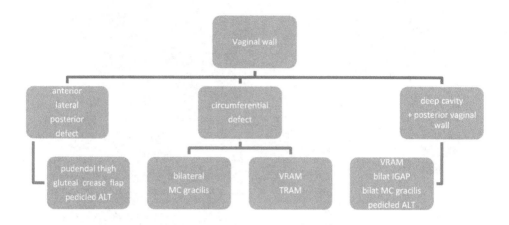

Fig. 6. Algorithm for vaginal wall reconstruction. ALT: anterolateral thigh flap. MC: myocutaneous, VRAM: vertical rectus abdominis muscle flap, TRAM: transverse rectus abdominis musculocutaneous flap, bilat IGAP: bilateral inferior gluteal artery perforator flap.

1.3 Large composite defects of the perineal wall

Most colorectal carcinomas with limited soft-tissue defects of the perineal wall are treated with primary closure of the neighboring tissue layers. However, tissue breakdown often occurs and poses a difficult reconstructive option because of scarring and tissue contracture.

Therefore, there is a tendency for closure of the perineal wall with locoregional, well-vascularized tissues, taking into consideration the fair outcome obtained with more extensive extirpation of colorectal cancer. Reconstructive options must address the dead space while inhibiting the herniation of the abdominal organs and introduce well-vascularized fasciocutaneous tissues in the perineal wall to prevent skin breakdown and fistulization (Fig. 7).

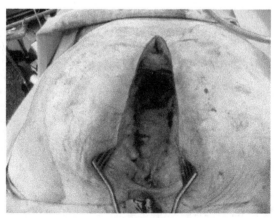

Fig. 7. A deep perineal defect requires obliteration of the pelvic cavity.

In addition, advanced colorectal cancer frequently involves the posterior vaginal wall, and carcinoma of the bladder may extend into the anterior vaginal wall, which further complicates the reconstruction.

Complications after surgical closure for extended abdominoperineal resection (APRA) and infralevatoric pelvic exenterations (TIPE) arise from non-collapsible dead space, the use of irradiated skin for closure and infection. Surgical reconstructive options should address these factors and also focus on donor-site morbidity and quality-of-life parameters concerning sexual function and body integrity.

Identification of the problem

There is a close relationship among the colorectal tissues, the vagina and the urinary bladder. A complex, dynamic support system of ligaments coordinates the topography and function of these organs. As a result, after surgical resection of a tumor in this region, the loss of integrity and function of one organ may result in the collapse, prolapse or herniation of the remaining organs into the rigid cone-shaped pelvis. If a herniation of bowels into the pelvic cavity exists, radiation therapy may result in dramatic fistulizations that are difficult to treat without new colectomies. Therefore, it is imperative that the introitus of the pelvic cavity is sealed in an efficient fashion and that the pelvic cavity is filled with well-vascularized tissues that may also provide closure of the perineal wall with tissues resilient against radiotherapy. For small defects, a primary closure may still be considered. However, for medium-sized and large defects a composite reconstruction is mandatory.

The preferred method to restore these complex defects should be selected based on the anatomical features of the defect, i.e., the required width of the perineal skin, the anticipated volume needed to fill the perineal cavity, the vaginal defect (partial or circumferential), and previous interventions that may have influenced the donor sites. Based on these reconstructive aims, donor tissues are selected based on their intrinsic features such as pedicle length, quality and width of skin, tissue bulk and donor-site morbidity.

The abdominal wall and thigh area harbor a multitude of locoregional flaps that have been reported as used in the context of perineal and vaginal reconstruction. In comparison with free flaps, treatment with pedicled locoregional flaps is preferred, especially for medium-sized defects. Even for large, complex defects, there is a renewed interest in using locoregional pedicled flaps to restore the perineal wall because of our better understanding of the vascular perfusion of these flaps by their perforators. Harvesting of composite locoregional flaps therefore does not necessarily lead to significant donor-site morbidity if certain technical refinements are included in the flap harvest. Free flaps therefore are only indicated after pelvic exenterations or extended defects when no locoregional tissues are available because of previous interventions.

Reconstructive options

Long bilateral myocutaneous gracilis flaps have been considered as the workhorse for large defects of the perineal wall. However because of the lack of tissue bulk, these flaps do not fill a deep cavity efficiently, and the longitudinally aligned skin island is randomly vascularized in its distal section. Furthermore, to obtain a symmetric alignment of tissues, a bilateral flap is mandatory. For smaller perineal wounds including a circumferential vaginal defect, however, a bilateral myocutaneous gracilis flap is still useful. The donor site is small, although the scars may widen. The distal skin island is not always reliable, but vascularization may be improved by incorporating more fascia.

The vertical rectus abdominis musculocutaneous flap displays robust vascularization and is characterized by large tissue bulk. The flap can be harvested on its inferior epigastric vascular pedicle. The skin island is oriented vertically aligning the median laparotomy incision. An anterior fascia-sparing approach is advised to diminish donor-site morbidity. This maneuver allows for minor resection of the anterior fascia, thereby removing the need for a mesh graft to restore the abdominal wall fascia. This strategy is highly recommended, especially for infected wounds. In addition, the proximal skin island can be extended as far as the posterior axillary line as proposed by Taylor et al. More recently, vascular angiographic studies demonstrated that multiple linking vessels exist between vertical and extended oblique skin territories, even at a subdermal level, which allows the surgeon to leave the deep fascia in the transition zone intact and to diminish donor-site morbidity when harvesting a large flap(Butler et al, 2008). The VRAM flap can be used in the perineal area via an anterior suprapubic or trans-groin approach using a subcutaneous tunnel at the pivot point (Fig. 8). This external rotation is useful when a defect in the groin needs to be restored simultaneously, for instance, after an extensive lymph node resection. Because of the external arc of rotation, the proximal segment of the flap allows the restoration of the groin

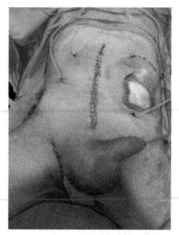

Fig. 8. VRAM flap externally rotated into the defect via a subcutaneous tunnel in the right groin. Part of the rectus abdominis muscle fills the deeper defect in the groin after lymphadenectomy.

area and the distal segment of the perineal defect. However because of the potentially increased donor-site morbidity for such defects, a pedicled anterolateral thigh flap may be the best option. Depending on the length-width ratio of the thigh, the anterolateral thigh flap may have sufficient length to fill the perineal cavity with well-vascularized tissues. When harvested distally on the thigh, the flap even may reach up posteriorly towards a partial sacrectomy defect. A vastus lateralis segment can be incorporated with the anterolateral thigh flap and offer supplementary tissue bulk when required. The major disadvantage of the anterolateral thigh flap is that the number and location of perforators to the skin paddle are not constant. Originally described as a septocutaneous perforator flap, musculocutaneous perforators are encountered in more than 60% of cases, which lengthens the time of harvest. In addition, the perforators quite often originate on the medial descending branch of the lateral circumflex vascular pedicle instead of the more conventional lateral descending branch. For these reasons, CT angiography is suggested to anticipate the topography of perforators in a fashion similar to that used for a DIEP perforator flap in breast reconstruction.

After an extended abdominoperineal rectum amputation, there is a wide and deep open pelvic introitus and a cavity that reaches the perineal wall. Adequate filling is mandatory to prevent the bowels from descending and exposure by radiotherapy. A transperitoneal course of the VRAM flap allows it to obliterate this pelvic cavity and to fill the dead space (Fig. 9). Usually, a traditional fascia-sparing VRAM flap is long enough to efficiently reach the posterior vaginal wall and the perineal wall down to the intergluteal crease (Fig. 10). If the defect travels more posteriorly, an extended VRAM is required.

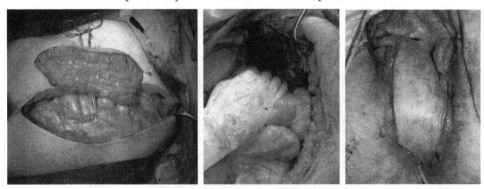

Fig. 9. Left: harvest of the VRAM vertical rectus abdominis musculocutaneous flap by fascia sparing approach. Middle: the VRAM flap is transferred via transabdominal approach into the pelvic cavity. Mark the deep inferior epigastric vascular pedicle at the upper right side under the retractor. Right: the VRAM flap has been tunneled to the perineum and only sutured distally. After verification that no traction is exerted on the vascular pedicle proximally, the skin island is remodeled according to the requirements for restoring the posterior vaginal wall and the perineal wall.

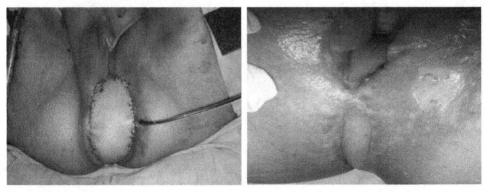

Fig. 10. Left: reconstruction of the perineal and posterior vaginal wall by transpelvic VRAM flap. Right: VRAM flap after 55 Gy local irradiation. The posterior vaginal lining remained soft, with a preserved circular vaginal configuration. The surrounding skin suffered from irradiation with significant erythema and skin erosions.

Inferior gluteal artery-based perforator flaps (IGAP) are a good option to close the perineal defect when less volume is needed to fill the dead space in the perineal cavity. If the patient is positioned in the prone position or when previous surgery or a badly planned positioning of the colostomy and urostomy after a Bricker derivation excludes the use of a VRAM flap, a unilateral or bilateral IGAP flap is a good option. Based on perforators of the inferior gluteal vascular pedicle, the adipocutaneous flap can be harvested with a wide arc of rotation.

The superomedial segment of the IGAP flap rotates into the defect and is de-epithelialized (Fig. 11). An end-to-side suture of the contralateral gluteal skin to the IGAP flap allows closure and filling of the defect. In obese patients, the obtained tissue bulk of an IGAP flap can be substantial. Fig. 12 represents our current algorithm for large perineal defects (Vranckx et al, 2011)

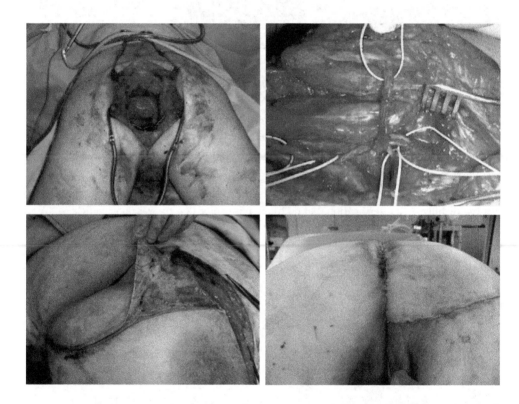

Fig. 11. Upper left: deep cavity after extended abdominoperineal rectum amputation. Upper right: an IGAP inferior gluteal artery perforator-based flap is harvested. One perforator is selected and further dissected to achieve optimal rotation. Lower left: the required segment has been de-epithelialized. Lower right: the de-epithelialized segment is sutured to the deep borders of the pelvic cavity. Skin closure is performed with an end-to-side suture to recreate the gluteal crease.

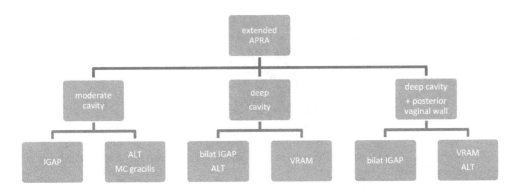

Fig. 12. Algorithm of the treatment of defects after extended abdominoperineal rectum amputation. A distinction is made between defects with a moderate pelvic cavity and deep cavities versus defects that require reconstruction of the posterior vaginal wall. IGAP: inferior gluteal artery perforator flap; ALT: anterolateral thigh flap: MC gracilis: myocutaneous gracilis flap; VRAM: vertical rectus abdominis myocutaneous flap.

2. Reconstruction of the abdominal wall

2.1 Pathophysiology

The abdominal wall is lined superiorly by the xiphoid process and the costal cartilage of ribs 7-12. The inferolateral border is lined by the inguinal ligament and medially by the pubis tubercle and pubic bone. A line from the midaxilla to the anterior superior iliac spine of the iliac crest delineates the lateral borders. The diamond-shaped abdominal wall consists of the peritoneum, three fascial layers and four significant muscles, a subcutaneous layer of variable thickness, Scarpa's fascia and the skin. The fascia layers of the external and oblique muscles and the transverse abdominis muscle fuse at the lateral border of the rectus abdominis muscle and form the deep fascia layer. The arcuate line halfway between the umbilicus and the pubic symphysis denotes the change in the composition of the rectus sheath. Above the arcuate line, the anterior fascia layer consists of the external and internal oblique muscle aponeuroses; below the arcuate line, the three aponeurotic layers form the anterior rectus sheet. Motor innervation to these muscles comes from the intercostal and subcostal nerves for the rectus abdominis muscle as well as from the iliohypogastric nerve for the external oblique muscle or the ilioinguinal nerve for the internal oblique muscle. The nerves should be preserved not only for sensation but especially to maintain the motor function of the abdominal wall. The structural integrity of all of these layers is important in the majority of biomechanical body movements, especially walking, bending, climbing and posture, and is also elementary in supporting the visceral functions of digestion, micturition, defecation, respiration and expectoration. Tumor extirpation and trauma are the most common causes of full-thickness abdominal wall defects. Necrotizing fasciitis, irradiation and burns may cause rather extensive superficial defects (Fig. 13).

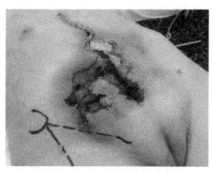

Fig. 13. Left: Irradiation wound after laparotomy for abdominal wall sarcoma with resection and primary closure.

Reconstruction of the abdominal wall focuses on the restoration of structural integrity and function and the prevention of visceral eventration. The available options depend on multiple parameters such as the location and size of the defect, BMI of the patient, scars from previous interventions, irradiation and presence of a colostomy or urostomy (Gottlieb et al., 1990). Matheset al. described the types of defects based on the defect components: type I defects with hernia defects and intact stable skin coverage and type II defects with hernia and unstable or absent skin coverage (Mathes et al., 2000). Defects were also assigned to zones: zone 1A represents the upper midline of the abdomen, zone 1B the lower midline area, zone 2 the upper quadrant and zone 3 the lower quadrant (Fig. 14).

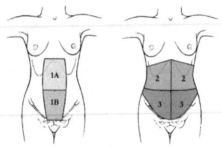

Fig. 14. Reconstructive zones of the abdomen. (Mathes . et al. Ann. Surg. 232; 586-596.)

Hurwitz described seven anatomic reconstructive subunits (Hurwitz & Hollins, 1994). Rohrich at al. described a six-subunit scheme delineating the midline and lateral upper, middle and lower thirds and proposed a treatment algorithm based on these zones (Rohrich et al., 2000). The most difficult zones to treat are zone IA or upper-midline defects because locoregional flaps from the thigh or the back are located distally. To treat such patients, zone-free flaps with vascular anastomosis to the deep inferior epigastric, superior epigastric or internal mammary vascular pedicle have been suggested. Most defects are type I incisional hernias with stable skin coverage and only require mesh coverage (Pless TK & Pless JE, 1993). There are currently many different types of meshes available. The risk of infection plays an important role in selection of the appropriate treatment strategy. Polypropylene is commonly used for fascia repair. This mesh induces an intense fibrovascular infiltration and incorporates into the surrounding tissues, leading to a strong repair, but it is also associated with adhesions to the intra-abdominal viscera with consequent frequent formation of enterocutaneous fistulas. Non-absorbable synthetic meshes are largely intolerant to an infected environment such as the environment that persists after the resection of abdominal wall tumors. New-generation biologic meshes (such as human acellular dermal matrix, which is derived from human cadaveric dermis) can be utilized in a contaminated milieu (Fig. 15). They are the first choice in the treatment of complex wounds after chronic exposure to provide the fascia layers with sufficient strength and adequate skin coverage (Breuing et al., 2010).

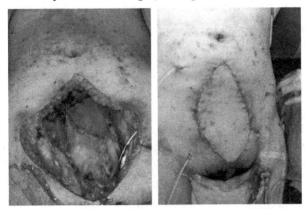

Fig. 15. Left: Biologic mesh restores the fascia gap before closure with a pedicled anterolateral thigh flap (right).

The treatment of type-II defects depends largely on the central tissue gap. The overall failure of treatment is often attributed to primary closure under tension, which causes midline necrosis of the abdominal wall. Primary closure should therefore be limited to patients with small defects and few associated risk factors for poor wound healing. Immediate reconstruction is the strategy of choice in primary extirpation surgery or eventration repair. A delayed repair is advisable when the wound is infected or when the patient is unstable and the defect is extensive. Vacuum-assisted closure can be of great value, and abdominal dressings have been developed to assist in progressive wound conditioning and prevent the abdominal muscular layers from retracting(Fig. 16).

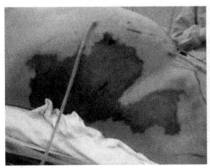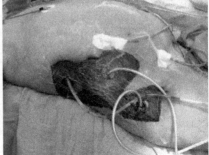

Fig. 16. Left. Vacuum-assisted closure device on zone III of the abdomen and on the lateral thighs after serial debridements for necrotizing fasciitis as a result of colon anastomotic leakage and resulting fistula to the skin.

In type II composite defects, *component release techniques* are the most frequently used approach to treatment (Ramirez et al., 1990). However, when excessive traction is exerted on the midline tissues, morbidity after a traditional Ramirez procedure is significant. With current perforator dissection techniques, relevant perforators to the abdominal wall skin are preserved during a component release procedure. Sufficient vascularization to the abdominal wall tissues ensures that closure can be performed under tension despite substantial undermining forces (Shestaq et al., 2000).

Large and composite defects after tumor extirpation and in the presence of a colostomy and urostomy still pose a surgical challenge. These defects require the introduction of tissues to bridge the gap. Local full-thickness abdominal wall rhomboid flaps and extended abdominal wall flaps may achieve closure of the defect but at the cost of further abdominal wall weakening. Pedicled uni-or bilateral *tensor fascia lata flaps* have long been used as a standard approach to restore the abdominal wall defect because thigh flaps leave the remaining abdominal wall intact (Williams et al., 1998). For meso-and epigastric defects, however, the harvest should include distal fascia to achieve sufficient length. Distally, the fascia is thin and less vascularized, and it does not restore function and aesthetic appearance, especially in more obese patients and defects located in the upper midline or supralateral zones.

The *rectus femoris myocutaneous flap* introduces more voluminous tissues and allows the closure of the donor site. The rectus femoris muscle is the most significant quadriceps muscle, and its harvest may diminish knee extension. In addition, the donor scar located anteriorly on the thigh is conspicuous when a large skin paddle has been incorporated. Because the transition zone of the quadriceps muscle and tendinous segment at the midline of the thigh should be kept intact to preserve the leverage of the quadriceps during knee extension, the harvest should stop at the distal two-thirds of the mid-thigh, which does not allow a sufficient length to reach upper-midline defects.

The anterolateral thigh is a common donor zone for free flaps used in lower-limb and head and neck reconstruction (Wei et al., 2002). Recent reports describe its use in perineal reconstructions (Yu et al. 2002, Luo et al., 2000). Donor-site morbidity is minimal if a perforator-based *anterolateral thigh flap* is harvested (Lipa et al., 2005, Tsuji et al., 2008). The vascularization pattern of this flap allows for a distal harvest on the thigh based on available perforators. A multitude of flaps can be designed based on these perforators. A useful combination in the anterolateral thigh is that of the skin paddle and the vastus lateralis muscle, which can be used in extensive defects (Posh et al., 2005). Sasaki and Kimata used free anterolateral thigh flaps in combination with a tensor fascia lata musculocutaneous flap to restore a large abdominal wall defect (Sasaki K. et al., 1998, Kimata et al., 1999) and concluded that the ALT flap with or without the TFL was superior to the TFL alone for the reconstruction of large abdominal wall defects.However, the anterolateral thigh flap can be raised distally on the thigh. The vascular pedicle is long and allows the harvesting of a large pedicled flap. To reach the abdominal wall as a pedicled flap, tunneling should be performed under the rectus femoris and sartorius muscles. During this maneuver, it is critical to not harm other femoral nerve branches to avoid a further decline in quadriceps function (Fig. 17). Thus far, the use of the anterolateral thigh flap for abdominal wall reconstruction is anecdotal, but those authors who have used the ALT in this setting claim that the ALT can reach all abdominal wall regions as a pedicled flap (Lannon et al., 2011, Vranckx et al., 2011).

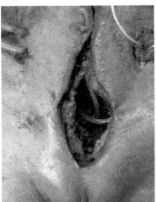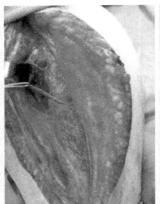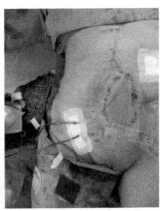

Fig. 17. ALT perforator flap for abdominal wall reconstruction. Left: abdominal wall full-thickness defect. Mid: anterolateral thigh flap harvested with the skin paddle perfused on one large perforator branch, which is followed to the origin of the descending branch into the lateral circumflex femoral vascular pedicle. At the same time, a segment of vastus lateralis is harvested with its femoral motor nerve intact. Right: flap closes the defect with like-with-like tissues.

The abdominal wall participates intensively in posture and has a synergistic function in a multitude of movements. Functional restoration of the abdominal wall is therefore an ultimate aim in reconstructive surgery. Dynamic activities may be restored using a layered wound closure method to identify and separate all muscle components (Pless T & Pless J, 2005). For large defects with extensive tissue loss, coaptation of the external oblique muscle continuity must be included, and dynamic tissues must be introduced into the defect. Koshima demonstrated that a pedicled rectus femoris muscle flap restored contractile activities in the abdomen (Koshima Iet al. 1999). Sasaki used a free TFL flap (Sasaki et al., 1998) and Ninkovic used a free, innervated latissimus dorsi flap (Ninkovic et al., 1998) to restore the contractile activities in the abdominal wall. They achieved excellent dynamic results. However, free flaps require a lag time during which the abdominal wall is weakened and herniation may (re)occur. Vranckx uses pedicled musculocutaneous anterolateral thigh flaps to restore the abdominal wall defect in a like-with-like fashion (Fig. 18). Femoral nerve branches to the harvested vastus lateralis muscle are left intact during the transfer. The muscle segment restores and bridges the muscular gap. The thigh fascia with the tractus iliotibialis is sutured to the fascial boundaries of the defect. The anterolateral thigh skin paddle restores the abdominal wall skin defect (Vranckx et al., 2010). The authors achieved excellent dynamic results over a 1-year follow up as determined by dynamometric analysis. Future aims should further focus on the dynamic restoration of abdominal wall defects using donor tissues with minimal donor-site morbidity (Fig. 18).

Conclusion. The reconstruction of complex abdominal wall defects is a veritable challenge. The aim of the restoration is the preservation of abdominal wall integrity and function while avoiding the herniation of the abdominal wall content. Type I defects consisting of herniation with adequate skin coverage require fascia repair, and various techniques are described. For small to moderate Type II full-thickness defects, perforator-preserving component-release techniques are efficient as long as excessive traction on the midline is avoided. For large composite defects, tissues should be introduced into the defect to restore the integrity of the abdominal wall. A dynamic instead of static reconstruction is the ultimate aim.

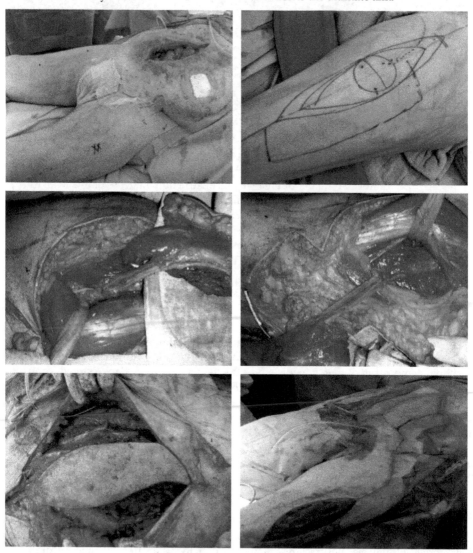

Fig. 18. Upper left: Abdominal wall defect in zones IA and IB. The most proximal part reaches the xyphoid process. Upper right: Anterolateral thigh flap with vastus lateralis segment harvested from the left thigh. Mid-left: The pedicle is dissected to its origin just lateral of the rectus femoris muscle. Mid-right: the ALT/VL flap is tunneled under the rectus femoris muscle to medialize the pivot point of the pedicle. Lower left: the ALT/VL flap covers the whole defect up to the xyphoid process with ease without any traction on the muscle, fascia or skin paddle (nb. xyphoid process at the right side of the picture). Lower right. After suturing of the flap into the defect. The donor site just before skin grafting.

3. References

Abbott DE., Halverson AL., Wayne JD., et al. *The oblique rectus abdominal myocutaneous flap for complex pelvic wound reconstruction.* Dis.Colon Rectum; 51:1237-1241, 2008

Breuing K., Butler CE., Ferzoco S., et al. *Ventral Hernia Working Group. Incisional ventral hernia's: review of litterature and recommendations regarding the grading and technique of repair.* Surgery 148: 544-558, 2010

Butler CE., Gundeslioglu AO., Rodriguez-Bigas MA. *Outcome of immediate vertical rectus abdominis myocutaneous flap reconstruction for irradiated abdominoperineal resection defects.*J.Am.Col.Surg.; 206: 694-703, 2008

Friji MT., Suri MP., Shankhdhar VK., Ahmad QG., Yadav PS. *Pedicled anterolateral thigh flap: a versatile flap for difficult regional soft tissue reconstruction.* Ann.Plast.Surg., 64, 458-61.; 2010

Glatt BS., Disa Jj. Et al. *Reconstruction of extensive partial or total sacrectomy defects with a transabdominal vertical rectus abdominis myocutaneous flap.* Ann. Plast.Surg; 56: 526-531, 2006

Gottlieb JR., Engrav LH., Walkinshaw MD et al. *Upper abdominal wall defects: immediate or staged reconstruction?* Plast.Reconstr.Surg; 86:281, 1990

Hurwitz DJ., Hollins RR. *Reconstruction of the abdominal wall and groin.* In M.Cohen (Ed), *Mastery of Plastic and Reconstructive surgery,* Vol 1, 1st Ed. Boston: Little, Brown, 1994

Kimata Y., Uchiyama K.,Sekido M et al. *Anterolateral thigh flap for abdominal wall reconstruction.* Plast.Reconstr.Surg.103: 1191-1197, 1999

Koshima I., Moriguchi T., Inagawa K., Urushibara K. *Dynamic reconstruction of the abdominal wall using a reinnervated free rectus femoris muscle transfer.* Ann.Plast.Surg.43:199-203, 1999

Lannon DA., Ross GL., Addison PD., Novak CB., Lipa JE., Neligan PC. *Versatility of the pedicled anterolateral thigh flap and its use in complex abdominal and pelvic reconstruction.* Plast.Reconstr.Surg., 127, 677-88,2011

Lannon DA.,Ross GL., Addisson PD., Novak CB.,Lipa JE., Neligan PC. *Versatility of the pedicled anterolateral thigh flap and its use in complex abdominal and pelvic reconstructions.*Plast.Reconstr.Surg. ;127,677-88, 2011

Lefevre JH., Parc Y et al. *Abdomino-perineal resecton for anal cancer.* Ann.Surg.; 250: 707-711, 2009

Lesavoy MA., Carter EJ. *Vaginal reconstruction.* In Raz S, ed: Female Urology, 2nd ed. Philadelphia,WB Saunders;605-616,1996

Lipa JE., Novak CB., Binhammer PA. *Patient-reported donorsite morbidity following anterolateral thigh free flaps.* J.Reconstr.Microsurg. 21; 365-370,2005

Luo S., Raffoul W., Piaget F., Egloff DV. *Anterolateral thigh fasciocutaneous flap in the difficult perineogenital reconstruction.* Plast.Reconstr.Surg. 105:171-173,2000

Mathes SJ., Steinwald PM.,Foster RD.,Hofffman WY.,Anthony JP. *Complex abdominal wall reconstruction: a comparison of flap and mesh closure.* Ann.Surg. 232: 586-96,2000

Ninkovic M., Kronberger P., Harpf C. et al. *Free innervated latissimus dorsi musculocutaneous flap for reconstruction of full-thickness abdominal wall defects.* Plast.Reconstr.Surg.; 101:971,1998

Nisar PJ., Scott HJ. *Myocutaneous flap reconstruction of the pelvis after abdominoperineal excision.* Colorectal Dis.; 11, 806-816, 2009

Park JY., Choi HJ et al. *The role of pelvic exenteration and reconstruction for treatment of advanced or recurrent gynaecologic malignancies: analysis of risk factor predicting recurrence and survival.* J.Surg. Oncol.; 96, 560-568,2007

Pless TK., Pless JE. *Giant ventral hernia's and their repair. A 10 year follow-up study.* Scand.HJ.Plast. Reconst.Surg.Hand.Surg.; 27:311,1993

Posh NA., Mureau MA., Flood SJ, Hofer SO. *The combined free partial vastus lateralis with anterolateral thigh flap reconstruction of extensive composite defects.*Br.J.Plast.Surg. 58: 1095-1103,2005

Pusic AL., Mehrara BJ. *Vaginal reconstruction: an algorithm approach to deect classification and flap reconstruction.* J. Surg. Oncol.; 94: 515-521, 2006

Ramirez OM., Ruas E., Dellon AL: *Component separation method for closure of abdominal wall defects: an anatomic and clinical study.* Plast.Reconstr.Surg.; 86:519,1990

Reddy VR., Stevenson TR, Whetzel TP. *A 10-year experience with the gracilis myofasciocutaneous flap.* Plast.Reconstr. Surg.; 117: 635-639, 2006

Rohrich RJ., Lowe JB., Hackney FL., Bowman JL.,Hobar PC. *An algorithm for abdominal wall reconstruction.* Plast. Reconstr. Surg.105: 202-216,2000

Sasaki K., Nozaki M., Nakazawa H., Kikuchi Y.,Huang T. *Reconstruction of a large abdominal wall defect using a combined free tensor fascia lata musculocutaneous flap and anterolateral thigh flap.* Plast.Reconstr. Surg. 102: 2244-2252,1998

Shestaq KC., Edington HJD., Johnson RR. *The separation of anatomic components technique for the reconstruction of massive midline abdominal wall defects: anatomy,surgical technique, applications and limitations revisited.* Plast. Reconstr. Surg. 105: 731-38,2000

Taylor GI, Corlett R., Boyd JB. *The extended deep inferior epigastric flap: a clinical technique.* Plast.Reconstr.Surg. 72:751-765, 1983.

Tobin GR, Day TG. *Vaginal and pelvic reconstruction with distally based rectus abdominis myocutaneous flaps.* Plast.Reconstr.Surg.; 81: 62-73, 1988

Tsuji N., Suga H., Uda K., et al. *Functional evaluation of anterolateral thigh flap donor sites: isokinetic torque comparisons for knee function.* Microsurgery 28: 233-7,2008

Villa M., Saint-Cyr M., Wong C., Butler CE. *Extended vertical rectus abdominis myocutaneous flap for perlvic reconstruction: three-dimensional and four-diensional computed tomography angiographic perfusion study and clonical outcome analysis.*Plast. Reconstr. Surg. 127:200, 2011

Vranckx J.J., Veys B., D'Hoore A., Joniau S.,Nanhekhan L., Fabré G., Segers K., Van Brussel M., Vandevoort M., *Reconstruction of perineum after extended APRA and infralevatoric pelvic exenteration.* Proceedings WSRM2011, World Society of Reconstructive Microsurgery,pp. 59-64, ISBN 978-88-7587-612-8, Helsinki(Finland), June 29-July 2, 2011

Vranckx JJ., Miserez M., D'Hoore A., Nanhekhan L., SegersK., Fabré G., Vandevoort M. *Dynamic reconstruction of full thickness abdominal wall defects by innervated musculocutaneous flaps from the anterolateral thigh.* Proceedings WSRM2011, World Society of Reconstructive Microsurgery,pp. 65-69, ISBN 978-88-7587-612-8, Helsinki(Finland), June 29-July 2, 2011

Wagstaff MJD., Rozen WM et al. *Perineal and posterior vaginal wall reconstruction with superior and inferior gluteal artery perforator flaps.* Microsurgery; 29: 626-629, 2009

Wei FC., Jain V., Celik N., et al. *Have we found an ideal soft-tissue flap? An experience with 672 anterolateral thigh flaps.* Plast.Reconstr. Surg. 109: 2219-2226,2002

Whetzel TP., Lechtman AN. *The gracilis myofasciocutaneous flap: vascular anatomy and clinical application.* PLAst.Reconstr. Surg.; 99: 1642-1652, 1997

Williams JK., carlson GW.,de Chalain T., Howell R., Coleman JJ. *Role of the tensor fascia latae in abdominal wall reconstruction.*Plast.Reconstr.Surg.101:713-8,1998

Yu P., Sanger JR.,Matloub HS.,Gosain A., Larson D. *Anterolateral thigh fasciocutaneous island flaps in perineoscrotal reconstruction.* Plast.Reconstr.Surg. 109; 610-6,2002

7

Consequences of Radiotherapy for Breast Reconstruction

Nicola S. Russell, Marion Scharpfenecker,
Saske Hoving and Leonie A.E. Woerdeman
The Netherlands Cancer Institute – Antoni van Leeuwenhoek Hospital, Amsterdam
The Netherlands

1. Introduction

What is the problem? The late effects of radiotherapy, which manifest from six months onwards, can have long-lasting and generally progressive and irreversible effects on normal tissues. In this chapter we will discuss the clinical effects of radiotherapy on breast reconstruction, but many of the aspects will also be relevant for other areas of reconstructive surgery for cancer. A literature review has been performed to determine the clinical impact of radiotherapy on breast reconstruction following mastectomy for breast cancer. The evidence base for clinical decision-making regarding the best scheduling of treatments and reconstruction technique will be examined. To explain the long term effects of radiotherapy on normal tissues, the underlying biological processes that radiation induces will be discussed, on the basis of our pre-clinical and translational research in this area. In particular, the effects on blood vessels and lymph vessels, inflammation and fibrosis will be highlighted, as these are relevant to reconstructive surgery following radiotherapy. Biological intervention strategies for future research to minimize the negative effects of radiotherapy on normal tissues will be described.

2. Impact of radiotherapy on clinical outcome in reconstructive surgery

In this section we describe the results of a literature search performed through Medline and by following up on studies listed in the reference section of published papers. This is therefore not a complete review on all available studies on the subject. However, we have tried to focus on the current knowledge pertaining to the indications for breast reconstruction and radiotherapy in breast cancer patients following mastectomy, and the issues involved when the two treatments are combined.

2.1 For which patients is radiotherapy and breast reconstruction an issue?

Despite of the fact that many breast cancer treatment guidelines state that reconstruction should be discussed with patients before undergoing mastectomy (for example the early breast cancer treatment guidance: UK National Institute for Clinical Excellence NICE guidelines 2009; Dutch national guidelines 2011), often only a minority of mastectomy patients undergo the procedure. From our own experience, we know that in the

Netherlands, about 25% of patients treated in a specialized cancer centre undergo a breast reconstruction, whereas this figure is below 10% in patients treated in general hospitals. In Denmark, Hvilsom et al. (2011a) investigated the socioeconomic factors that influence the likelihood of undergoing an immediate or delayed breast reconstruction after mastectomy. Overall, 14% of patients had undergone a reconstruction. They found that the offer of breast reconstruction was unequally distributed, and living in an area where the hospital has a plastic surgery department significantly increased the odds of undergoing a reconstruction. In younger patients up to 45 years of age, educational level had no influence on the chances of reconstruction, but at older ages the longer the education, the higher the chances of reconstruction. Alderman et al. (2008) have assessed the impact of discussion of breast reconstruction with patients by their surgeon on the decision-making process for their cancer in 1844 respondents in the USA, and found a similar pattern to that seen in Europe. Only 33% of patients had discussed the possibility of reconstruction with their general surgeon. Most patients were aware of breast reconstruction, but choose not to undergo the procedure. Many patients had limited knowledge of the procedure and a negative perception of what it entailed. This was related to ethnic background and educational level. Also, the uptake of delayed reconstruction is often low due to lack of information regarding the procedure and concerns about safety (Alderman et al. 2011).

2.2 Indications for breast reconstruction

Studies have suggested that breast reconstruction following mastectomy can have a positive effect on well-being and revalidation, although this has not been demonstrated in all studies, and most are small, single institution retrospective assessments that are therefore liable to bias. For example, Rowland et al. (2000) reported that women with a breast reconstruction had a higher rate of dissatisfaction with their sexual functioning compared to women after breast conserving therapy or mastectomy without reconstruction. Harcourt et al. (2003) performed a prospective multicentre study with 103 women to assess women's decision making for or against reconstruction. Their results showed that women report improved psychological distress functioning in the year following their breast cancer surgery, whether this was mastectomy alone, or with immediate or a delayed reconstruction. However, they also reported that women were conscious of an altered body image at one year post-operatively irrespective of whether they had a reconstruction or not. They concluded that breast reconstruction does not necessarily confer psychological benefits compared to mastectomy alone. In contrast, Al-Ghazal et al. (2000a) retrospectively assessed psychological morbidity and satisfaction of cosmetic outcome in patients who had been treated with breast conserving therapy, mastectomy or mastectomy with reconstruction. Although the greatest morbidity was observed in the mastectomy group, this was less in the reconstruction group, with the best results for the breast conservation group.

There is also some evidence from retrospective studies that a direct or immediate reconstruction is preferable to a secondary or delayed reconstruction (Al-Ghazal et al. 2000b; Fernandez-Delgado et al. 2008). Metcalfe et al. (2011) performed a prospective study in 190 women with questionnaires pre-operatively and at one year of follow-up. Women who were undergoing delayed breast reconstruction had significantly higher levels of body stigma, body concerns, and transparency than women who were undergoing mastectomy alone (i.e. without a reconstruction), or a mastectomy with an immediate reconstruction. Of these women, 158 (83.2%) completed the one year follow-up. There were, however, no significant differences in any of the psychosocial functioning scores between the three groups.

In a Cochrane database systematic review of immediate versus delayed reconstruction, D'Souza et al. (2011) identified only one randomized clinical trial on the subject, with 64 women, carried out from 1978-1980, i.e. more than 30 years ago (Dean et al. 1983). This study had methodological flaws and a high risk of bias. They concluded that there was some evidence that immediate reconstruction reduced the psychiatric morbidity at three months postoperative compared to delayed or no reconstruction.

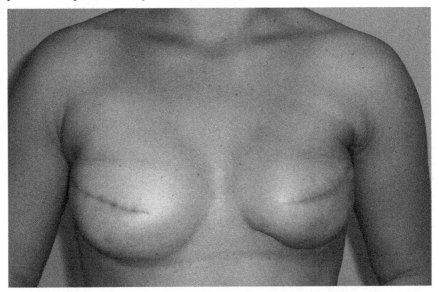

Fig. 1. Bilateral skin sparing mastectomy and immediate breast reconstruction; left sided irradiation post reconstruction showing retraction of the reconstruction compared to the unirradiated right side.

2.3 Oncological safety of breast reconstruction

There are concerns that patients may have a potentially higher risk of local recurrence after a skin-sparing mastectomy compared to a modified radical mastectomy. In one retrospective study of 133 cases with a median follow-up of at least five years, the local recurrence rate was higher in the subcutaneous mastectomy group, but the survival was not significantly different (Horiguchi et al. 2001). In contrast, Carlson et al. (2001) reported that immediate reconstruction with an implant had a higher local control rate than reconstruction with autologous tissue. However, these results were not confirmed in other studies. Nedumpara et al. (2011) reported on a series of 691 consecutive patients undergoing mastectomy, of whom 136 (20%) underwent immediate breast reconstruction (either with latissimus dorsi flap or subpectoral implant). The median follow-up was 55 months. For the whole group or within prognostic categories, they found no differences in local recurrence, distant metastases or survival between the group treated with mastectomy alone and the group with direct reconstruction. Lanitis et al. (2010) performed a meta-analysis of nine observational studies in which skin-sparing mastectomy was compared to non skin-sparing mastectomy. The local recurrence rate was reported in seven of these trials (including a total of 3436 patients) but there was no difference between the two types of mastectomy for this end-point. There is no evidence that the detection of recurrences or that the recurrence rate is affected by breast reconstruction (Gerber et al. 2009; Slavin & Goldwyn 1988). The indications for post mastectomy radiotherapy, or other adjuvant therapy, are therefore not influenced by whether a patient has had reconstructive surgery or not.

In conclusion, there is some evidence that an immediate breast reconstruction is to be preferred to a delayed reconstruction, and that this is safe from an oncologic perspective. However, most guidelines caution the use of immediate breast reconstruction if radiotherapy is scheduled, or if there is a high chance of an indication for radiotherapy, for reasons discussed below (breast cancer treatment guidance: UK NICE guidelines 2009; Dutch national guidelines 2011). Unfortunately, the radiotherapy indication is not always certain pre-operatively.

2.4 Indications for post-mastectomy radiotherapy

Post-mastectomy radiotherapy reduces the local recurrence rate and improves survival (Clarke et al. 2005; Kyndi et al. 2009; Overgaard et al. 2007; Ragaz et al. 2005). It is offered to high risk patients (stage III and IV) and to patients with intermediate risk (stage II) in selected cases, but practice varies widely (Marks et al. 2008). The role of post-mastectomy radiotherapy to the chest wall area in this group is the subject of an ongoing international clinical trial (Russell et al. 2009a) and translational research (Cheng et al. 2006a; Cheng et al. 2006b). For the patient group with intermediate stage disease there is often uncertainty pre-operatively whether radiotherapy will be indicated. Often the pathological nodal status is an important determinant, and this is only certain after histological examination of the operation specimen has been performed (Vinh-Hung et al. 2009). This makes decision making regarding performing an immediate reconstruction difficult. From published reports of clinical studies, it is clear that radiotherapy has a negative effect on the results of reconstructive surgery, and is a risk factor for a worse cosmetic result, as discussed below.

2.5 Implant based versus autologous reconstruction and radiotherapy

When reviewing the literature regarding radiation effects on breast reconstructions, it is important to bear in mind the limitations of the studies reported, especially the reporting of complications. Many studies are inconsistent in the definitions of complications or adverse outcomes, details on follow-up duration, and risk factors (Potter et al. 2011). In particular, the follow-up duration is relevant for radiotherapy effects, as these are progressive at later time points (Turesson 1989). A selection of the larger published studies is discussed below.

Some authors report very poor outcomes for breast reconstruction after radiotherapy. Jhaveri et al. (2008) have retrospectively assessed complications and cosmetic outcome of implant-based versus autologous immediate reconstruction in 92 patients who subsequently underwent radiotherapy. The median follow-up was 38 months. The rate of severe complications (IV antibiotics, surgical intervention, removal or replacement of the reconstruction) was 33.3% in the implant group versus 0% in the autologous group, a highly significant difference. An acceptable cosmetic outcome was obtained in 51% of the patients in the implant group.

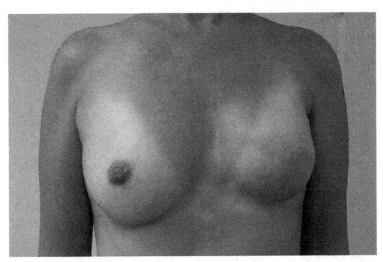

Fig. 2. Left-sideds skin sparing mastectomy and direct reconstruction with implant followed by irradiation. Right breast untreated.

Chawla et al. (2002) reported on a series of 48 patients who were treated with radiotherapy and reconstruction. The two year complication rate was much higher in the implant reconstruction group (53%) compared to the TRAM (transverse rectus abdominis musculocutaneous) reconstruction group (12%). No other factors were predictive.

Kronowitz & Robb (2009) have performed an extensive literature review of radiation therapy and breast reconstruction. For immediate reconstruction with an implant, they concluded that radiotherapy is associated with a 40% complication rate and capsular contracture and 15% extrusion rate of the implant. Also reconstructions with autologous tissue were found to have an increased rate of fibrosis and contracture if radiation is delivered to the reconstruction site after the reconstruction (figures 1-4).

Hvilsom et al. (2011b) have reported on the results of implant-based reconstruction for breast cancer from a prospective database registry of plastic surgery between 1999 and 2006. The study concerned the risks of capsular contracture and re-operation for 717 patients undergoing one-stage or two-stage delayed breast reconstructions with implants, but without autologous tissue. They found that radiotherapy was associated with a significantly increased risk of capsular contracture. The adjusted hazard ratio for capsular contracture with a one-stage procedure (performed with expandable implants) was 3.3 (95% confidence interval: 0.9 - 12.4) with a ten year risk of 20.5% in the radiotherapy group versus 7.0% in the unirradiated group. With a two-stage procedure (with temporary expanders followed by a scheduled second implant exchange) the adjusted hazard ratio was even higher at 7.2 % (95% confidence interval: 2.4 - 21.4), with ten year risks of 17.1% versus 8.2%. Not surprisingly, patients who received radiotherapy were also more likely to have nodal metastases and chemotherapy compared to patients without radiotherapy. There was a non-significant increase in re-operation rate in the irradiated patients. The majority of severe capsular contractures and re-operations occurred in the first two years, regardless of whether radiotherapy was given or not. This is somewhat intriguing, considering the continuing long-term development of fibrosis following radiotherapy, as discussed later in this chapter.

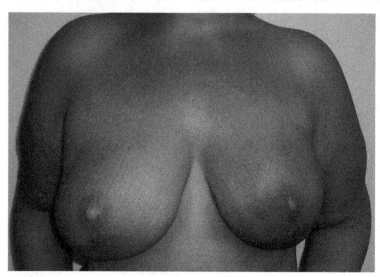

Fig. 3. Bilateral DIEP reconstruction, followed by radiotherapy to the left side. Note the volume loss on the left side (after 3 years follow-up). There was also some fat necrosis in both DIEP flaps, more extensive on the left side.

In contrast, other authors report generally satisfactory results for patients undergoing breast reconstruction and radiotherapy. Cordeiro et al. (2004) reported on a retrospective study of immediate breast reconstruction with a tissue expander and a permanent implant before starting post-operative radiotherapy. Sixty-eight of 687 patients received radiotherapy, with a mean follow-up of 34 months and they were compared to 75 unirradiated patients. Although 68% of the irradiated patients developed capsular contracture, compared to 40% in the unirradiated group, 80% of the irradiated group had acceptable (good to excellent) aesthetic results, compared to 88% of the unirradiated group, a non-significant difference. Patient satisfaction with the reconstruction was 67% in the irradiated group compared to 88% in the unirradiated group. They concluded that implant reconstruction should be considered for patients undergoing postoperative radiotherapy, especially those who may not be candidates for autologous reconstruction. Behranwala et al. (2006) assessed capsular contracture, cosmesis and symmetry at four years after implant-based reconstruction in 114 patients of whom 44 were also treated with radiotherapy. The incidence of capsule formation was 39% in the irradiated group compared to only 14% in the unirradiated group. Capsular contraction was associated with worse scores for symmetry, photographic assessments, and pain. They concluded however that although the chances of capsular contraction were three times higher in the radiotherapy group, 60% of patients do not get capsule formation four years after radiotherapy, and so this should be considered a viable option for breast reconstruction in selected cases.

Krueger et al. (2001) compared the complication risk and failure rate of implant/expander reconstruction in nineteen patients with radiotherapy with those of 62 patients without radiotherapy. With a median follow-up of 31 months, complications occurred in thirteen of the irradiated patients (68%) compared to 19 of the unirradiated patients (31%). Reconstruction failure was experienced by twelve patients in the whole group (15%) and was significantly related to experiencing a complication and to radiotherapy. Interestingly, they also performed a satisfaction study amongst the patients in the study with a seven point questionnaire and a five point Likert scale. Sixty-six patients completed the survey. A lower percentage of patients (10%) reported satisfaction with the result if they experienced a reconstruction failure compared to 23% of patients expressing satisfaction if the reconstruction was successful. Tamoxifen use was associated with a decreased esthetic satisfaction, but rather unexpectedly radiotherapy was not. Although this was a relatively small study, the results suggest that if patients have a successful reconstruction with an implant technique, radiotherapy does not adversely affect their satisfaction, if they are well informed about the possible disadvantages.

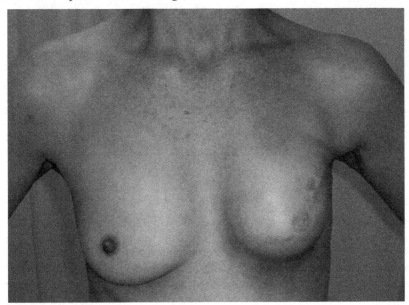

Fig. 4. Skin–sparing mastectomy with implant followed by chest wall irradiation on the left side.

Hussien et al. (2004) performed a retrospective audit over a time period in which the use of adjuvant post-mastectomy radiotherapy increased. They noted an increased tendency to the use of autologous tissue reconstruction in the more recently treated cohort, ascribed to better preoperative prediction of which patients have a radiotherapy indication postoperatively. Autologous tissue reconstruction seems to produce better results in patients who require radiation (figures 5 and 6). In one series there was an increased complication rate and slightly poorer but acceptable cosmetic outcome if radiotherapy was given prior to the reconstruction (Kroll et al. 1994). However, in other series, minimal disadvantage was seen for radiotherapy in the results of autologous reconstructions whether they were with a free-flap or pedicled technique (Slavin & Goldwyn 1988; Williams et al. 1995). Williams et al. (1995) reported on 108 patients who underwent TRAM reconstruction after radiotherapy. With this technique both the recipient bed and the vascular pedicle is included in the radiation field. They compared the irradiated patients to 572 patients who had not been irradiated. Overall there were comparable complication rates; fat necrosis (17% versus 10%) was the only outcome that was significantly worse result after irradiation (figure 3). Obesity was also associated with higher rates of fat necrosis. Another series (Soong et al. 2004) also reported good tolerance of post-mastectomy radiotherapy after autologous reconstruction, without any flap necrosis or flap loss, with 85% of the patients rating the cosmesis as good to excellent.

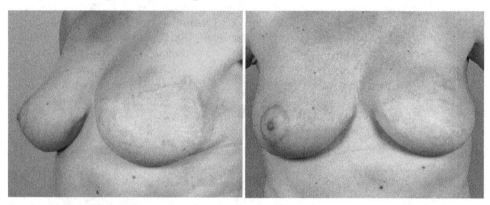

Fig. 5. Results of deep inferior epigastric perforator (DIEP) free-flap reconstruction after chest wall radiotherapy to the left side. On the right side a reduction mammoplasty has been performed.

2.6 Sequencing of reconstruction and radiotherapy

Whether the timing of radiotherapy delivery before or after implant reconstruction influences the complication rate has been investigated by Javaid et al. (2006) who performed a systematic review of published studies including at least 20 patients. There were no randomized trials on the topic identified. Four studies directly compared the results of reconstruction performed before or after radiotherapy, and two of these reported worse outcomes associated with post-reconstruction radiotherapy. Anderson et al. (2009) could not find significant differences in complication rate for patients irradiated after permanent implant reconstruction compared to patients irradiated with a temporary tissue expander, followed by insertion of the permanent implant. For both groups the complication rate was low. There was a slight increase in expander loss compared to permanent implant loss, and slightly better cosmetic outcome in the expander group (excellent / good in 90% versus 80% in the permanent implant group), but both comparisons were non-significant. The same group also reported low complication rates for radiotherapy after reconstruction, whether this was with implant or autologous techniques. The five year major complication rate, defined as requiring corrective surgery or loss of the reconstruction, was 0% in the TRAM group, compared to 5% in the implant group. The sequencing of radiotherapy and reconstruction was not a significant factor influencing the complication rate, nor was the type of reconstruction or other patient-related factors. The only factor that influenced the complication rate was the use of customized bolus material for the radiotherapy treatment. However, due to the long-term effects of radiation on tissue, in particular on connective tissue and microvasculature, it is unlikely that the timing of the radiotherapy in relation to the reconstructive surgery will have much impact on the fibrosis risk or implant loss, as discussed later on in this chapter. For patients undergoing reconstruction with a flap technique, there is some evidence that the results are impaired if radiation is given following the reconstruction due to fibrosis and contracture of the tissue. Thus, waiting until after radiotherapy has been completed before performing a flap-based reconstruction would have a logical preference. This is despite the fact that patients therefore have to undergo a delayed reconstruction (figures 3, 5 and 6).

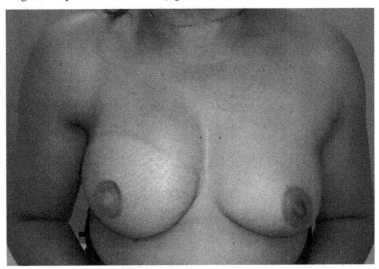

Fig. 6. DIEP free-flap reconstruction on the right side following radiotherapy to the right chest wall.

Performing a free flap-based reconstruction in a previously irradiated area may help improve perfusion and lymphatic drainage (Chang & Kim 2010) (figure 7). Tran et al. (2001) assessed two cohorts of patients after TRAM flap reconstruction performed over a ten year period. Early and late complications were compared. There was no difference in the early complication rate, but there was a great increase in the late complication rate in the immediate reconstruction group compared to the delayed reconstruction group (87% versus 9%). Twenty-eight percent of the immediate reconstruction group required additional surgery to correct for distortion due to flap shrinkage. In contrast, Zimmerman et al. (1998) assessed the results of immediate TRAM flap reconstruction followed by radiation therapy in 21 patients. Most patients thought that there was no effect on cosmetic outcome from the radiotherapy, and a few patients even thought that it was improved due to the radiation. Williams et al. (1997) compared the results of radiation given before or after TRAM flap reconstruction. They concluded that the timing of the radiotherapy did not influence the rate of complications, only the type of complication: fibrosis if radiation was given after the reconstruction, and fat necrosis if radiation was given beforehand. Gill et al. (2004) have presented the ten-year retrospective results of 758 DIEP (deep inferior epigastric perforator) flap breast reconstructions. In their analysis of risk factors for complications, post-reconstruction radiotherapy had the highest odds ratio of 5.40 (CI 2.95-9.92) and level of significance, the only other significant factors were current smoking (odds ratio = 2.24) and hypertension (odds ratio = 1.60). Pre-reconstruction radiotherapy and other factors consisting of age over 60 years, chemotherapy, diabetes mellitus, obesity, abdominal scar and two venous anastomoses were not associated with an increased odds ratio for complications. The specific complications associated with post reconstruction radiotherapy were fat necrosis and partial flap loss.

2.7 Strategies to avoid problems when radiotherapy and breast reconstruction are combined

To reduce the risk of complications after breast reconstruction when there is also an indication for radiotherapy the following strategy can be applied. First, a good prediction is needed of which patients require radiotherapy. This cannot be defined with certainty in some patients with intermediate risk breast cancer. Better determination of which patients with intermediate risk breast cancer will benefit from radiotherapy is currently the subject of an international, randomized clinical trial (Russell et al. 2009a). There is some evidence that patients who require radiation have fewer complications if reconstruction is performed with autologous tissue after radiotherapy rather than with an implant alone, and if the radiotherapy is completed before the reconstruction (Woerdeman et al. 2004, 2006) (figures 5-8). Also, careful attention to radiotherapy technique can help to improve the dose distribution and cause less side effects (Anderson et al. 2004). Furthermore, breast reconstruction performed after radiotherapy can also help to reduce radiotherapy side effects such as lymph oedema (Chang & Kim 2010) (figure 7).

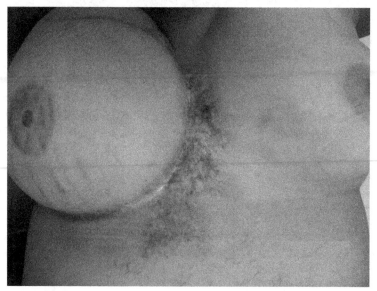

Fig. 7. DIEP reconstruction after radiotherapy. Note the extensive telangiectasia and fibrosis in the radiation field to the internal mammary chain nodes.

3. Late biological effects of radiation on normal tissues

Radiotherapy can affect normal tissues at very long time intervals after the initial treatment. This can cause increased morbidity and mortality, especially cardiovascular morbidity and secondary tumour induction, also in breast cancer patients (Darby et al. 2005; Giordano et al. 2005; Patt et al. 2005; Roychouduri et al. 2007). However, these serious effects occur in only a small proportion of patients. There are also less serious effects of radiotherapy that affect a greater proportion of patients and include tissue changes such as fibrosis, oedema and microvascular changes, which can negatively impact on (plastic) surgery and reconstruction, as discussed above. To explain the sometimes very long latency - spanning months to decades - of the normal tissue effects of radiotherapy one has to diverge from the paradigm that radiation only affects cells at the level of DNA damage at the time of radiation. There is increasing evidence for long-term changes in the micro-environment and cell-cell interactions in irradiated tissues. Biological responses to irradiation evolve and amplify, mostly in a non-linear fashion, altering cell differentiation and senescence, and inducing cytokine signals that affect unirradiated cells or generate a state of chronic genomic instability. The sum of these events, occurring in different organs and tissues, is highly modulated by genotype, and predicates the health risks. The non-mutagenic effects of radiation on stroma and tissues contributes significantly to the late clinical consequences of radiotherapy, long after the patient has been cured of the original cancer for which they were treated. This includes fibrosis and late vascular damage, but also contributes to the development of radiation-induced cancer (Barcellos-Hoff 2010). These late changes due to radiotherapy are subject to wide inter-individual variation, depending on genetic differences, but also other treatments and co-morbidities (Safwat et al. 2002). Some of the individual components of late normal tissue effects of radiotherapy relevant for the plastic surgeon are discussed below.

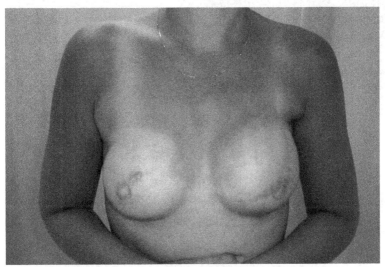

Fig. 8. Skin sparing mastectomy with implant on the right and reconstruction with implant and thoracodorsalis pedicled lap after radiotherapy on the left. No radiotherapy given on the right side.

3.1 Radiation-induced fibrosis

The fibroblast is the main target cell responsible for the fibrotic response after radiation exposure. Fibroblasts which survive the cell killing effects of radiation, undergo an accelerated ripening and differentiation. The differentiated fibroblasts are post-mitotic and thus unable to divide (Herskind et al. 1998a; Akudugu et al. 2006, 78:17-26); Herskind et al. 2000; Russell et al. 2000) (figure 9). This has consequences for wound healing after surgical procedures, as active fibroblast differentiation is required for successful wound healing (Akudugu et al. 2006).

Mature, post-mitotic fibroblasts have large nuclei and cytoplasmic compartments, and are capable of producing large amounts of collagen fibers. The increase in collagen production shows a dose response relationship in that the higher the radiation dose, the more collagen production is observed (Lara et al. 1996). *Ex-vivo* studies of primary fibroblast cultures have shown that there is a wide inter-patient variation in the response of fibroblasts to irradiation; both in the intrinsic cellular radiosensitivity (cell killing) as in the degree of induction of terminal differentiation (Herskind et al. 1998a; Herskind et al. 2000; Johansen et al. 1994; Lara et al. 1996).

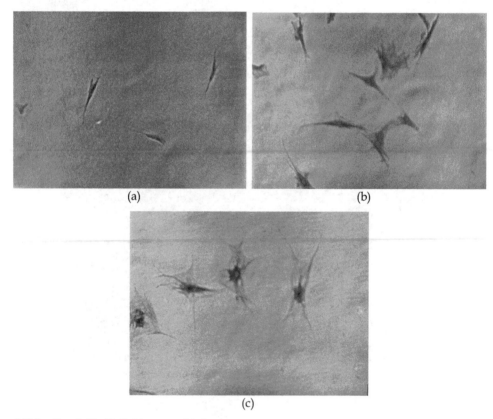

(a)   (b)

(c)

a) Unirradiated: 30 - 50 divisions possible *in vitro*.
b) After *in vitro* irradiation: 2-3 divisions possible.
c) Two weeks after 2 Gy *in vitro* irradiation: post-mitotic differentiation.

Fig. 9. Fibroblasts derived from unirradiated skin of breast cancer patients in primary tissue culture.

This is also reflected by clinical observation: for a standard radiation dose there is a large variation in the degree of fibrosis development observed between different patients after radiation treatment for breast cancer, both after breast conserving treatment and after mastectomy (Bentzen et al. 1989; Bentzen et al. 1993; Borger et al. 1994; Collette et al. 2008) (figure 10). This inter-individual difference remains even after all known technical and clinical factors which can affect fibrosis development are taken into account (Borger 1994). However, it has not as yet proved feasible to predict the degree of fibrosis developing in individual patients on the basis of biological parameters such as intrinsic fibroblast radiosensitivity or radiation-induced fibroblast differentiation *in vitro* (Russell et al. 1998, 2000, 2002, Peacock et al. 2000).

Radiation causes a massive increase in the production, activation, and signaling of the cytokine transforming growth factor-beta (TGF-β) (Rube et al. 2000). The effects of TGF-β on fibroblasts have been studied *in vitro* and *in vivo* (Illsley et al. 2000*)*. It is postulated that these differences in radiation response may be at least in part due to genetic variations in genes regulating TGF-β production or signaling. For example, specific Single Nucleotide Polymorphisms (SNPs) have been associated with increased risk of radiation induced-fibrosis in some studies, although this has not been confirmed in larger series (Andreassen et al. 2005; Andreassen & Alsner 2009). Interfering with TGF-β signalling reduces the degree of radiation-induced fibrosis *in mice* (Scharpfenecker et al. 2009) and may be a therapeutic intervention in the future which could be applied to radiation-induced fibrosis, but this research is as yet in a very preliminary stage.

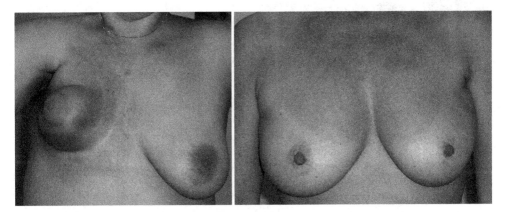

Fig. 10. Clinically there is wide variation in the degrees of fibrosis development, here after breast conserving therapy. Left: Extreme fibrosis 2 years following treatment; right clinically no fibrosis ten years after treatment of the left breast.

The variation between patients in the fibrotic response to radiation also impacts on the results of breast reconstruction, especially in the degree of capsule contracture with implant-based reconstructions. The biological differences between patients in the degree of fibrosis development after irradiation can explain why there are such wide estimates for the rate of clinically relevant capsule contracture seen with implant-based reconstructions reported in the literature, as discussed in section 2.

3.2 Radiation-induced microvascular damage

Vascular injury is a major cause of late radiation morbidity developing slowly and progressively over many years. Vascular lesions manifest in microvessels as telangiectasia which are characterised as dilated, tortuous and thin-walled blood vessels. Telangiectasia develop in skin, mucous membranes and also internal organs. In skin, telangiectasia appear after radiotherapy for breast cancer in 80% of the patients, but only become clinically apparent after several months to years following the radiation treatment with a mean latency of 4.7 years, and with a considerable inter-patient variation in the rate of onset and extent. For all patients, the levels increase with increasing follow-up time (Tucker et al. 1992; Turesson 1989; Turesson 1990). Skin telangiectasia may be dismissed as only having cosmetic consequences; yet they are a cause of dissatisfaction, especially if located in the décolleté, or neck (figure 11).

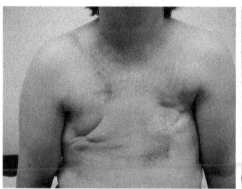 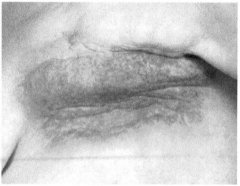

Left: telangiectasia of the skin following irradiation to the periclavicular area.
Right: telangiectaia following chest wall irradiation. Note also the increase in fibrosis.

Fig. 11. Clinical appearance of microvascular damage in the skin.

Further, radiation-induced damage in the skin may contribute to graft failure after free-flap reconstructive surgery because of impaired perfusion of the tissue. Also, telangiectatic lymph vessels cause lymph oedema and affect quality of life. Perturbations of the lymphatic network after irradiation are illustrated by the finding of altered lymph drainage patterns on sentinel node procedure performed for breast cancer that develops secondary to irradiation for Hodgkin's lymphoma up to decades earlier (van der Ploeg et al. 2009) (figure 12).

As with the development of fibrosis, TGF-β signalling (in concert with other growth factors) also plays an important role in the development of telangiectasia and the recovery of the microvasculature following radiation (Herskind et al. 1998b; Kruse et al. 2009). The importance of properly regulated TGF-β signaling in sustaining normal homeostasis of the microvasculature is illustrated by patients with the syndrome hereditary hemorrhagic telangiectasia (HHT). HHT patients have a mutation in either the TGF-β receptor called Activin receptor–like kinase-1 (ALK-1) or the accessory receptor endoglin (Jacobson 2000). HHT patients develop telangiectasia of the skin, or internal organs probably precipitated by trauma. This can lead to severe blood loss from mucous membranes, for example from nose bleeds. However, recovery of endothelial cell damage after irradiation is different to that after other types of trauma, because of the sustained increase in TGF-β levels in the irradiated tissue over many months and years following irradiation (Ehrhart et al. 1997).

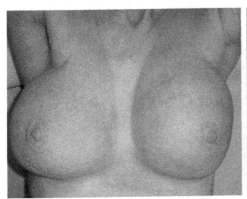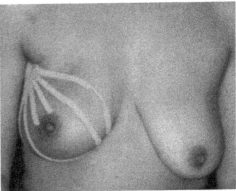

Fig. 12. Left: lympho-vascular damage causing chronic lymph oedema of the breasts after bilateral irradiation; right: kinesiotaping for lymphoedema of the right breast after breast conserving therapy.

Preclinical studies in the mouse kidney (chosen as a model as it is rich in microvessels) have shown that ALK-1 and endoglin are upregulated after irradiation (Scharpfenecker et al. 2009). This is accompanied by increased telangiectasia formation and fibrosis development. Accordingly, in skin punch biopsies taken from irradiated breast cancer patients, an increase in endoglin RNA was observed in the irradiated skin with macroscopically visible telangiectasia compared to non-irradiated skin from a contralateral site (unpublished data). Paradoxically, reduced receptor levels in heterozygous mice (that serve as a model for the human HHT syndrome) seem to protect from development of late normal tissue damage, as fibrosis and telangiectasia development are delayed in these mice after kidney irradiation. The mechanism of how the two TGF-β receptors modulate repair after irradiation is not clear, but our data suggest that they regulate the expression of vascular endothelial growth factor (VEGF), which is crucial for endothelial cell survival and repair.

In pre-clinical murine models, we have observed that the development of telangiectasia (after a lag period of several months following the radiation treatment) is associated with an inflammatory cell infiltrate, composed predominantly of macrophages.

Macrophages may contribute to the development of normal tissue damage, especially fibrosis, but also to vascular damage, by producing excessive amounts of cytokines and pro-fibrotic factors thereby preventing proper repair of the damaged tissue. Studies in our pre-clinical murine system suggest that both endoglin and ALK-1 regulate the secretion of some of these pro-inflammatory / pro-fibrotic factors, thereby modulating tissue repair (Scharpfenecker et al. 2011).

In another study performed by our group, biopsies from irradiated and unirradiated skin taken from cancer patients undergoing plastic surgical reconstructions were analysed by immunohistochemistry. The number of lymphatic vessels was increased in 67% of the irradiated biopsies (unpublished data, figure 13). Irradiated biopsies also contained significantly more macrophages than the respective non-irradiated controls (unpublished data, figure 14). Seventy-five percent of the patients with increased lymphatic score also displayed an increase in macrophage numbers.

Inhibition of the release of mononuclear cells from the bone marrow is a strategy currently under investigation to prevent tumour re-growth following radiation, through inhibition of vasculogenesis (Ahn & Brown, 2009). We are currently conducting a clinical trial to investigate whether biphosphonate administration in breast cancer patients can reduce telangiectasia formation in the skin. Biphosphonates are frequently indicated in breast cancer patients to treat both osteoporosis resulting van endocrine therapy, and also for patients with osseous metastases to reduce the risk of fractures. They are also being investigated in trials as adjuvant treatment to improve the disease free survival. Biphosphonates are powerful inhibitors of metalloproteinase-9 (MMP-9), an enzyme that promotes the release of mononuclear cells from the bone marrow. In this way, biphosphonates might modulate monocyte infiltration into the irradiated tissue, thereby reducing late toxicity.

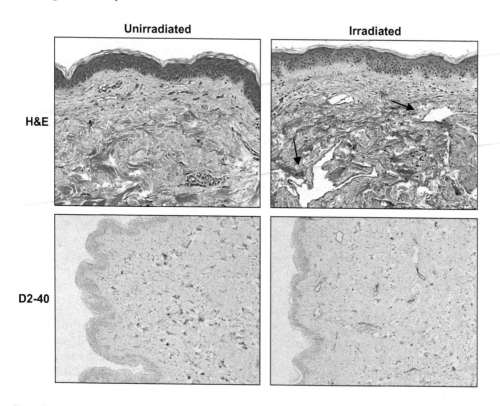

Fig. 13. Increase in the number and diameter of lymphatic vessels following irradiation. Upper panels: haematoxylin and eosin staining of histological sections of skin. Arrows show telangiectatic lymph vessels. Lower panels: brown D2-40 staining for lymphatic vessels.

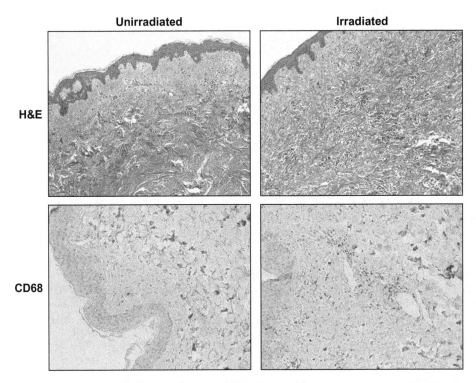

Fig. 14. Increase in macrophage infiltration in irradiated skin compared to non-irradiated skin. H&E: haematoxylin and Eosin; CD 68: immunohistochemical marker for macrophages (brown stain).

3.3 Changes to muscular arteries following radiation and atherosclerosis

Clinical studies have demonstrated and increased risk of atherosclerosis in the radiation field. For example in patients treated for head and neck cancer, there is an increased risk of ischemic stroke, and in patients receiving mediastinal irradiation an increase in coronary vascular disease and myocardial infarction (Aleman et al. 2003; Dorresteijn et al. 2002; Dorresteijn et al. 2005; Hooning et al. 2007). In a study performed on irradiated muscular arteries and control vessels in breast cancer patients and head and neck cancer patients undergoing free-flap reconstructive surgery, we observed an increase in the intima media thickness (IMT) in the irradiated vessels compared to the unirradiated vessels in the breast cancer patients. In the head and neck cancer patients we observed an increase in the glycoprotein content of media the irradiated vessels compared to the unirradiated control vessels (Russell et al. 2009b, figure 15). Although there was a significant increase in the IMT of the internal mammary arteries that had previously been irradiated, the absolute thickness was still very limited. This is compatible with the finding that the internal mammary arteries are rather resistant to developing atherosclerosis, (indeed they are the vessels of choice for coronary artery grafting), and to our knowledge, no reports of graft failure in breast reconstruction have been ascribed to atherosclerosis in the internal mammary artery.

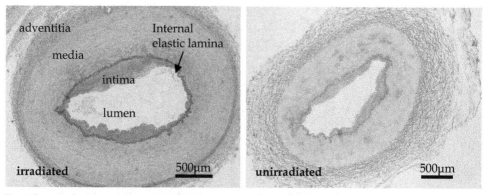

Fig. 15. Histological cross section of the irradiated facial artery of a patient with head and neck cancer undergoing free-flap reconstruction (left panel) showing increased intima thickness, compared to the radial artery of the same patient used as the donor vessel.

In animal models, radiation-induced atherosclerosis displays a more inflammatory and thrombosis-prone plaque phenotype compared to age or cholesterol-induced lesions. In addition, radiation-induced atherosclerosis is resistant to pharmacological interventions that reduce age-related atherosclerosis such as aspirin or statins (Stewart et al. 2006; Hoving et al. 2008, 2010 & 2011, manuscript submitted). There has been a report of atherosclerosis in donor vessels of free flaps precluding the use of the flap, but this was in a patient with head and neck cancer and not after radiation to the artery (de Bree et al. 2004).

3.4 Atrophy of skin and subcutaneous tissues following irradiation

Radiotherapy can also cause atrophy of tissues, which usually manifests over several years. This is due to cellular loss (mitotic death) caused directly by the irradiation, but also secondary to poor perfusion related to the vascular damage. Atrophy due to mitotic cells death manifests at a rate which is dependent on the normal cell turnover in an organ or tissue. In tissues with a slow natural turnover such as connective tissue, it may be months or years before a cell goes into mitosis after radiotherapy, only then does the DNA damage cause mitotic failure. Some cell types, such as fibroblasts can survive for decennia in a tissue after radiation (Peacock & Yarnold, personal communication) and remain metabolically active, for example in collagen production. However, a longer time points there is an increased chance that the cells will eventually go into apoptosis or a failed mitosis and die, causing atrophy of the tissue or organ, with functional or structural loss as a result. Thinning of the dermis layer of the skin after radiotherapy is well documented (Rezvani et al. 2000).

Atrophy of skin can cause thinning and discolouration over implants used for breast reconstruction (figures 16 and 17). Volume loss of breast tissue is commonly seen after breast conserving therapy, and can be attributed to a combination of atrophy, fibrotic contracture and fat necrosis (figure 18). If tissue atrophy becomes even more pronounced, then even necrotic tissue breakdown can occur, but this is luckily a quite rare and late event after radiotherapy. Extra stress on tissues due to a surgical intervention, anaemia or diabetes can precipitate the development of necrosis.

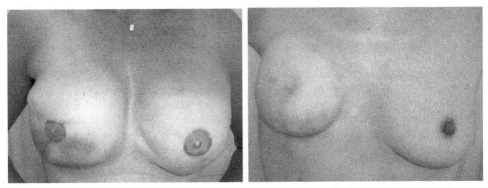

Fig. 16. Clinical manifestation of atrophy after radiotherapy: in both patients there is the appearance of atrophy of skin overlying an implant after irradiation to the right side.

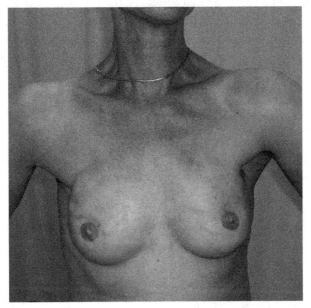

Fig. 17. Bilateral skin-sparing mastectomy 25 years after mantle field irradiation for Hodgkin lymphoma (radiation–induced breast cancer). Note muscle atrophy in neck and chest wall area.

4. Conclusions

Breast reconstruction and radiotherapy are two treatment modalities commonly employed to combat the health consequences of breast cancer; on one hand reducing the esthetic and psychological impact, and on the other hand reducing the risk of local recurrence and increasing survival. From our literature review, it is clear that clinicians have limited high level evidence on which to base clinical decisions regarding the optimal type and timing of reconstruction and radiotherapy. For this chapter, we have limited our review to the effects of radiotherapy on breast reconstruction. Aspects such as the impact of breast reconstruction on radiotherapy delivery, or the use of plastic surgical techniques to restore the contour of the breast after breast conserving therapy have not been considered. Due to the large variation in the quality of the studies published, and the use of non-standardized end-points and follow-up duration, the results should be interpreted with caution. Although general conclusions can be drawn, for example that radiotherapy increases the risk of fibrosis, it is unwise to quote an exact percentage when advising individual patients on the optimal treatment strategy. Not only are the results influenced by individual clinical and surgical factors, but there is a very wide variation in the rate and extent of the development of late radiotherapy effects, both between patients and even within individual patients depending on follow-up duration, radiation technique and scheduling, and other treatments, medication and co-morbidity. This is one of the reasons why series of treatment outcome reported in the literature can seem to have contradictory conclusions. It has not as yet proven possible to predict, on a biological basis, which patients are more predisposed to develop more extreme radiation-induced late effects than others.

We have examined the underlying radiobiological causes of the clinical manifestations of late radiation-induced changes in normal tissues. The most relevant effects for breast reconstruction are the increased development of fibrosis and the micro-vascular and micro-lymphovascular abnormalities, which in turn lead to secondary effects such as micro-thrombi, tissue hypoxia and necrosis. In the current context, fat necrosis is the most common problem. Necrosis of other tissue types solely due to radiotherapy is usually a very late event occurring several decades after the radiation exposure. The increased risk of atherosclerosis in muscular arteries following radiotherapy is not a clinical problem in the breast cancer population in as far as the effects on reconstructive surgery are concerned, although for other cancer patient groups, such as those with head and neck cancer, radiation accelerated atherosclerosis can impact reconstructive surgery, also because of the predisposition to vascular pathology due to other risk factors such as male sex and smoking in these patients.

Research by our group and others has shown that the late biological effects of radiation on connective tissue and vessels and other cells is not determined solely at the time of radiation exposure, but can be modulated by factors months or even years later. Late effects in normal tissues after irradiation are due to a gradual process of tissue modulation and repair and mis-repair that can result in pathological states such as fibrosis and telangiectasia. Cytokines such as TGF-β, VEGF, MMP-9 can all vary in levels and interactions over time, and this might be influenced by genetic variation between patients. Also, we have evidence that inflammatory cell infiltration in the irradiated area contributes to both the fibrotic response and telangiectasia formation.

For future research, it is exactly this continuing process of tissue changes following radiation that open up opportunities for therapeutic interventions. Modulating cytokines or inflammatory cell activity to reduce the development of fibrosis or micro-vascular damage, at time points long after the patient has been cured of the cancer for which she received the radiation is an attractive strategy. This is currently under investigation in early clinical trials, both by our group and others. By improving the therapeutic ratio of radiotherapy (increased cure but less side effects), the quality of skin and subcutaneous tissues should improve and aid plastic surgeons in achieving the optimal restorative results for their patients with breast cancer and other types of cancer.

5. Acknowledgements

We thank the Dutch Cancer Society KWF for financially supporting the original research described in this chapter (grants NKI-2005 3373; NKI 2005-3380 and NKI 2009-4480). We gratefully acknowledge Mrs. E. J. C. Luza-Helling for a generous personal donation. We thank Ms. Suzanne Bakker, Head of the Central Cancer Library at the Netherlands Cancer Institute for help with the literature search and references.

6. References

Ahn GO, and Brown JM. 2009. Influence of bone marrow-derived hematopoietic cells on the tumor response to radiotherapy: experimental models and clinical perspectives. *Cell Cycle* 8 (7): 970-976.

Akudugu JM, Bell RS, Catton C, Davis AM, Griffin AM, O'Sullivan B, Waldron JN, Ferguson PC, Wunder JS, and Hill RP. 2006. Wound healing morbidity in STS patients treated with preoperative radiotherapy in relation to in vitro skin fibroblast radiosensitivity, proliferative capacity and TGF-beta activity. *Radiotherapy and Oncology:* 78 (1): 17-26.

Al-Ghazal SK, Fallowfield L, and Blamey RW. 2000. Comparison of psychological aspects and patient satisfaction following breast conserving surgery, simple mastectomy and breast reconstruction. *Eur. J. Cancer* 36 (15): 1938-1943.

Al-Ghazal SK, Sully L, Fallowfield L, and Blamey RW. 2000. The psychological impact of immediate rather than delayed breast reconstruction. *Eur. J. Surg. Oncol.* 26 (1): 17-19.

Alderman AK, Hawley ST, Morrow M, Salem B, Hamilton A, Graff JJ, and Katz S. 2011. Receipt of delayed breast reconstruction after mastectomy: do women revisit the decision? *Ann. Surg. Oncol.* 18 (6): 1748-1756.

Alderman AK, Hawley ST, Waljee J, Mujahid M, Morrow M, and Katz SJ. 2008. Understanding the impact of breast reconstruction on the surgical decision-making process for breast cancer. *Cancer* 112 (3): 489-494.

Aleman BM, van den Belt-Dusebout AW, Klokman WJ, Van't Veer MB, Bartelink H, and van Leeuwen FE. 2003. Long-term cause-specific mortality of patients treated for Hodgkin's disease. *J. Clin. Oncol.* 21 (18): 3431-3439.

Anderson PR, Freedman G, Nicolaou N, Sharma N, Li T, Topham N, and Morrow M. 2009. Postmastectomy chest wall radiation to a temporary tissue expander or permanent breast implant--is there a difference in complication rates? *Int. J. Radiat. Oncol. Biol. Phys.* 74 (1): 81-85.

Anderson PR, Hanlon AL, Fowble BL, McNeeley SW, and Freedman GM. 2004. Low complication rates are achievable after postmastectomy breast reconstruction and radiation therapy. *Int. J. Radiat. Oncol. Biol. Phys.* 59 (4): 1080-1087.

Andreassen CN, Alsner J, Overgaard J, Herskind C, Haviland J, Owen R, Homewood J, Bliss J, and Yarnold J. 2005. TGFB1 polymorphisms are associated with risk of late normal tissue complications in the breast after radiotherapy for early breast cancer. *Radiotherapy and Oncology* 75 (1): 18-21.

Andreassen CN, and Alsner J. 2009. Genetic variants and normal tissue toxicity after radiotherapy: a systematic review. *Radiotherapy and Oncology* 92 (3): 299-309.

Barcellos-Hoff MH. 2010. Stromal mediation of radiation carcinogenesis. *J. Mammary. Gland. Biol. Neoplasia.* 15 (4): 381-387.

Behranwala KA, Dua RS, Ross GM, Ward A, A'hern R, and Gui GP. 2006. The influence of radiotherapy on capsule formation and aesthetic outcome after immediate breast reconstruction using biodimensional anatomical expander implants. *J. Plast. Reconstr. Aesthet. Surg.* 59 (10): 1043-1051.

Bentzen SM, Overgaard M, and Overgaard J. 1993. Clinical correlations between late normal tissue endpoints after radiotherapy: implications for predictive assays of radiosensitivity. *Eur. J. Cancer* 29A (10): 1373-1376.

Bentzen SM, Overgaard M, Thames HD, Christensen JJ, and Overgaard J. 1989. Early and late normal-tissue injury after postmastectomy radiotherapy alone or combined with chemotherapy. *Int. J. Radiat. Biol.* 56 (5): 711-715.

Borger JH, Kemperman H, Smitt HS, Hart A, van DJ, Lebesque J, and Bartelink H. 1994. Dose and volume effects on fibrosis after breast conservation therapy. *Int. J. Radiat. Oncol. Biol. Phys.* 30 (5): 1073-1081.

Breast cancer treatment guidance for the UK: national Institute for Clinical Excellence NICE. Available from: http://guidance.nice.org.uk/CG80/NICEGuidance/doc/English

Breast cancer treatment guidance for the Netherlands: Nationaal Borstkanker Overleg Nederland NABON / Comprehensive Cancer Center Netherlands IKNL. Available from:
http://www.oncoline.nl/uploaded/docs/mammacarcinoom/Richtlijn%20mamm acarcinoom_concept%202011.pdf

Carlson GW, Losken A, Moore B, Thornton J, Elliott M, Bolitho G, and Denson DD. 2001. Results of immediate breast reconstruction after skin-sparing mastectomy. *Ann. Plast. Surg.* 46 (3): 222-228.

Chang DW, and Kim S. 2010. Breast reconstruction and lymphedema. *Plast. Reconstr. Surg.* 125 (1): 19-23.

Chawla AK, Kachnic LA, Taghian AG, Niemierko A, Zapton DT, and Powell SN. 2002. Radiotherapy and breast reconstruction: complications and cosmesis with TRAM versus tissue expander/implant. *Int. J. Radiat. Oncol. Biol. Phys.* 54 (2): 520-526.

Cheng SH, Horng CF, Clarke JL, Tsou MH, Tsai SY, Chen CM, Jian JJ, Liu MC, West M, Huang AT, and Prosnitz LR. 2006. Prognostic index score and clinical prediction model of local regional recurrence after mastectomy in breast cancer patients. *Int. J. Radiat. Oncol. Biol. Phys.* 64 (5): 1401-1409.

Cheng SH, Horng CF, West M, Huang E, Pittman J, Tsou MH, Dressman H, Chen CM, Tsai SY, Jian JJ, Liu MC, Nevins JR, and Huang AT. 2006. Genomic prediction of locoregional recurrence after mastectomy in breast cancer. *J. Clin. Oncol.* 24 (28): 4594-4602.

Clarke M, Collins R, Darby S, Davies C, Elphinstone P, Evans E, Godwin J, Gray R, Hicks C, James S, MacKinnon E, McGale P, McHugh T, Peto R, Taylor C, and Wang Y. 2005.

Effects of radiotherapy and of differences in the extent of surgery for early breast cancer on local recurrence and 15-year survival: an overview of the randomised trials. *Lancet* 366 (9503): 2087-2106.

Collette S, Collette L, Budiharto T, Horiot JC, Poortmans PM, Struikmans H, Van Den BW, Fourquet A, Jager JJ, Hoogenraad W, Mueller RP, Kurtz J, Morgan DA, Dubois JB, Salamon E, Mirimanoff R, Bolla M, Van Der HM, Warlam-Rodenhuis CC, and Bartelink H. 2008. Predictors of the risk of fibrosis at 10 years after breast conserving therapy for early breast cancer: a study based on the EORTC Trial 22881-10882 'boost versus no boost'. *Eur. J. Cancer* 44 (17): 2587-2599.

Cordeiro PG, Pusic AL, Disa JJ, McCormick B, and VanZee K. 2004. Irradiation after immediate tissue expander/implant breast reconstruction: outcomes, complications, aesthetic results, and satisfaction among 156 patients. *Plast. Reconstr. Surg.* 113 (3): 877-881.

D'Souza N, Darmanin G, and Fedorowicz Z. 2011. Immediate versus delayed reconstruction following surgery for breast cancer. *Cochrane. Database. Syst. Rev.* 7: CD008674.

Darby SC, McGale P, Taylor CW, and Peto R. 2005. Long-term mortality from heart disease and lung cancer after radiotherapy for early breast cancer: prospective cohort study of about 300,000 women in US SEER cancer registries. *Lancet Oncol* 6 (8): 557-565.

de Bree R, Quak JJ, Kummer JA, Simsek S, and Leemans CR. 2004. Severe atherosclerosis of the radial artery in a free radial forearm flap precluding its use. *Oral Oncol.* 40 (1): 99-102.

Dean C, Chetty U, and Forrest AP. 1983. Effects of immediate breast reconstruction on psychosocial morbidity after mastectomy. *Lancet* 1 (8322): 459-462.

Dorresteijn LD, Kappelle AC, Boogerd W, Klokman WJ, Balm AJ, Keus RB, van Leeuwen FE, and Bartelink H. 2002. Increased risk of ischemic stroke after radiotherapy on the neck in patients younger than 60 years. *J. Clin. Oncol.* 20 (1): 282-288.

Dorresteijn LD, Kappelle AC, Scholz NM, Munneke M, Scholma JT, Balm AJ, Bartelink H, and Boogerd W. 2005. Increased carotid wall thickening after radiotherapy on the neck. *Eur. J. Cancer* 41 (7): 1026-1030.

Ehrhart EJ, Segarini P, Tsang ML, Carroll AG, and Barcellos-Hoff MH. 1997. Latent transforming growth factor beta1 activation in situ: quantitative and functional evidence after low-dose gamma-irradiation. *FASEB J.* 11 (12): 991-1002.

Fernandez-Delgado J, Lopez-Pedraza MJ, Blasco JA, ndradas-Aragones E, Sanchez-Mendez JI, Sordo-Miralles G, and Reza MM. 2008. Satisfaction with and psychological impact of immediate and deferred breast reconstruction. *Ann. Oncol.* 19 (8): 1430-1434.

Gerber B, Krause A, Dieterich M, Kundt G, and Reimer T. 2009. The oncological safety of skin sparing mastectomy with conservation of the nipple-areola complex and autologous reconstruction: an extended follow-up study. *Ann. Surg.* 249 (3): 461-468.

Gill PS, Hunt JP, Guerra AB, Dellacroce FJ, Sullivan SK, Boraski J, Metzinger SE, Dupin CL, and Allen RJ. 2004. A 10-year retrospective review of 758 DIEP flaps for breast reconstruction. *Plast. Reconstr. Surg.* 113 (4): 1153-1160.

Giordano SH, Kuo YF, Freeman JL, Buchholz TA, Hortobagyi GN, and Goodwin JS. 2005. Risk of cardiac death after adjuvant radiotherapy for breast cancer. *J. Natl. Cancer. Inst.* 97 (6): 419-424.

Harcourt DM, Rumsey NJ, Ambler NR, Cawthorn SJ, Reid CD, Maddox PR, Kenealy JM, Rainsbury RM, and Umpleby HC. 2003. The psychological effect of mastectomy with or without breast reconstruction: a prospective, multicenter study. *Plast. Reconstr. Surg.* 111 (3): 1060-1068.

Herskind C, Bentzen SM, Overgaard J, Overgaard M, Bamberg M, and Rodemann HP. 1998a. Differentiation state of skin fibroblast cultures versus risk of subcutaneous fibrosis after radiotherapy. *Radiotherapy and Oncology* 47 (3): 263-269.

Herskind C, Bamberg M, and Rodemann HP. 1998b. The role of cytokines in the development of normal-tissue reactions after radiotherapy. *Strahlenther. Onkol.* 174 Suppl 3: 12-15.

Herskind C, Johansen J, Bentzen SM, Overgaard M, Overgaard J, Bamberg M, and Rodemann HP. 2000. Fibroblast differentiation in subcutaneous fibrosis after postmastectomy radiotherapy. *Acta Oncol.* 39 (3): 383-388.

Hooning MJ, Botma A, Aleman BM, Baaijens MH, Bartelink H, Klijn JG, Taylor CW, and van Leeuwen FE. 2007. Long-term risk of cardiovascular disease in 10-year survivors of breast cancer. *Journal of the National Cancer Institute* 99 (5): 365-375.

Horiguchi J, Iino JHY, Takei H, Koibuchi Y, Iijima K, Ikeda F, Ochiai R, Uchida K, Yoshida M, Yokoe T, and Morishita Y. 2001. A comparative study of subcutaneous mastectomy with radical mastectomy. *Anticancer Res.* 21 (4B): 2963-2967.

Hoving S, Heeneman S, Gijbels MJ, te Poele JA, Bolla M, Pol JF, Simons MY, Russell NS, Daemen MJ, and Stewart FA. 2010. NO-donating aspirin and aspirin partially inhibit age-related atherosclerosis but not radiation-induced atherosclerosis in ApoE null mice. *PLoS. One.* 5 (9): e12874.

Hoving S, Heeneman S, Gijbels MJ, te Poele JA, Russell NS, Daemen MJ, and Stewart FA. 2008. Single-dose and fractionated irradiation promote initiation and progression of atherosclerosis and induce an inflammatory plaque phenotype in ApoE(-/-) mice. *Int. J. Radiat. Oncol. Biol. Phys.* 71 (3): 848-857.

Hussien M, Salah B, Malyon A, and Wieler-Mithoff EM. 2004. The effect of radiotherapy on the use of immediate breast reconstruction. *Eur. J. Surg. Oncol.* 30 (5): 490-494.

Hvilsom GB, Holmich LR, Frederiksen K, Steding-Jessen M, Friis S, and Dalton SO. (2011a). Socioeconomic position and breast reconstruction in Danish women. *Acta Oncol.* 50 (2): 265-273.

Hvilsom GB, Holmich LR, Steding-Jessen M, Frederiksen K, Henriksen TF, Lipworth L, McLaughlin J, Elberg JJ, Damsgaard TE, and Friis S. (2011b). Delayed Breast Implant Reconstruction: Is Radiation Therapy Associated With Capsular Contracture or Reoperations? *Ann. Plast. Surg.* [Epub ahead of print], add: 2011, May 2

Illsley MC, Peacock JH, McAnulty RJ, and Yarnold JR. 2000. Increased collagen production in fibroblasts cultured from irradiated skin and effect of TGF beta(1)- clinical study. *Br. J. Cancer* 83 (5): 650-654.

Jacobson BS. 2000. Hereditary hemorrhagic telangiectasia: A model for blood vessel growth and enlargement. *Am. J. Pathol.* 156 (3): 737-742.

Javaid M, Song F, Leinster S, Dickson MG, and James NK. 2006. Radiation effects on the cosmetic outcomes of immediate and delayed autologous breast reconstruction: an argument about timing. *J. Plast. Reconstr. Aesthet. Surg.* 59 (1): 16-26.

Jhaveri JD, Rush SC, Kostroff K, Derisi D, Farber LA, Maurer VE, and Bosworth JL. 2008. Clinical outcomes of postmastectomy radiation therapy after immediate breast reconstruction. *Int. J. Radiat. Oncol. Biol. Phys.* 72 (3): 859-865.

Johansen J, Bentzen SM, Overgaard J, and Overgaard M. 1994. Evidence for a positive correlation between in vitro radiosensitivity of normal human skin fibroblasts and the occurrence of subcutaneous fibrosis after radiotherapy. *Int. J. Radiat. Biol.* 66 (4): 407-412.

Kroll SS, Schusterman MA, Reece GP, Miller MJ, and Smith B. 1994. Breast reconstruction with myocutaneous flaps in previously irradiated patients. *Plast. Reconstr. Surg.* 93 (3): 460-469.

Kronowitz SJ, and Robb GL. 2009. Radiation therapy and breast reconstruction: a critical review of the literature. *Plast. Reconstr. Surg.* 124 (2): 395-408.

Krueger EA, Wilkins EG, Strawderman M, Cederna P, Goldfarb S, Vicini FA, and Pierce LJ. 2001. Complications and patient satisfaction following expander/implant breast reconstruction with and without radiotherapy. *Int. J. Radiat. Oncol. Biol. Phys.* 49 (3): 713-721.

Kruse JJ, Floot BG, te Poele JA, Russell NS, and Stewart FA. 2009. Radiation-induced activation of TGF-beta signaling pathways in relation to vascular damage in mouse kidneys. *Radiat. Res.* 171 (2): 188-197.

Kyndi M, Overgaard M, Nielsen HM, Sorensen FB, Knudsen H, and Overgaard J. 2009. High local recurrence risk is not associated with large survival reduction after postmastectomy radiotherapy in high-risk breast cancer: a subgroup analysis of DBCG 82 b&c. *Radiotherapy and Oncology* 90 (1): 74-79.

Lanitis S, Tekkis PP, Sgourakis G, Dimopoulos N, Al MR, and Hadjiminas DJ. 2010. Comparison of skin-sparing mastectomy versus non-skin-sparing mastectomy for breast cancer: a meta-analysis of observational studies. *Ann. Surg.* 251 (4): 632-639.

Lara PC, Russell NS, Smolders IJ, Bartelink H, Begg AC, and Coco-Martin JM. 1996. Radiation-induced differentiation of human skin fibroblasts: relationship with cell survival and collagen production. *Int. J. Radiat. Biol.* 70 (6): 683-692.

Marks LB, Zeng J, and Prosnitz LR. 2008. One to three versus four or more positive nodes and postmastectomy radiotherapy: time to end the debate. *J. Clin. Oncol.* 26 (13): 2075-2077.

Metcalfe KA, Semple J, Quan ML, Vadaparampil ST, Holloway C, Brown M, Bower B, Sun P, and Narod SA. 2011. Changes in Psychosocial Functioning 1 Year After Mastectomy Alone, Delayed Breast Reconstruction, or Immediate Breast Reconstruction. *Ann. Surg. Oncol.* 2011, June 15 [Epub ahead of print]

Nedumpara T, Jonker L, and Williams MR. 2011. Impact of immediate breast reconstruction on breast cancer recurrence and survival. *Breast.* 20(5): 437-433

Overgaard M, Nielsen HM, and Overgaard J. 2007. Is the benefit of postmastectomy irradiation limited to patients with four or more positive nodes, as recommended in international consensus reports? A subgroup analysis of the DBCG 82 b&c randomized trials. *Radiotherapy and Oncology* 82 (3): 247-253.

Patt DA, Goodwin JS, Kuo YF, Freeman JL, Zhang DD, Buchholz TA, Hortobagyi GN, and Giordano SH. 2005. Cardiac morbidity of adjuvant radiotherapy for breast cancer. *J. Clin. Oncol.* 23 (30): 7475-7482.

Peacock J, Ashton A, Bliss J, Bush C, Eady J, Jackson C, Owen R, Regan J, and Yarnold J. 2000. Cellular radiosensitivity and complication risk after curative radiotherapy. *Radiotherapy and Oncology* 55 (2): 173-178.

Potter S, Brigic A, Whiting PF, Cawthorn SJ, Avery KN, Donovan JL, and Blazeby JM. 2011. Reporting clinical outcomes of breast reconstruction: a systematic review. *Journal of the National Cancer Institute* 103 (1): 31-46.

Ragaz J, Olivotto IA, Spinelli JJ, Phillips N, Jackson SM, Wilson KS, Knowling MA, Coppin CM, Weir L, Gelmon K, Le N, Durand R, Coldman AJ, and Manji M. 2005. Locoregional radiation therapy in patients with high-risk breast cancer receiving adjuvant chemotherapy: 20-year results of the British Columbia randomized trial. *Journal of the National Cancer Institute* 97 (2): 116-126.

Rezvani M, Hopewell JW, Wilkinson JH, Bray S, Morris GM, and Charles MW. 2000. Time- and dose-related changes in the thickness of skin in the pig after irradiation with single doses of thulium-170 beta particles. *Radiat. Res.* 153 (1): 104-109.

Rowland JH, Desmond KA, Meyerowitz BE, Belin TR, Wyatt GE, and Ganz PA. 2000. Role of breast reconstructive surgery in physical and emotional outcomes among breast cancer survivors. *Journal of the National Cancer Institute* 92 (17): 1422-1429.

Roychouduri R, Robinson D, Putcha V, Cuzick J, Darby S, and Moller H. 2007. Increased cardiovascular mortality more than fifteen years after radiotherapy for breast cancer: a population-based study. *BMC. Cancer* 7 (1): 9.

Rube CE, Uthe D, Schmid KW, Richter KD, Wessel J, Schuck A, Willich N, and Rube C. 2000. Dose-dependent induction of transforming growth factor beta (TGF-beta) in the lung tissue of fibrosis-prone mice after thoracic irradiation. *Int. J. Radiat. Oncol. Biol. Phys.* 47 (4): 1033-1042.

Russell NS, Grummels A, Hart AA, Smolders IJ, Borger J, Bartelink H, and Begg AC. 1998. Low predictive value of intrinsic fibroblast radiosensitivity for fibrosis development following radiotherapy for breast cancer. *Int. J. Radiat. Biol.* 73 (6): 661-670.

Russell NS, Lara PC, Grummels A, Hart AA, Coco-Martin JM, Bartelink H, and Begg AC. 2000. In vitro differentiation characteristics of human skin fibroblasts: correlations with radiotherapy-induced breast fibrosis in patients. *Int. J. Radiat. Biol.* 76 (2): 231-240.

Russell NS, and Begg AC. 2002. Editorial radiotherapy and oncology 2002: predictive assays for normal tissue damage. *Radiotherapy and Oncology* 64 (2): 125-129.

Russell NS, Kunkler IH, van TG, Canney PA, Thomas J, Bartlett J, van d, V, Belkacemi Y, Yarnold JR, and Barrett-Lee PJ. 2009a. Postmastectomy radiotherapy: will the selective use of postmastectomy radiotherapy study end the debate? *J. Clin. Oncol.* 27 (6): 996-997.

Russell NS, Hoving S, Heeneman S, Hage JJ, Woerdeman LA, de BR, Lohuis PJ, Smeele L, Cleutjens J, Valenkamp A, Dorresteijn LD, Dalesio O, Daemen MJ, and Stewart FA.

2009b. Novel insights into pathological changes in muscular arteries of radiotherapy patients. *Radiotherapy and Oncology* 92 (3): 477-483.

Safwat A, Bentzen SM, Turesson I, and Hendry JH. 2002. Deterministic rather than stochastic factors explain most of the variation in the expression of skin telangiectasia after radiotherapy. *Int. J. Radiat. Oncol. Biol. Phys.* 52 (1): 198-204.

Scharpfenecker M, Floot B, Russell NS, Ten DP, and Stewart FA. 2009. Endoglin haploinsufficiency reduces radiation-induced fibrosis and telangiectasia formation in mouse kidneys. *Radiotherapy and Oncology* 92 (3): 484-491.

Scharpfenecker M, Floot B, Korlaar R, Russell NS, and Stewart FA. 2011. ALK1 heterozygosity delays development of late normal tissue damage in the irradiated mouse kidney. *Radiotherapy and Oncology* 99 (3): 349-355.

Slavin SA, and Goldwyn RM. 1988. The midabdominal rectus abdominis myocutaneous flap: review of 236 flaps. *Plast. Reconstr. Surg.* 81 (2): 189-199.

Soong IS, Yau TK, Ho CM, Lim BH, Leung S, Yeung RM, Sze WM, and Lee AW. 2004. Post-mastectomy radiotherapy after immediate autologous breast reconstruction in primary treatment of breast cancers. *Clin. Oncol. (R. Coll. Radiol.)* 16 (4): 283-289.

Stewart FA, Heeneman S, Te PJ, Kruse J, Russell NS, Gijbels M, and Daemen M. 2006. Ionizing radiation accelerates the development of atherosclerotic lesions in ApoE-/- mice and predisposes to an inflammatory plaque phenotype prone to hemorrhage. *Am. J. Pathol.* 168 (2): 649-658.

Tran NV, Chang DW, Gupta A, Kroll SS, and Robb GL. 2001. Comparison of immediate and delayed free TRAM flap breast reconstruction in patients receiving postmastectomy radiation therapy. *Plast. Reconstr. Surg.* 108 (1): 78-82.

Tucker SL, Turesson I, and Thames HD. 1992. Evidence for individual differences in the radiosensitivity of human skin. *Eur. J. Cancer* 28A (11): 1783-1791.

Turesson I. 1989. The progression rate of late radiation effects in normal tissue and its impact on dose-response relationships. *Radiotherapy and Oncology* 15 (3): 217-226.

Turesson I. 1990. Individual variation and dose dependency in the progression rate of skin telangiectasia. *Int. J. Radiat. Oncol. Biol. Phys.* 19 (6): 1569-1574.

van der Ploeg IM, Russell NS, Nieweg OE, Oldenburg HS, Kroon BB, Olmos RA, and Rutgers EJ. 2009. Lymphatic drainage patterns in breast cancer patients who previously underwent mantle field radiation. *Annals of surgical oncology* 16 (8): 2295-2299.

Vinh-Hung V, Nguyen NP, Cserni G, Truong P, Woodward W, Verkooijen HM, Promish D, Ueno NT, Tai P, Nieto Y, Joseph S, Janni W, Vicini F, Royce M, Storme G, Wallace AM, Vlastos G, Bouchardy C, and Hortobagyi GN. 2009. Prognostic value of nodal ratios in node-positive breast cancer: a compiled update. *Future. Oncol.* 5 (10): 1585-1603.

Williams JK, Bostwick J, III, Bried JT, Mackay G, Landry J, and Benton J. 1995. TRAM flap breast reconstruction after radiation treatment. *Ann. Surg.* 221 (6): 756-764.

Williams JK, Carlson GW, Bostwick J, III, Bried JT, and Mackay G. 1997. The effects of radiation treatment after TRAM flap breast reconstruction. *Plast. Reconstr. Surg.* 100 (5): 1153-1160.

Woerdeman LA, Hage JJ, Smeulders MJ, Rutgers EJ, and van der Horst CM. 2006. Skin-sparing mastectomy and immediate breast reconstruction by use of implants: an assessment of risk factors for complications and cancer control in 120 patients. *Plast. Reconstr. Surg.* 118 (2): 321-330.

Woerdeman LA, van Schijndel AW, Hage JJ, and Smeulders MJ. 2004. Verifying surgical results and risk factors of the lateral thoracodorsal flap. *Plast. Reconstr. Surg.* 113 (1): 196-203.

Zimmerman RP, Mark RJ, Kim AI, Walton T, Sayah D, Juillard GF, and Nguyen M. 1998. Radiation tolerance of transverse rectus abdominis myocutaneous-free flaps used in immediate breast reconstruction. *Am. J. Clin. Oncol.* 21 (4): 381-385.

Part 3

New Technologies and Future Scope in Plastic Surgery

8

Three Dimensional Tissue Models for Research in Oncology

Sarah Nietzer, Gudrun Dandekar, Milena Wasik and Heike Walles
Chair of Tissue Engineering and Regenerative Medicine
University Wuerzburg/Fraunhofer Institute for
Interfacial Engineering and Biotechnology IGB
Germany

1. Introduction

Cancer is a leading cause of death world-wide with 7.6 million deaths in 2008 which is estimated to rise up to 11 million in 2030. The main cancer types include lung, stomach, liver, colorectal and breast cancer (World Health Organization [WHO], 2011). One of three persons in developed countries dies of cancer, and the expected survival time of newly diagnosed cancer patients (e.g. pancreatic carcinoma) is often less than five years (Kamb, 2005).

In the last three decades great advances in understanding the molecular bases of cancer biology have been made. But up to now cancer therapy is still often empirical, based on inhibiting DNA synthesis and cellular division with a high rate of clinical failure. There is an unprecedented number of new substances in clinical trials. However, the number of highly efficacious drugs approved by the regulatory authorities remains low and there is still a desperate medical need for new drugs which are successful for long-term survival of patients. Costs for bringing a drug to market are estimated to be over US$ 1 billion (Figure 1). This makes the low success rate for oncology products of about 10 percent even more disappointing (Hait, 2010). Patients, the pharmaceutical and biotechnology community invest enormous efforts to validate new therapeutics only to watch them fail in humans due to the lack of suitable model systems. Today commonly used cancer models include native human tumor cell lines (e.g. HCT116 colon) or engineered cell lines (FLT3.dependent BaF/3 cells). Cancer cell lines provide a certain degree of standardization and are easy to handle, but the establishment of cell lines is difficult and often they lack key features of the tumor they should model. Improvements for the generation of new cancer cell lines are recently made by the introduction of three-dimensional (3D) culture systems, the selection of tumor initiating cells and the use of specialized media. To create a more complex tumor environment cell lines can be grown subcutaneously (e.g. PC-3 prostate) or orthotopic (e.g. PC-3 prostate, implanted in prostate) in immuno-compromised mice (Kamb, 2005; Caponigro & Sellers, 2011). In immuno-compromised mice human cancer cell lines produce tumor-like tissues that show a slight resemblance to clinical tumors concerning histological architecture and they fail to recapitulate key aspects of human tumorigenicity such as invasion and metastasis. A more complex tumor tissue is formed after implantation of whole fragments of human tumors into a mouse. Also mouse tumors can be implanted syngeneically (e.g. B16 melanoma), induced (radiation induced skin tumors) or genetically engineered (e.g. RIP-Tag mouse pancreatic islet) (Kamb, 2005). An advantage of mouse models is that mechanistic studies can be done in genetically engineered mouse models. As a novel strategy in the development of engineered mouse models, chimeric animals are created that arise from blastocysts which are injected with engineered stem cells that harbour tissue specific inducible oncogenes. These chimeric animals develop tumors in the context of normal tissues and could reflect clinical observations accurately such as e.g. distinct tumor regression upon anti-EGFR treatment dependent on the mutated oncogene (Zhou et al., 2010). Improvements of animal models have been made by using mice with humanized haematopoietic and immune systems or by using genetic mouse models that include tumor progression and metastasis. But the success of these models remains to be determined (Hait, 2010). In 2001 a retrospective study of drug candidates showed only a weak correlation between the responses of xenografted tumors to these drugs and the clinical outcome (Weinberg, 2006). To counteract this problem preclinical strategies and tumor models have to be developed with a robust predictive value for the clinical outcome of anti-cancer agents.

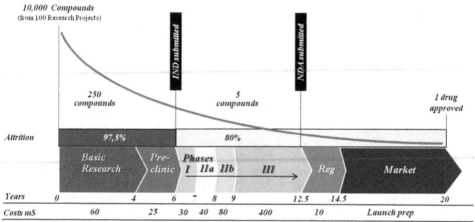

Source: PhRMA, Pharmaceutical Industry Profile 2007; http://link.brightcove.com/services/link/bcpid1541043091/bctid1541121027

Fig. 1. Time Schedule of the Pharma Drug Development Process. There is an urgent need for novel drugs and strategies to fight cancer. However, the development of a single new anti-cancer agent is very costly (up to 1 billion US$). Moreover, only very few compounds are successful: During long lasting testing of many compounds more and more substances become selected as being ineffective until in the end one compound out of 10.000 becomes one single approved drug. Reg: Regulation.

To understand the demands tumor models have to fulfil in the first part of this chapter, we are going to give (i) a survey of the historical development of preclinical models, (ii) explain different classes of mechanisms of anti-cancer drugs including some examples and problems of cytotoxicity, and (iii) summarize the limitations that face preclinical models right now.

1.1 History of preclinical tumor models

The first cancer models were established over 60 years ago and were derived from carcinogen-induced mouse tumors, primarily sarcomas and lymphomas (Chabner & Roberts, 2005). Observed effects of mustard gas on lymphoid and myeloid cell lineages in soldiers were reinvestigated in a transplantable lymphoma model by Gilman and Philips in 1946 (Gilman & Philips, 1946; as cited in Caponigro & Sellers 2011). This contributed to the introduction of *in vitro* and *in vivo* models for first successful clinical trials with antineoplastic agents. In the following 30 years these transplantable models were used to determine the potential efficacy and toxicity of drugs. In 1957 Heidelberger introduced 5-fluoruracil, an inhibitor of the pyrimidine biosynthesis pathway, still a key component in many cancer treatment regimens today, based on the observation that rat hepatomas show an extremly high level of uracil uptake (Heidelberger et al., 1957; as cited in Caponigro & Sellers, 2011). Many chemotherapeutic agents used today, such as anti-mitotic vinca alkaloids, actinomycin D and platinum salts were discovered or developed during one of the first large-scale programmes of the Cancer Chemotherapy National Service Center at the US National Cancer Institute. During this program which started in 1955, mouse lymphoma models were investigated (Chabner & Roberts, 2005). In the late 1980s, a new concept for the application of preclinical models to validate novel therapeutics called NCI60 (National Cancer Institute, 60 human tumor cell lines) also included solid tumors in large-scale screening platforms. This effort required the use of new technologies, such as performing cell culture in microtiter well plates, the development of high-throughput cytotoxicity assays, and the establishment of a bioinformatic infrastructure to analyze the large data sets being generated (Caponigro & Sellers, 2011). These models provided important insights in different mechanisms of cancer cell growth and its inhibition. Recently the role of NCI60 changed more to a service screen for cancer scientists (Shoemaker, 2006). Even though up to now also many tumor cell lines were created from solid tumors, leukemia-lymphoma cell lines remain a key tumor model system reflecting the original tumor with high precision due to its detailed oncogenomic documentation. But here also some hematopoietic entities are underrepresented and resist the establishment of cancer cell lines (Drexler & Macleod, 2010). New technologies from tissue engineering should also help to generate models with immortalized primary cells that maintain differentiation.

1.2 Mechanisms of anti-cancer drugs

To optimize the application of preclinical tumor models it is important to understand the different ways and mechanisms in which anti-cancer drugs act. These mechanisms can be divided into three classes: The first class of agents improves personal therapeutic accuracy by targeting genetic dependencies, such as mutations in oncogenes responsible for cancer progression. Recent successful examples include imatinib (Gleevec/Glivec; Novartis), which targets the activated BCR-ABL gene fusion product in chronic myeloid leukaemia (CML) or in gastro-intestinal stromal tumors (GIST) (Kamb, 2005). It is also under investigation for application in other cancers as NSCLC. Other biomarkers for patients with NSCLC were determined recently and include an activating mutation in the Epidermal-Growth-Factor-Receptor (EGFR) gene which is recommended to be tested before a treatment with therapeutics such as gefitinib or erlotinib is started (Cadranel et al., 2011). Colon cancer patients with a mutation in the k-ras gene are excluded from antibody therapy against the

EGFR because the targeted pathway is constitutively activated in these patients without any influence of the receptor on this activation. Further success in targeted therapy is shown by a high clinical response rate of malignant melanoma patients (phase I) to inhibitors of B-RAF kinase activity (Bollag et al., 2010). Also the treatment with trastuzumab in metastatic breast cancer patients with amplified/overexpressed epidermal growth factor receptor 2 (HER2 or ERBB2) showed some success (Vogel et al., 2002). Furthermore mutated downstream components of the ras-dependend mitogen-activated protein (MAP) kinase signalling pathway, a major regulator of cell survival and proliferation, are attractive targets for therapeutic intervention (Fremin & Meloche, 2010). The development of imatinib was driven on by mechanistically experimenting with different engineered cancer cell lines and was confirmed in xenografted mouse experiments deducing treatment success from the inhibition of Abl-protein tyrosine kinase and PDGF receptor activation (Buchdunger et al., 1996). This indicates that also mechanistically designed experiments using cancer cell lines and animal tumor models can lead to clinical success.

Drugs of the second class of therapeutics target host-tumor interactions, such as hormones and secreted factors upon which the tumors depend. They can be developed on the basis of hormonal suppression in non-tumor bearing animals. Examples for efficacious therapies are aromatase inhibitors for the treatment of oestrogen receptor-positive breast cancer (Baum et al., 2002; Caponigro & Sellers, 2011). And recently, abiraterone, an inhibitor of CYP17A, revealed some progress in the treatment of castration–resistant prostate cancer by complete blocking of androgen synthesis. Prostate cancer depends to 80 percent on androgen the biosynthesis of which is catalyzed in the last step by the P450 enzyme CYP17A both in testes and in adrenals (Hartmann et al., 2002; Reid et al., 2010). Understanding the molecular epidemiology of human tumors should help to promote the development of agents against such host factors.

Agents of the third class of drugs often affect fundamental cellular processes on which cancer cells rely more strongly than normal cells. The target population of these therapeutic agents is often determined by using the trial-and-error method, a fact that leads to high failure rates (Caponigro & Sellers, 2011). Among these drugs of the third class there are common cytotoxic chemotherapeuticals such as nucleoside analogues, DNA-modifying chemicals and natural products with a narrow therapeutic window that were initially introduced in the 1940s (Kamb, 2005). As a therapeutic guideline, safe starting doses are estimated from animal toxicology studies escalating up to the maximum tolerated dose (MTD), which is defined as the highest dose which can be tolerated without any unmanageable side effects. In xenograft animal models the efficacy of each drug is estimated from the ratio of tumor volumes in treated animals and control animals. The toxicity is estimated from the loss of weight of the animals which should be no more than 10 percent during the course of a treatment over two weeks (Kamb, 2005). These standard animal experiments correspond only approximately to human responses to new substances (Hartung, 2009). Limitations of animal models reside mainly in the differences between animals and humans concerning body weight, life span, metabolism and drug uptake mechanisms. Results from toxicology studies of different animal species show only a concordance in the case of 53-60 percent of all tested chemicals (Schardein et al., 1985). The toxic effect in humans can be predicted correctly only for 43-63 percent of all the tested pharmaceuticals (Olson et al., 2000). In clinical trials made by the pharmaceutical industry, 20 percent of the drug candidates showed toxic effects in humans whereas these effects were not detected in animal models (false-negative results). The number of false-positive results concerning chemicals which are not toxic in humans but could show to be toxic in animals is estimated from reproductive toxicity testing in 63 percent of all investigated drugs (Hartung, 2009). Data from phase III trials suggest that preclinical models overestimate the efficacy of candidate molecules, especially of cytotoxic agents (Caponigro & Sellers, 2011). Starting in 1990, over 10.000 compounds per year have been screened in model systems derived from eight different solid tumors. Unique patterns of cytotoxicity should help to unravel their mechanism of action (Caponigro & Sellers, 2011). Typical cytotoxic mechanisms are operated via the inhibition of microtubules and topoisomerases. Novel therapeutic mechanisms, such as the inhibition of the proteasome by bortezomib (Velcade; Millennium Pharmaceuticals) were recently introduced concerning the treatment of multiple myeloma (Adams, 2002). But attention should also be paid to inter-individual variations in drug metabolism. For instance, irinotecan is a standard drug in treatment of advanced colorectal cancer but 10 percent of the caucasian population show low enzyme activity of an important catabolic enzyme and therefore suffer from greater side effects based on the toxicity of the drug. Here also individual biomarker tests could reduce the problem of superfluous side effects caused by toxicity, because patients with this specific genotype should be treated in a different way than people with another genotype (Schilsky, 2010). However, with regard to toxicity, it has to be taken into account that cancer is mainly a disease of older persons. This augments the problem of drug-toxicity because the detoxification becomes more difficult in elderly people.

1.3 Limitations of preclinical tumor models

There is a number of typical limitations of preclinical models: Certainly, the number of models available does not reflect the number of distinct tumors. Moreover, the molecular characterization of models is often inadequate and hence the alignment to human cancers is impossible. The observed effects such as tumor growth rate reduction do not necessarily correlate with the tumor regression observed in the patient. Moreover, *in vitro* models undergo various selection pressures and biases such as the dependence on oncogenic key pathways. The preclinical models do not reflect stromal-tumor interactions. As an exception, human cells transplanted in mice exhibit stromal interactions and to a certain content angiogenesis. However, these observations still suffer from cross-species differences. Furthermore, murine models often actively reject human tumors and hence it is difficult to study tumor initiating cells in the murine organism. In contrast, the anti-tumor immunity is low to absent in immuno-compromised animals. Finally, the costly and time-consuming *in vivo* testing limits high-throughput screening of substances (Caponigro & Sellers, 2011). Tissue engineering could offer new strategies for overcoming the mentioned limitations of conventional tumor models and could even improve cost effectiveness and accuracy.

2. Overview about tissue engineering

Tissue engineering is an interdisciplinary field that applies the principles of engineering and the life sciences to the development of biological substitutes that restore, maintain, or improve tissue function (Lavik & Langer, 2004). Potentially, it can create replacement structures from biodegradable scaffolds and autologous cells for reconstructive surgery (Stock & Vacanti, 2001). According to the U.S. Department of Health and Human Services, meanwhile 110.586 people in the USA are waiting for an organ, and due to the shortage of available donor material, an average of 20 potential candidates for organ transplantation die each day in the USA. This could be prevented with an artificial alternative for donor tissue suitable for transplantation and reconstructive surgery.

The basic conception of tissue engineering is the cultivation of cells on biocompatible scaffolds or matrices, so that they can organize and develop a tissue structure. These scaffolds can be composed of synthetic materials like hydroxylapatite (HA) and polyurethane (PU) or of biological materials like collagen or decellularized organs. The advantage of synthetic materials is the easier availability, but they are not suitable to generate all kinds of tissues. Solid materials like HA are suited very well for the culture of e.g. osseous tissue for oral and casualty surgery. Human osteoblasts build 3D structures on HA-matrices and are able to calcify without special growth factors [zellwerk.biz]. PU-matrices have the advantage of biodegradability which means that the matrix disintegrates in the body gradually and only the newly grown tissue remains. Moreover, PU scaffolds can be formed easily before implantation, so that body parts like e.g. ear cups can be reconstructed by using computer tomography (CT) data and can then be implanted after having been reseeded with cells. By using collagen/fibronectin gel skin equivalents can be cultured which resemble naturally human skin with its two-layered composition very closely (Fraunhofer IGB, Stuttgart, Germany). In this model (Figure 2), the dermis is built up by using primary dermal fibroblasts deriving from skin biopsies which are embedded into a collagen gel. This dermis is used as a basis for the epidermal ceratinocytes which are seeded into a fibronectin gel and build up the epidermis. This patent-registered skin model (Patent-Nr. EP 1 290 145B1) is accredited for the control of biocompatibility of medical products (DIN ISO 10993-5). But for dermal reconstructive surgery (e.g. in the case of burns), a graft consisting of decellularized bovine skin is used. This kind of matrix consists of collagen which is virginally structured and is therefore better suitable for being used as a tissue replacement. During the healing procedure, the body's own fibroblasts produce a collagen matrix whereas the transplanted matrix becomes resorbated (Kolokythas et al., 2008).

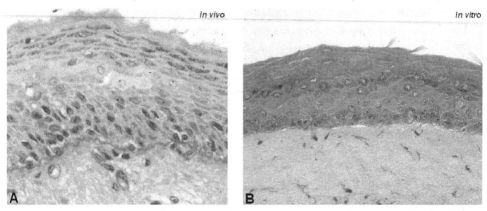

Fig. 2. Cross section of native skin (A) and skin equivalent (B), hematoxylin and eosin (HE) stain. Both samples show a two-layered construction with epidermis (upper part) and dermis (bottom). The basal lamina is seen as a thin red line between epidermis and dermis in the natural skin (A).

Due to the possibility of reseeding the matrices with autologous cells, immune responses are reduced or even prevented (Stock & Vacanti, 2001). One example is found among others in the area of cardiovascular tissue engineering: The fibrin gel for the production of heart valve scaffolds derives from the patient's blood. Autologous myofibroblasts are injected into this gel and after growing the tissue becomes lined with autologous endothelial cells (Jockenhoevel et al., 2001). Therefore no heterologous cells are needed. Another advantage of the *in vitro* grown tissue is the ability to expand in the body of the patient. This is very important in the case of paediatric surgery because implants which are able to grow do not need to be replaced and therefore no additional operations are needed (Jockenhoevel et al., 2001). For this reason tissue engineering is a very important technology in the field of regenerative medicine. Decellularized matrices are also often used for the replacement of the viscera like kidney, liver and lung due to their elasticity. Homografts deriving from a different organism (e.g. pig) and allografts deriving from an individual of the same species (human) are used for generating these matrices.

In vitro applied bioartificial human tissue models allow the generation of functional 3D cell-systems mimicking the microenvironment of potential human target tissues which eventually reflect the *in vivo* behaviour of tested cells more precisely than currently applied cell-based test systems. Their application in drug research may help to make drug development safer and more efficient and reduce research and development expenses. Additionally, they represent promising models for individualized oncologic therapy by revealing new insights into mechanisms of organogenesis and expression of malignancy (Walles et al., 2007).

3. Generation of vascularized *in vitro* tissues

Our tissue model technology is based on decellularized porcine small bowl segments and preserved tubular structures of the capillary network within the collagen matrix which is functionally associated with one small vein and artery (biological vascularised scaffold [BioVaSc]) (Mertsching et al., 2005). To obtain this biological scaffold BioVaSc (Figure 3) with a preserved feeding artery, a draining vein, and a functional capillary network for graft supply, we developed a special harvesting procedure in the pigs. Our decellularization procedure left behind a dense layer of cross linked collagen and elastin fibers evolved from the stratum compactum, the small intestinal submucosa (SIS), the tunica serosa, and the tunica muscularis externa with its arterial and venous network. HE staining was used to survey the cellular state of each processed matrix (Mertsching et al., 2005). Our decellularization process resulted in remaining acellular tubular network of 20 to 200 µm diameter (Fig. 4 A, B) connected to the venous and arterial pedicle, respectively, with a basal membrane and elastica interna. Semi quantitative DNA detection was applied as molecular marker for scaffold decellularization. Its results confirmed our histological findings. Our scaffold thickness was 0.2±0.01 mm. First clinical experience shows, that the BioVaSc is well tolerated and supports an extensive tissue maturation process following implantation (Mertsching et al., 2009). The functional reseeding of the remaining tubular structures of the vascular network within our biological scaffold with endothelial cells was the main objective of this study. Microvascular endothelial cells (mECs) were identified as the ideal endothelial cell (EC) type in respect to genetic and functional stability during isolation, proliferation and seeding in the vascular structures. To control the differentiation of the endothelial cells, we evaluated the endothelial specific markers CD31, VE-Cadherin and Flk-1 by immunohistochemistry and western blot analysis. Anyway the mECs generate an active antithrombotic surface that facilitates transit of plasma and cellular constituents (Mertsching et al., 2009). For proper function of the endothelium, integrity is required, i.e. mainly ensured by endothelial cell-to-cell junctions. A functional vascular endothelial lining is of paramount importance to avoid graft thrombosis and failure.

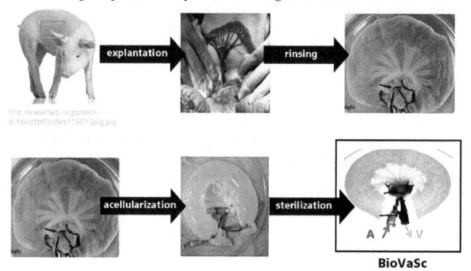

BioVaSc

Fig. 3. Standardized method to generate a biological vascularised scaffold (BioVaSc) for the engineering of complex vascularised tissues. A part of the porcine jejunum is isolated including the feeding artery and vein and the connecting capillary bed. After intensive rinsing the cells are removed chemically. The acelluarisation process is finished after a γ-radiation to sterilize the BioVaSc.

Three weeks after endovascular seeding and permanent perfusion, the luminal surface of the supplying artery and vein is lined with a cellular monolayer staining positive for CD31, which mediates adhesion between cells that express CD31. Its expression is limited to endothelial cells, platelets, leukocytes, and their precursors and it has been shown to be highly specific and sensitive for vascular endothelial cells. Within the scaffold matrix, CD31 positive structures are unequally distributed. No positive reaction was detected in acellular controls, excluding non-specific antibody-reactions with the matrix and remaining porcine endothelial cells in the scaffold (Mertsching et al., 2009). Analogical findings were obtained for VE-Cadherin and Flk-1. VE-Cadherin is an endothelial-specific trans-membrane protein that promotes hemophilic cell adhesion mechanically connecting endothelial cells providing the structural base for interendothelial mechanical stability. It plays a morphogenic role in vascular development by participating in contact inhibition of VEGF signalling and its expression is required for the normal organization of the vasculature in the embryo (Carmeliet et al., 1999). Flk-1 is a high-affinity VEGF-2 receptor and is found on differentiated endothelial progenitor cells. It produces a positive endothelial proliferation signal during developmental blood vessel formation. Western blot analysis confirmed the immunohistochemical findings. The simultaneous expression of three specific endothelial markers on our reseeded biological scaffold indicates the successful EC seeding of the vascular structures. Vitality of vascularized scaffold was analyzed by 2`-[18F]-fluoro-2`-desoxy-glucose (FDG) positron emission tomography (PET) using a dedicated fullring scanner facilitating general graft survey with no need for tissue dissection. As viable cells take up FDG, localized vitality can be in principle visualized by PET. To increase the resolution of detected activity distribution, additional thin layer scanning was performed. PET images showed 3D activity accumulation within the proximity of the reseeded arterial pedicle. Only radioactive background was seen in acellular controls. PET imaging allows quantification of the PET signal. Maximum uptake ratios for the reseeded biological matrix (perfused with buffer-medium) were 11±0.7 vs. 2±0.9 for the non-seeded matrix. In addition to this, PET scanning revealed the functional integrity of the endothelial vascular lining, thereby supporting our immunohistochemical morphological findings. Cellular FDG uptake can be stimulated by insulin exposure and we applied this principle as an additional test for functional cellular vitality. Insulin stimulation amplified the FDG PET uptake in reseeded matrices by a factor of 4.2±1.1. No increase was detectable in acellular controls. These findings amplify our previous findings that the reseeded matrices are populated with viable EC (Mertsching et al., 2005).

The approaches presented here enable the generation of a functional artificial vascular network in a porcine scaffold (Fig. 4 A-D). The generated biological vascularized scaffold may serve as a universal scaffold for tissue engineering.

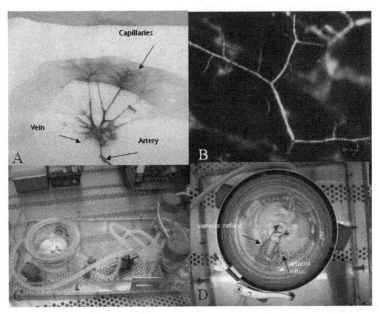

Fig. 4. A) The vascularized scaffold (BioVaSc) with blue stained capillary network. B) Seeded capillaries of the matrix with fluorescence marked liver endothelial cells. C) A bioartificial human tissue model in the specific developed bioreactor enclosed in the closed perfusion stet-up. D) 3D human vascularised tumor test system with arterial and venous access.

Pharmaceutical research is hampered by limited predictive value of routinely applied *in vitro* and *in vivo* drug screening models for clinical efficacy. In drug development, the common approach of pharmaceutical industry is to screen small-molecule libraries for function and toxicity in biochemical based or ligand binding high-throughput assays (Sundberg, 2000). In general enzymes and two-dimensional (2D) cell lines are used in those cell-based assays. The obtained results are of limited biological relevance, since the 2D cell systems do not adequately mimic the 3D environment in healthy and tumour tissues (Sundberg, 2000).

4. Engineered tumor tissues for applied research

Our BioVaSc can additionally be populated with tumor cells to create *ex vivo* vascularized tumor-like structures. The system offers the option to administer the substances as well as nanomaterials in the arterial inflow and to study the influence of the tumor-like tissue macroscopically as well as on a cellular and molecular level. Human derived tumor cells are co-cultivated with the endothelial cells in such a way that they can form a physiological filtration barrier. The medium is conducted over capillaries seeded with endothelial cells to the tumor cells. Anti-angiogenic therapy molecules as antibodies are now tested in the system. This model offers the possibility to simulate physiological drug application and a human 3D test system to established nanomaterials/systems for cancer research/therapy.

Hackmann and Redelmeier have found out in 2006 that 92 percent of the new drugs fail in clinical studies although the animal experiments were successful (Hackam & Redelmeier, 2006; as cited in Schanz et al., 2010). And it is not least for ethical reasons that suitable alternatives should be found for animal experiments. Already established test tissues at Fraunhofer IGB are the intestine, liver, trachea and fascia models. The cultivation of the cells must take place in special bioreactors in which nutrients can be fed and metabolism products can be removed and which reflect the conditions in the human body in this way (Fig. 4 C, D). These test systems will be transferred into tumor test systems. The heterologous cellular micro-environment of a tumor can be copied by co-culture of tumor cells with stroma cells like fibroblasts. This is important, because the cancerogenesis is influenced by interactions of stroma, epithelium and components of the extracellular matrix (Micke & Ostman, 2004). The main application will be the testing of patient-specific therapies like drugs, chemotherapy, and immunotherapy. In this manner one can test new therapies and drugs outside the patient, but within human (perhaps autologous) tissue before they find use in the cancer therapy.

Why do we need tumor test systems? Up to now there are no suitable human *in vitro* models of cancer available as described in "the biology of cancer" (Weinberg, 2006). But why do we need as many "nature identical" tumor models generated from human cells? The first reason is that new therapies and new drugs are needed to fight cancer by inhibiting tumor growth, angiogenesis as well as tumor metastasis. To test the effects of many different substances on these processes of tumor development, a time-saving and standardized method is used. The widely used animal xenograft animal models show some advantages for being used as a test system e.g. the interaction between tumor and the whole living organism including blood circulation. The immune system can be studied as well as psychophysiological consequences of medication which can be analyzed during behavioural studies of the animals. But on the other hand there are many pros for the *in vitro* tumor models: the generation of such *in vitro* tumors is not as time-consuming as the breeding and fostering of animals used for xenograft transplantation, a circumstance which is very interesting for high-throughput screening of drugs and diverse therapeutical methods from a wide pool of possible cancer treatments. Moreover, *in vitro* tumor models do not contain any unrelated cells from other species which interact with the human cell population and can bias the results. And, last but not least, the *in vitro* tumor models can be standardized better than any living organism can be. Additionally, synthetic human tumors cultured in 3D do not suffer psychologically from treatment and for this reason can be supported from an ethical point of view for first drug screening.

Another important field is the so-called "personalized medicine", a very individual tumor treatment for each patient. As not only each patient but also each tumor can be seen as an individual, it is very important to individualize treatment, too. A big aim for the future is the cultivation of primary cells deriving from the special tumor of the individual patient. These primary tumor cells can be used to build up artificial tumors *in vitro* which can also be medicated *in vitro* and which can be used for analyzing the characteristic features of this special disease e.g. the genetic background of the tumor cells, their interaction with surrounding tissue cells and their responsiveness to various treatments. All these studies can be done in parallel by using an array of these *in vitro* tumor models. By using these models it could be possible to circumvent side effects of inefficient treatments and it could be possible to adjust tumor treatment within a short period of time because of the parallel investigation possibilities. For the investigation of tumor-stroma interactions these *in vitro* tumor models are also very useful. Activated cancer-associated fibroblasts e.g. are involved in tumor progression and are a possible target for anti-cancer therapies (Kalluri & Zeisberg, 2006). Dermal fibroblasts can be isolated quite easily from skin biopsies and can be employed to mimic these interactions between tumor cells and connective tissue in the human body. Also the interaction between endothelial cells and the tumor cells can be investigated in an artificial tumor especially when it is grown and cultured in a bioreactor with an artificial "blood stream". In this dynamic system it is possible to study the angiogenesis of the tumor and to identify signals between tumor cells and endothelial cells as well as to test the ability of drugs to inhibit these interactions. Also signal pathways involved in tumor development can be analyzed in these artificial tumors generated by co-cultivation of tumor cells and stroma cells as well as extracellular matrix components involved in carcinogenesis (Micke & Ostman, 2004).

5. Examples for 3D tissue models for research in oncology

An *in vitro* model of malignant melanoma was created by using of the 3D skin model developed by the Fraunhofer company (EP 01953961.8-2405). Different types of melanoma cells can be used to create skin tumors on or in this dermal equivalent.

Malignant melanomas often differ in invasiveness as well as tumor expansion. There must be various subtypes of melanomas and for this reason it is important to investigate the features of this special tumor which a single patient suffers from. To characterize the pathogenical background of different tumors and to test various medical therapies *in vitro*, this 3D skin model developed by the Fraunhofer IGB (EP 01953961.8-2405) can be used. Additionally, it can be useful in testing pharmaceutical penetration and resorption of different drugs. The test tissue was generated as described in [Walles et al., 2007]: Human primary fibroblasts derived from human foreskin (1×10^4 cells/cm^2) were seeded in a rodent collagen-I gel (isolated from rat tail) resulting in a dermal-like cell-matrix construct. Human ceratinocytes (1×10^5 cells/cm^2) were seeded on the surface of the cell-matrix construct and incubated for 5 days in cell culture medium (submerged cell culture). The "epidermal" ceratinocyte layer of the tissue surface was exposed to the air for another 12-14 days to induce ceratinization (air-lift culture). The resulting tissue was composed of a stable connective tissue rich of cells (= dermis) with a ceratinizing surface.

Now different human melanoma cell lines were inoculated into the dermal layer and showed their characteristic growth behavior in these *in vitro* models (Figure 5).

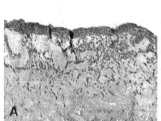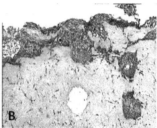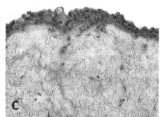

Fig. 5. Bioartificial human *in vitro* skin model for malignant melanoma spread. A) Superficial spreading melanoma (SSM) diffusely infiltrating the skin equivalent. B) Nodular melanoma (NM) forming tumor nests. C) Lentigo maligna melanoma (LMM) spreading superficially without invasion of the skin equivalent. (Adapted from Walles et al., 2007)

Additionally, an interaction between tumor tissue and endothelial cells could be shown when they were co-cultivated in this model (Walles et al., 2007). For this reason, also endothelial cell differentiation as well as angiogenesis can be analyzed with this model as well as the development of medical devices, e.g. a laser assisted diagnostic device for melanoma can be developed using such an *in vitro* model (Mertsching et al., 2008).

Because lung cancer is the most common cancer in terms of both incidence and mortality (Jemal et al., 2011) it is very important to develop new and better therapeutic approaches. An *in vitro* model of lung adenocarcinoma was created by using the BioVaSc reseeded with A549 tumor cells as well as primary dermal fibroblasts in co-culture. A549 cells are a lung cancer cell line derived from adenocarcinomic human alveolar basal epithelial cells. Results showed that the primary fibroblasts influenced the growth of the tumor cells concerning growth behavior and morphology and formed nodular structures in some areas (Wasik, 2011). Immortalized cell lines derived from tumor cells are a good basic material to build up standardized *in vitro* tumors because primary cells derived from tumor biopsies are not as uniform as these cell clones. There are different matrices which can be used as a substrate for the 3D cell culture e.g. inserts of polycarbonate.

Another important field of cancer research is colon cancer because it is the second most common cancer disease in Germany and kills about 600.000 people annually worldwide [globocan.iarc.fr]. An *in vitro* model for colon adenocarcinoma which was also created by using the BioVaSc reseeded with cells of different cancer cell lines derived from colon adenocarcinomas (Caco-2 and SW480) as well as dermal primary fibroblasts and mECs which were co-cultured with the cancer cells. In this model, the SW480 cells show nodular growth in co-culture with primary fibroblasts and exhibit a more malignant morphology than Caco-2 cells. To test the influence of substances on tumor growth and invasiveness, *in vitro* models built up from human colon carcinoma cells are in very dire need because animal xenograft models have some drawbacks especially concerning such studies of the gut: mice or rats have a very different diet compared to man and in consequence of this their gut not only a "miniature edition" but it is different in some ways compared to the human one e.g. the gut flora is very different or food does not stay as long in the gut as in humans. First models are built up by using various colon carcinoma cell lines e.g. the well-established cell lines Caco-2 and SW480. Budding results could be seen concerning the more aggressive SW480 cells which invade the matrix in monoculture and showed nodular structures in co-culture with fibroblasts (own data, unpublished). But more read outs for tumor features of these *in vitro* "tumors" are needed e.g. proliferation quantification as well as verification of an upcoming epithelial mesenchymal transition (EMT).

6. Conclusion

Conventional preclinical tumor models were proved to be successful in some limited settings when the cell models, the human xenografts or the mouse model include mutations, amplifications or translocations of the original malignancy that was to be treated in the clinic. Also important aspects such as pharmacokinetic behaviour, tissue distribution and percentage of free compounds in plasma can be determined in conventional animal tumor models. However, there is a tendency to overestimate the real clinical impact of any compound measured by reduction of the tumor mass in xenograft models. Nowadays genetically engineered mouse models are ever more sophisticated but still habour additional unknown changes which challenge the translation to the patient (Kamb, 2005). Other drawbacks of conventional models remain, such as the insufficient number of experiments for proper statistics, the time-consuming generation of animal models and the low number of cell lines that do not represent the tumors' heterogeneity (Kamb, 2005).

Cancer is foremost a genetic disease, making the analysis of correlation between compound activity and molecular changes important (Caponigro & Sellers, 2011). Averagely about 80 genes are affected in different common tumor types as breast and colon cancer (Todaro et al., 2010) which makes clear that 60 cancer cell lines can not accurately reflect the diversity of over 100 histologically distinct tumor types. Progress in drug development requires the identification of essential and compensating functions that are specific to cancer cells and their translation in a proper tumor model.

At present many projects try to identify gene signatures in screens of large sets of cell lines that predict sensitivity and resistance to specific targeted drugs. For example, the Novartis Institutes for BioMedical Research in collaboration with other investigators assembled in the "Cell Line Encyclopedia Project" expression profiles, copy-number alterations and dose-response data of over 1000 cell lines (Caponigro & Sellers, 2011). Other promising approaches for targeted drug development are current genome-profiling projects such as the National Cancer Institute's "Cancer Genome Atlas" and the Sanger's Institute's "Cancer Genome Project" (Schilsky, 2010). However, while relating targeted anti-cancer drug efficacy and toxicity it is important to consider physiology. In organisms from *E. coli* to mouse three quarters of the individual genes are non-essential or only essential in a particular genetic or epigenetic background. This explains why tumors often not depend on the target for viability (Kamb, 2005).

Another approach for successful cancer therapy is the testing of different drug combinations in sufficiently large sets of *in vitro* models where many compounds can be tested in one cell line or one combination in many different cell lines. In some cases combination therapy could also overcome acquired drug resistance.

In future it would be a desirable goal to create *in vitro* tumor models by using primary cells derived from the patient's tumor biopsies to get to test various therapeutic approaches on autologous test systems *in vitro* before application. Therefore this personalized medicine would be the best to avoid side effects of ineffective treatments and to save time and therefore lives because many therapeutic methods can be tested in parallel *in vitro* on their effectiveness in fighting this special tumor before being given to the patient. For successful personalized medicine further biomarkers such as k-ras in anti-EGFR colon cancer therapy have to be identified and diagnostic tests have to be co-developed with new drugs (Hait, 2010). To accelerate the development and approval of targeted cancer therapies, clinical investigators, scientists, drug developers and regulatory experts joined by the Brookings Institution and have recently proposed a novel strategy for drug and biomarker co-development called "targeted approval" (Schilsky, 2010). Tumor models with higher efficiency and accuracy should be generated with cell lines harbouring certain mutations that are targeted by drugs the impact of which is predicted by bioinformatic analysis of genomic and epigenomic screens.

It has been proven that personalized medicine could also improve cost efficiency in prescription practice: Stratification of patient population that should be treated with certain agents such as the use of anti-EGFR drugs only in k-ras wild-type colorectal cancer patients. This could save the US health care system about US$ 700 million annually (Schilsky, 2010). Not only is the development of novel drugs expensive but also the drugs themselves and the following treatment protocols. The National Institute of Health of the United States estimated the overall cost of cancer care in 2007 to US$ 219.2 billion. Cost-utility studies for cancer started initially in the 1990s and extended to 14 percent in 2007, which gives hope to improve cost-effectiveness in cancer in future (Greenberg et al., 2010).

In general new approaches have to be considered to bring more successful anti-cancer agents to market. If a strong genetic and epidemiological indication exists for any drug more caution should be applied before excluding these rashly from the clinic (Kamb, 2005). Toxicity models should balance sensitivity (false-negative rate) with selectivity (false-positive rate) (Kamb, 2005). Treatment-related deaths in Phase I oncology have fallen down to a fraction of a percentage point (Roberts et al., 2004) and therefore regulatory agencies should reconsider the criteria for advancement into the clinic to improve the throughput of drug testing in humans. However, there is a need for global regulation to judge which criteria form the basis of approval of drugs which are active but have no significant side effects (Hait, 2010).

Last but not least there is hope to improve clinical applications also due to impressive and well-coordinated ventures occurring worldwide that could go along with the generation of more complex and accurate preclinical 3D tumor models in the field of tissue engineering to fight cancer.

7. References

Adams, J. (2002). Development of the proteasome inhibitor PS-341. *The oncologist*, Vol.7, No.1, pp. 9-16

Baum, M.; Budzar, A. U. et al. (2002). Anastrozole alone or in combination with tamoxifen versus tamoxifen alone for adjuvant treatment of postmenopausal women with early breast cancer: first results of the ATAC randomised trial. *Lancet*, Vol.359, No.9324, pp. 2131-2139

Bollag, G.; Hirth, P. et al. (2010). Clinical efficacy of a RAF inhibitor needs broad target blockade in BRAF-mutant melanoma. *Nature*, Vol.467, No.7315, pp. 596-599

Buchdunger, E.; Zimmermann, J. et al. (1996). Inhibition of the Abl protein-tyrosine kinase in vitro and in vivo by a 2-phenylaminopyrimidine derivative. *Cancer research,* Vol.56, No.1, pp. 100-104

Cadranel, J.; Zalcman, G. et al. (2011). Genetic profiling and epidermal growth factor receptor-directed therapy in nonsmall cell lung cancer. *The European respiratory journal: official journal of the European Society for Clinical Respiratory Physiology,* Vol.37, No.1, pp. 183-193

Caponigro, G. & Sellers, W. R. (2011). Advances in the preclinical testing of cancer therapeutic hypotheses. Nature reviews. *Drug discovery,* Vol.10, No.3, pp. 179-187

Carmeliet, P. ; Lampugnani, M. G. et al. (1999). Targeted deficiency or cytosolic truncation of the VE-cadherin gene in mice impairs VEGF-mediated endothelial survival and angiogenesis. *Cell,* Vol.98, No.2, pp. 147-157

Chabner, B. A. & Roberts, T. G. Jr. (2005). Timeline: Chemotherapy and the war on cancer. Nature reviews. *Cancer,* Vol.5, No.1, pp. 65-72

Drexler, H. G. & Macleod, R. A. (2010). History of leukemia-lymphoma cell lines. *Human cell: official journal of Human Cell Research Society,* Vol.23, No.3, pp. 75-82

Fremin, C. & Meloche, S. (2010). From basic research to clinical development of MEK1/2 inhibitors for cancer therapy. *Journal of Hematology & Oncology,* Vol.3, No.8, pp. 1-11

Gilman, A. & Philips, F. S. (1946). The Biological Actions and Therapeutic Applications of the B-Chloroethyl Amines and Sulfides. *Science,* Vol.103, No.2675, pp. 409-436

Greenberg, D.; Earle, C. et al. (2010). When is cancer care cost-effective? A systematic overview of cost-utility analyses in oncology. *Journal of the National Cancer Institute,* Vol.102, No.2, pp. 82-88

Hackam, D. G. & Redelmeier, D. A. (2006). Translation of research evidence from animals to humans. *JAMA: the journal of the American Medical Association,* Vol.296, No.14, pp. 1731-1732

Hait, W. N. (2010). Anticancer drug development: the grand challenges. *Nature reviews. Drug discovery,* Vol.9, No.4, pp. 253-254

Hartmann, R. W.; Ehmer, P. B. et al. (2002). Inhibition of CYP 17, a new strategy for the treatment of prostate cancer. *Archiv der Pharmazie,* Vol.335, No.4, pp. 119-128

Hartung, T. (2009). Toxicology for the twenty-first century. *Nature,* Vol.460, No.7252, pp. 208-212

Heidelberger, C.; Chaudhuri, N. K. et al. (1957). Fluorinated pyrimidines, a new class of tumour-inhibitory compounds. *Nature,* Vol.179, No.4561, pp. 663-666

Jemal, A.; Bray, F. et al. (2011). Global cancer statistics. *CA: a cancer journal for clinicians,* Vol.61, No.2, pp. 69-90

Jockenhoevel, S.; Chalabi, K. et al. (2001). Tissue engineering: complete autologous valve conduit--a new moulding technique. *The Thoracic and cardiovascular surgeon,* Vol.49, No.5, pp. 287-290

Jockenhoevel, S.; Zund, G. et al. (2001). Fibrin gel -- advantages of a new scaffold in cardiovascular tissue engineering. *European journal of cardio-thoracic surgery: official journal of the European Association for Cardio-thoracic Surgery,* Vol.19, No.4, pp. 424-430

Kalluri, R. & Zeisberg M. (2006). Fibroblasts in cancer. *Nat Rev Cancer,* Vol.6, No.5, pp. 392-401

Kamb, A. (2005). What's wrong with our cancer models? *Nature reviews. Drug discovery,* Vol.4, No.2, pp. 161-165

Kolokythas, P.; Aust, M. C. et al. (2008). [Dermal subsitute with the collagen-elastin matrix Matriderm in burn injuries: a comprehensive review]. *Handchirurgie, Mikrochirurgie, plastische Chirurgie: Organ der Deutschsprachigen Arbeitsgemeinschaft für Handchirurgie: Organ der Deutschsprachigen Arbeitsgemeinschaft fur Mikrochirurgie der*

Peripheren Nerven und Gefässe: Organ der Vereinigung der Deutschen Plastischen Chirurgen, Vol.40, No.6, pp. 367-371

Lavik, E. & Langer, R. (2004). Tissue engineering: current state and perspectives. *Applied microbiology and biotechnology*, Vol.65, No.1, pp. 1-8

Mertsching, H.; Schanz, J. et al. (2009). Generation and transplantation of an autologous vascularized bioartificial human tissue. *Transplantation,* Vol.88, No.2, pp. 203-210

Mertsching, H.; Walles, T. et al. (2005). Engineering of a vascularized scaffold for artificial tissue and organ generation. *Biomaterials*, Vol.26, No.33, pp. 6610-6617

Mertsching, H.; Weimer, M. et al. (2008). Human skin equivalent as an alternative to animal testing. *GMS Krankenhaushygiene interdisziplinar*, Vol. 3, No.1, Doc11

Micke, P. & Ostman, A. (2004). Tumour-stroma interaction: cancer-associated fibroblasts as novel targets in anti-cancer therapy? *Lung cancer*, Vol.45, Suppl.2, pp. S163-175

Olson, H.; Betton, G. et al. (2000). Concordance of the toxicity of pharmaceuticals in humans and in animals. *Regulatory toxicology and pharmacology: RTP*, Vol.32, No.1, pp. 56-67

Reid, A. H.; Attard, G. et al. (2010). Significant and sustained antitumor activity in post-docetaxel, castration-resistant prostate cancer with the CYP17 inhibitor abiraterone acetate. *Journal of clinical oncology: official journal of the American Society of Clinical Oncology*, Vol.28, No.9, pp. 1489-1495

Roberts, T. G. Jr.; Goulart, B. H. et al. (2004). Trends in the risks and benefits to patients with cancer participating in phase 1 clinical trials. *JAMA: the journal of the American Medical Association*, Vol.292, No.17, pp. 2130-2140

Schanz, J.; Pusch, J.; Hansmann, J. & Walles H. (2010). Vascularised human tissue models: a new approach for the refinement of biomedical research. *Journal of Biotechnology*, Vol.148, No.1, pp. 56-63

Schardein, J. L.; Schwetz, B. A. et al. (1985). Species sensitivities and prediction of teratogenic potential. *Environmental health perspectives,* Vol.61, pp. 55-67

Schilsky, R. L. (2010). Personalized medicine in oncology: the future is now. Nature reviews. *Drug discovery,* Vol.9, No.5, pp. 363-366

Shoemaker, R. H. (2006). The NCI60 human tumour cell line anticancer drug screen. Nature reviews. *Cancer,* Vol.6, No.10, pp. 813-823

Stock, U. A. & Vacanti, J. P. (2001). Tissue engineering: current state and prospects. *Annual review of medicine,* Vol.52, pp. 443-451

Sundberg, S. A. (2000). High-throughput and ultra-high-throughput screening: solution- and cell-based approaches. *Current opinion in biotechnology*, Vol.11, No.1, pp. 47-53

Todaro, M.; Francipane, M. G. et al. (2010). Colon cancer stem cells: promise of targeted therapy. *Gastroenterology*, Vol.138, No.6, pp. 2151-2162

Vogel, C. L.; Cobleigh, M. A. et al. (2002). Efficacy and safety of trastuzumab as a single agent in first-line treatment of HER2-overexpressing metastatic breast cancer. *Journal of clinical oncology: official journal of the American Society of Clinical Oncology,* Vol.20, No.3, pp. 719-726

Walles, T.; Weimer, M. et al. (2007). The potential of bioartificial tissues in oncology research and treatment. *Onkologie*, Vol.30, No.7, pp. 388-394

Wasik, M. (2011). Investigations of the differentiation of A549 lung carcinoma cells on a 3D collagen scaffold: a basis for the development of a tumor test system. Bachelor thesis. Wuerzburg, Germany

Weinberg, R. A. (2006). The Biology of Cancer. *Garland Science*. ISBN 0-8153-4076-1

Zhou, Y.; Rideout, W. M. et al. (2010). Chimeric mouse tumor models reveal differences in pathway activation between ERBB family- and KRAS-dependent lung adenocarcinomas. *Nature biotechnology*, Vol.28, No.1, pp. 71-78

9

Mathematical Modeling in Rehabilitation of Cleft Lip and Palate

Martha R. Ortiz-Posadas[1] and Leticia Vega-Alvarado[2]
[1]Electrical Engineering Department. Universidad Autónoma Metropolitana-Iztapalapa
[2]Centro de Ciencias Aplicadas y Desarrollo Tecnológico
Universidad Nacional Autónoma de México
México

1. Introduction

Mathematical modeling is the art of translating problems from an application area into tractable mathematical formulations whose theoretical and numerical analysis provides insight, answers, and guidance useful for the originating application. In recent years, mathematicians and medical researchers have combined their individual expertise to study diseases of the human body that are amenable to mathematical analysis. Mathematical models have been proposed in many areas of medicine. Indeed, mathematical modeling in medicine can exist at many scales from cellular processes to the delivery of healthcare. In specific, the importance of discovering the response of a patient to a determined treatment as a feedback for professionals in health care, since it allows them to determine the evolution of the prescribed therapeutics and, where appropriate, to continue or modify treatment.

For patients with cleft lip and palate, it is of great use to have available new models allowing the description of the initial and final condition of them. With this information it is possible to evaluate the evolution of their rehabilitation, which is a process that depends on patient's growth and development, it is a process that depends on time. These patients must be attended by a group of specialists from different areas such as surgery, orthodontics, psychology and speech therapy that form a multidisciplinary cleft lip and palate team, whose objective is to integrally rehabilitate the patients and lead them to normal bio-psychosocial conditions.

For developing a mathematical model of this clinical problem, we selected the logical combinatorial approach of pattern recognition theory which uses analogies (likelihood, similarity, etc.) between the objects (patients). The analogy concept is a fundamental methodological tool to be able to establish the relations between the objects and hence the likelihood that exist among them. The mathematical modeling involves the process of variable selection (which yields a description of the objects under study) and the knowledge of their relative importance (the one such variables have in this case). For this reason, we had to define the variables and their domains, the comparison criteria for each variable and an analogy function, which allows quantifying the similarity between patients (cleft descriptions). Finally we used a partial precedence algorithm called voting algorithm to classify patients under study. The work was developed in a joint collaboration with the multidisciplinary team for cleft lip and palate at the Tacubaya Pediatrics Hospital, which belongs to the Health Institute in Mexico City. The method was tested with a sample of 95 patients cared for by this team at the Reconstructive Surgery Service from this Hospital.

2. The clinical problem: Congenital malformation in the lip and/or palate

The clinical problem consists of congenital malformations in the lip and/or palate, which are called *cleft-primary palate and/or cleft-secondary palate* respectively. Primary palate is formed by the prolabium, the premaxilla, and columella (Kernahan & Stark, 1958). This is the visible part of these kinds of malformations. The secondary palate begins at the incisive foramen and extends posteriorly (Fig. 1). It includes the horizontal portion of the premaxilla, horizontal portion of the palatine bones, and soft palate (Kernahan & Stark, 1958). It is important to say that cleft of the primary palate can be present in a *unilateral* way, left or right, or in a *bilateral* way (Fig. 2). The latter is formed from the combination of two unilateral fissures. Worldwide incidence of these congenital abnormalities is around one per 500-700 of all births; the birth prevalence rate varies substantially across ethnic groups and geographical areas (WHO, 2007). For example, in the USA the prevalence is 6.35/10,000 live births for cleft palate only and 10.63/10,000 live births for cleft lip with or without cleft palate (Parker et al, 2010). In Mexico it is 0.81 per 1000 live born babies (Health Ministry of Mexico, 2008), meaning more than 90 000 cases in this country.

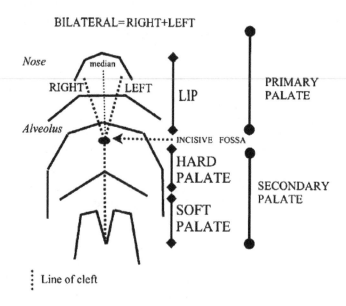

Fig. 1. Schematic representation of the lip and palate (Hodgkinson et al, 2005)

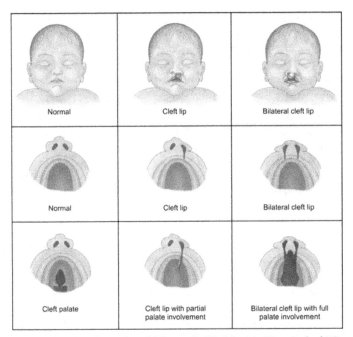

Normal	Cleft lip	Bilateral cleft lip
Normal	Cleft lip	Bilateral cleft lip
Cleft palate	Cleft lip with partial palate involvement	Bilateral cleft lip with full palate involvement

Fig. 2. Cleft lip and palate (unilateral and bilateral) (Children´s Hospital of Wisconsin, 2009)

3. Cleft palate clinical team

The management of patients with cleft lip and palate presents many challenges but also many rewards. In order to do an integral rehabilitation, patients are treated by a multidisciplinary cleft lip and palate team. This is a group of individuals from different specialist backgrounds who work closely together, not only to bring each specialist's particular expertise to the patient in the optimum way, but also to develop an understanding of the requirements and specialist skills of the other team members to enhance the delivery of the total package (Hodgkinson et al, 2005; Sze-Van et al, 2007). The multidisciplinary team encompassing four medical specialties: reconstructive surgery, orthodontics, speech therapy and psychology. These four specialties are described below.

3.1 Reconstructive surgery

Reconstructive surgery is performed on abnormal structures of the body caused by congenital defects, developmental abnormalities, trauma, infection, tumors or disease. It is generally performed to improve functions, but may also be done to approximate a normal appearance. Reconstructive surgery is generally covered by most health insurance policies, although coverage for specific procedures and levels of coverage may vary greatly. In facial surgeries, these can be performed to correct facial defects such as cleft lip, breathing problems, or chronic infections, such as those that affect the sinuses, or even snoring.

Closure of the cleft in the lip and palate requires a surgical procedure. There are a variety of surgical techniques and timings. Any surgical protocol has to satisfy several apparently contradictory requirements: 1) Cosmetic restoration of a normal appearance to the patient at an appropriate time. 2) Functional restoration of the lip and particularly the palate to provide normal eating and drinking, and produce a functionally adequate palate to allow the development of normal speech. 3) Optimum facial growth and development to prevent deformity developing in association with impaired growth.

Surgical closure of a cleft lip is performed as early in infancy as is compatible with a good long-term result; the contemporary consensus being 10 to 12 weeks of age. Correcting the lip earlier than this (immediately after birth) offers psychological advantages to the family and was briefly popular in the 1960s. However, it entails a greater risk of surgical morbidity and maxillary growth retardation, and the long-term esthetic results tend not to be unsatisfactory. Moreover, after 10 to 12 weeks other problems are more likely to be identified (if they exist), and the immune system is better developed to cope with infection (Witzel MA et al, 1984).

3.2 Ortodonthics

Orthodontic treatment (alignment of the teeth and their underlying supporting structures) can be used to intervene at almost any age from birth to teenage years, but the orthodontic cleft specialist must be cognizant of the burden of care for these patients. Examination of facial balance and proportions is essential in determining a treatment plan that combines surgery and orthodontics (Friede H et al, 1986; Semb G, 1991). Figure 3 shows some measures that are considered for orthodontic treatment. Primary surgery for cleft lip and palate is only the beginning of management for this condition; any congenital malformation and scars of corrective surgery during infancy affect physiological development of the skeleton and soft tissues, which gives rise to varying degrees of maxillary underdevelopment. The degree of maxillomandibular discrepancy determines the ultimate treatment plan. If the skeletal discrepancy is mild and esthetic concerns are minimal, dental compensation by orthodontic treatment alone may resolve the malocclusion. Alterations in the axial inclination of the teeth may adequately camouflage the skeletal relationship. In cases where the skeletal discrepancy is beyond the envelope of orthodontic camouflage or when an individual is suspected to outgrow the dental correction, orthognathic surgery may eventually become necessary to achieve normal occlusion. The most frequent skeletal malformations in secondary palate are hypoplasia and malposition in the three planes of the superior maxilla space. In these cases, combined orthodontic and surgical treatment is necessary (Keer WJ et al, 1992; Stellzig – Eisenhauer A et al, 2002).

3.3 Speech therapy

Children born with cleft lip and cleft palate may have problems in developing speech and language skills. It was reported that 25% developed normal speech spontaneously and 75% required episodes of speech and language therapy (Witzel, 1991). After cleft palate repair, all patients are referred to the speech therapists for speech evaluation. The speech and language therapists will evaluate the patient's ability to understand and use language and his speech resonance (oral and nasal tone quality). Most children with cleft lip and/or palate are slower in developing consonant sounds and in learning to talk. Speech therapy entails: teaching blowing skills, maintaining intraoral pressure, foster muscle training, stimulating speech development and the prevention of undesirable compensatory articulations. Formal training starts around 2 to 3 years of age.

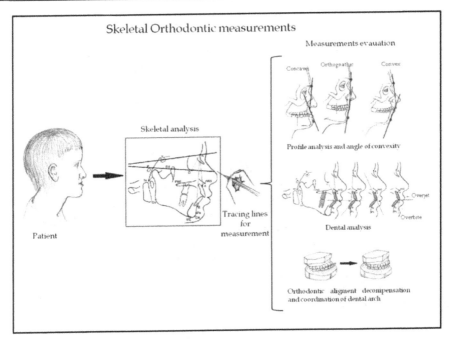

Fig. 3. An overview of orthodontic evaluation.

The speech and language therapist with the cleft team will contribute to assessment, diagnosis and treatment planning for children requiring further surgery for velopharyngeal insufficiency affecting speech outcome and symptomatic palatal fistulae. In addition, assessment is required for older children and adults who require maxillary advancement and those needing prosthetic management of velopharyngeal insufficiency where surgery is contraindicated (Fox VA et al, 2002).

3.4 Psychology

Parents are often very shocked when they learn their child has a facial disfigurement. They need reassurance, support and time to assimilate the information. In this sense, the psychological care of the patient with a cleft begins at the time of diagnosis, even if this is before birth. With more involvement of specialist psychologists within cleft teams the importance of this is becoming increasingly apparent.

Taking a lifespan perspective, the earliest interventions that may help to improve social competence and reduce distress begin in the perinatal stages of care when working with parents and significant family members. The next stage of opportunities for interventions arises as the child begins to function within the family and within external systems such as school and peer groups. As the child matures and faces the task of individuation from the family, there may be a need for psychological work. Lastly, adulthood provides its own set of challenges to the individual and there is potential for further psychological interventions throughout this period of life. While some of the psychological needs of patients and their families will require the knowledge and expertise of a clinical psychologist, many needs can be met by ensuring psychological thinking and planning takes place at all levels of care.

Although there has been an assumption that parents find it harder to bond with a baby with a facial disfigurement (Pruzinsky T, 1992; Langlois J, 1995), there is growing evidence that babies born with a cleft are not at particular risk of developing an insecure attachment (Coy K et al, 2002; Pelchat D et al, 2003). Indeed, forming a secure attachment to the parent may be one of the factors that helps buffer the child with a cleft. Hence it is the role of the cleft lip and palate team to try to facilitate secure infant attachments.

4. Introduction to the logical-combinatorial approach

In order to develop a mathematical model of this clinical problem, we selected the logical combinatorial approach of pattern recognition (Martínez-Trinidad & Guzman-Arenas, 2001). This approach works with the descriptions of the objects in terms of a combination of quantitative and qualitative variables. Variables can be processed by numeric functions in a differential manner, depending on their nature. Furthermore, it gives the possibility of "absent information" in some feature values in the objects descriptions. For classifying objects, there are several classification algorithms based on the concept of partial precedence, that is, partial analogies: an object can be alike to another object not in its totality. Those parts which do alike each other, can give information about possible regularities; of course not all of the same magnitude. These characteristics are suitable to model classification problems in medicine and that is why we selected this approach. The mathematical model is described below.

4.1 Mathematical model

Let U be a universe of objects, and let us consider a given finite sample $O = \{O1, . . ., Om\}$ of such (descriptions of the) objects. We shall denote by $X= \{x_1, . . ., x_n\}$ the set of features or variables used to study these objects. Each of these variables has associated a set of admissible values (its domain) $M_i = \{m_{i1}, m_{i2}, . . .\}\cup\{*\}$. Over M_i no algebraic, topologic or logic structure is assumed. These sets of values, in contrast to the other approaches, can be of any nature: variables can be quantitative and qualitative simultaneously. Each of these sets also contains a special symbol (*) denoting absence of information (missing data). Thus, incomplete information about some objects is allowed. This will turn out to be a fundamental feature of this pattern recognition paradigm. By a description of an object O we understand an n-tuple $I(O)=(x_1(O),... , x_n(O))$.

Let $C = \{C_1, ..., C_n\}$ be a set of functions called comparison criteria for each variable $x_i \in X$ defined as the Cartesian product of variable domain such as: $C_i: M_i \times M_i \rightarrow \Delta_i$; $i=1, . . ., n$ where Δ_i can be of any nature; it is an ordered set and can be finite or infinite. Comparison criteria can denote similarity or difference between two different values of the same variable x_i. The characteristics of each comparison criterion (C_i) depend on the problem that has been modeled. However, it is important to remark that every C_i is designed individually to reflect the nature and interpretation of each feature x_i. In this sense, the set C allows differentiation and non-uniform treatment of the features that describe the objects. Furthermore, it gives also the possibility of "absent information" in some feature values in the objects descriptions. It is important to mention that all comparison criteria must be defined jointly with the expert in order to incorporate his/her expertise in the problem modeling. In the context of medicine problems, the experts will be the physicians, surgeons, etc. with their knowledge and expertise, with the ability to provide the entire criterion about medical problem modeling (Martínez-Trinidad & Guzman-Arenas, 2001).

In general, medical problems imply a supervised classification problem, which consists in to recognize, given a set of objects grouped into classes, in which one (or more than one) of these classes, new objects belong. In this kind of problems, we assume that the universe **U** is structured in a finite number $K_1,\ldots,K_r$ of proper subsets, called classes, and from each of them we have a sample of descriptions of objects, the so-called training matrix TM={$K_1 \cup \ldots \cup K_r$}. The problem is to find the membership relations from a new object from **U** (outside the given samples) with the r classes. This relationship does not have to be all or nothing.

The logical combinatorial approach deals with spaces without algebraic (or of any other kind of) structure. The representation space is simply a Cartesian product, which also has the peculiarity of being heterogeneous, that is, each of the sets forming it can be of different nature: a set of real numbers, a set of labels, a set of truth values from a given logic, etc. An example of this appears in medical diagnosis problems, where descriptions take the form I(O)=(black, female, 45, 38.63, 1500, *, slight, 2), where * means absence of information. That is, objects are described in terms of qualitative and quantitative variables. Thus, the tools herein presented. Most significant algorithms of supervised classification in the logical combinatorial approach are those works based on partial precedence. As follows we describe the voting algorithm.

4.1.1 Voting algorithm

This algorithm comprising six steps: (1) defining the system of support sets; (2) defining the similarity function; (3) row evaluation, given a fixed support set; (4) class evaluation for a fixed support set; (5) class evaluation for all the system of support sets, and (6) resolution rule. Thus, to define a voting algorithm, is to define a set of parameters for each of the above six steps.

A support set is a non-empty subset $\omega = \{x_{i1},\ldots, x_{is}\}$ of features which shall be used to analyze the objects. We denote as ωO the sub-description in terms of the features of ω. Thus, a system of support sets denoted by Ω are several support sets which together will allow analysis of the objects to be classified, comparing them with objects in each one of the classes K_i, i=1, …, r. Note that said analysis is done paying attention to different parts or sub-descriptions of the objects, and not analyzing the complete descriptions. Examples of systems of support sets are combinations of variables with a fixed cardinality, the power set of features, etc.

The analogy between two objects is formalized by means of the concept of similarity function β. This function is based on the comparison criterion C_i generated for each variable x_i. It is important to mention that the similarity function can evaluate the similarity or difference between two objects, i.e., between their descriptions. $\beta(I(Oi), I(O_j))$ is defined by:

$$\beta((C_1(x_1(O_i), x_1(O_j)), \ldots, C_n(x_n(O_i), x_n(O_j))))$$

Let β_ω be a partial similarity function defined by: $\beta_\omega(I(O_i), I(O)) = \sum_{x_t \in \omega} \rho_t C_t(x_t(O_i), x_t(O))$, where ω represents a support set and ρ_t is the relevance parameter associated to each variable x_t defined by the expert.

When the systems of support sets and the similarity function have been defined, the voting process starts in the stage of row evaluation; that is, the similarity between the different parts (support sets) of the objects already classified and those to be classified is analyzed. Each row of TM (each object $O_i \in TM$) is compared with object O to be classified using the partial similarity function $\beta\omega$. This evaluation is a function of the similarity values among the different parts (support set) being compared. An example of this evaluation is:

$$\Gamma_\omega(O_i, O) = \rho(O_i)\rho(\omega)\beta(\omega I(O_i), \omega I(O))$$

Where $\rho(Oi)$ is the weight of the object Oi from TM, $\rho(\omega)$ is the weight of the support set ω and $\beta(\omega I(Op), \omega I(O))$ is the similarity value of the compared objects.

The class evaluation for a fixed support set ω consists in totaling the evaluations obtained for each of the objects TA with respect to the object O to be classified. This total evaluation is a function of the row evaluations already obtained. An example of this evaluation is:

$\Gamma_\omega^j(O) = \frac{1}{|K_j|}\Sigma_{t=1,...,|K_j|} \Gamma_\omega(O_i, O)$. The upper index refers to the class K_j.

In class evaluation for all the system of support sets, evaluations are totaled for all the system of support sets. Following our example, this step could be expressed as follows:

$$\Gamma_j(O) = \frac{1}{|\Omega|} \sum_{\omega \in \Omega} \Gamma_\omega^j(O)$$

Finally, the resolution rule is a function that establishes a criterion taking into account each voting thus obtained, and reaches a decision concerning the relations of the object to be classified with every class of the posed problem.

5. Mathematical modeling of the clinical problem

5.1 Cleft lip and palate mathematical model

5.1.1 Variables and comparison criteria

In order to describe the type of cleft it was necessary to define, in conjunction with the five surgeons team (with an expertise about 20 years in this clinical area), the variables related with the different anatomical structures affected (cleft, lip and nose). In this sense, eighteen variables were defined for cleft description. Comparison criterion for each variable was modeled and all are of difference. That is, the minimum value of its domain means that the compared values are equal (there is no difference), and the maximum value means that the compared values are different (Ortiz-Posadas et al, 2009).

Cleft. For describing cleft, two variables were defined,: 1) primary palate, and; 2) secondary palate. The variables (x_i), their domain (M_i) and the comparison criterion (C_i) are shown in Table 1. These malformations can have different characteristics with a direct consequence on surgical complexity. For this reason it was necessary to assign a relevance parameter (ρ) to the different clefts. For primary palate it was $\rho=0.65$ and for secondary palate $\rho=0.35$, this parameter clearly means that primary palate (the visible part) is more important than the second one. By the other hand, primary palate can take values into the interval [0, 100] and secondary palate into [0, 55]. Likewise, comparison criteria were defined as the absolute difference of the compared values divided by 100 (or 55) depending on the considered variable. This division is done with the objective to limit the result into [0, 1].

x_i	ρ_i	M_i	C_i
x_1. Primary palate (left and/or right)	0	Normal	
	1	Microform	
	3	Incomplete 1/3	
	6	Incomplete 2/3	$C_i = \dfrac{|x-y|}{100}$
	12	Complete with contact of segments	
	$12(1+m\times10^{-1})$ (m: milimeters)	Complete without contact of segments	
x_2. Secondary palate (left and/or right)	0	Normal	
	1	Submucous without bifid uvula (soft palate)	
	4	Submucous with bifid uvula (soft palate)	
	8	Incomplete 1/3 central (soft palate)	
	13	Incomplete 2/3 unilateral (soft palate + one palatal shelf)	
	14	Incomplete 2/3 bilateral (soft palate + both palatal shelves)	$C_i = \dfrac{|x-y|}{55}$
	25	Complete grade I unilateral	
	27	Incomplete 2/3 + Complete grade I	
	28	Complete grade I bilateral	
	34	Complete grade II unilateral	
	36	Incomplete 2/3 + Complete grade II	
	37	Complete grade II bilateral	
	50	Complete grade III unilateral	
	53	Incomplete 2/3 + Complete grade III	
	55	Complete grade III bilateral	

Table 1. Cleft variables, domain, relevance parameter and comparison criteria.

Lip. In this case 9 variables were defined. All these variables have the same 4-valued domain: yes, almost (less than optimal), barely (more deficient) and no. Their comparison criterion are of the fuzzy type, with a homogeneous scale, or rather, the difference between two consecutive values is equivalent (according to the surgeons team), and it is represented by a comparison matrix (Table 2). Notice that this matrix displays two important characteristics: 1) The main diagonal is equal to zero because there is no difference when equal values are compared; and 2) this matrix is symmetric. By the other side, all the variables considered do not have the same importance for the surgeon. Hence informational importance (relevance) was assigned by a relevance parameter (ρ_i) to each of them with the support of the clinical model, the specialist experience and the type of fissure. These variables are useful for evaluating the initial condition of the patient lip (before surgery), as well as after any surgical procedure.

x_i	ρ_i	M_i	C_i				
x_3. Symetry of lip height	0.16						
x_4. Normal lip height	0.15			yes	almost	barely	no
x_5. Muscular integrity	0.14	yes	yes	0	0.33	0.66	1.0
x_6. Skin integrity	0.15	almost	almost		0	0.33	0.66
x_7. Mucous membrane integrity	0.08	barely	barely			0	0.33
x_8. Symmetry of lip thickness	0.12	no	no				0
x_9. Symmetry of philtral ridges	0.10						
x_{10}. Normal sulcus depth	0.05						
x_{11}. Presence of cupid arch	0.05						

Table 2. Domain, comparison criteria and relevance parameter (r) for lip variables

Nose. In this case, seven variables with different domain were defined, as well as three different fuzzy comparison criteria (Table 3). In the same manner as in the lip, each criterion has a homogeneous scale and it is represented by a comparison matrix. These variables are useful for evaluating the initial condition of the patient nose, as well as after any surgical procedure

Variables of cleft-primary palate and cleft-secondary palate jointly with lip and nose variables define the initial space representation (ISR). With this set of variables it was possible to incorporate elements that are not considered in other approaches and allows to more fully describing the clefts.

5.1.2 Similarity function for cleft palate

This similarity function was defined taking into account the partial similarity related with the different structures considered in cleft evaluation. In this sense, three support sets were defined: the first, formed by the cleft variables set; the second, by the lip variables set, and the third, by the nose variables set.

Definition 1. Let $\Omega = \{\omega_{cleft}, \omega_{lip}, \omega_{nose}\}$ be the system of support sets for cleft lip and palate. Where $\omega_{cleft} = \{x_1, x_2\}$, $\omega_{lip} = \{x_3,..., x_{11}\}$ and $\omega_{nose} = \{x_{12},..., x_{18}\}$.

Definition 2. Let β_{cleft} the partial similarity function for cleft defined by:

$$\beta_{cleft}\left(I(P_i), I(P_j)\right) = 1 - \sum_{t=1}^{2} \rho_t C_t\left(x_t(P_i), x_t(P_j)\right) \tag{1}$$

Definition 3. Let β_{lip} the partial similarity function for lip, defined by:

$$\beta_{lip}\left(I(P_i), I(P_j)\right) = 1 - \sum_{t=3}^{11} \rho_t C_t\left(x_t(P_i), x_t(P_j)\right) \tag{2}$$

x_i	ρ_i	M_i		yes	almost	barely	no
x12. Symmetry of nasal floor	0.17						
x13. Symmetry of nostril archs	0.25	yes	yes	0	0.33	0.66	1
x14. Symmetry of notrils (vertical plane)	0.10	almost	almost		0	0.33	0.66
x15. Symmetry of nostrils (anteroposterior plane)	0.10	barely	barely			0	0.33
x16. Nasal septum deviation	0.11	no	no				0

x_i	ρ_i	M_i		norm	almost	barely	absent
x17 Length of columella	0.15	normal	norm	0	0.33	0.66	1
		almost	almost		0	0.33	0.66
		barely	barely			0	0.33
		absent	absent				0

x_i	ρ_i	M_i		greater	normal	minor
x18 Width of nasal base	0.12	greater	greater	0	0.5	1
		normal	normal		0	0.5
		minor	minor			0

Table 3. Lip variables, relevance parameter, domain and comparison criteria.

Definition 4. Let β_{nose} the partial similarity function for nose, defined by:

$$\beta_{nose}\left(I(P_i),I(P_j)\right) = 1 - \sum_{t=1}^{7} \rho_t C_t \left(x_t(P_i), x_t(P_j)\right) \tag{3}$$

Definition 5. Let β_{TC} the *total* similarity function for cleft lip and palate, defined by:

$$\beta_{TC}\left(I(P_i),I(P_j)\right) = \left(\begin{array}{l} 0.60\left[\beta_{cleft}\left(I(P_i),I(P_j)\right)\right] + \\ \quad +0.20\left[\beta_{lip}\left(I(P_i),I(P_j)\right)\right] + \\ \quad\quad +0.20\left[\beta_{nose}\left(I(P_i),I(P_j)\right)\right] \end{array} \right) \tag{4}$$

Where β_{cleft}, β_{lip}, β_{nose} are the similarity functions corresponding to the affected structures cleft, lip and nose, with a relevance parameter of 0.60, 0.20 y 0.20 respectively.

5.1.3 Evaluation of cleft similarity

To further illustrate the evaluation of cleft similarity, two patients with different clefts were evaluated with the proposed function. As it was mentioned, clefts may be unilateral or bilateral. The latter cannot be considered as the simple union of two unilateral clefts. For evaluating a bilateral one, it is necessary to do the addition of the evaluation of each unilateral cleft and then multiply this result by a 1.5 factor. This factor represents the bilateral condition according to the surgeons. Three patients with different clefts are described by the lip and nose variables and criteria defined (Table 4 and 5), as follows:

Patient 1 (Figure 4): This patient has a left complete cleft of the primary palate with 3mm of separation between the segments. The secondary palate is normal. Cleft evaluation is given by the function defined for complete cleft without contact of segments showed in Table 1 as followed: Evaluation$_{cleft}$ = 12[1 + (M×10-1)] = 12[1 + (3×10-1)] = 12(1.3) = 15.6 ~ 16.

Patient 2 (Figure 5): This patient has a bilateral cleft of the primary palate. The left side is incomplete (one-third), while the right side is complete with 3mm of segment separation. In this case, the cleft evaluation must be done attending each side. Considering Table 1, the score for the left side is 3. The right side is the same as above: 16. Total evaluation for this cleft is given by: Evaluation$_{cleft}$ =[3 (left primary)+16(right primary)]1.5 (bilateral)= 28.5 ~ 29.

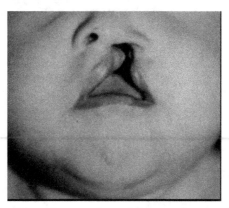

Fig. 4. Left complete cleft of the primary palate with 3mm of separation between the segments. Secondary palate is normal.

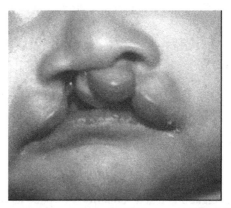

Fig. 5. Bilateral cleft of the primary palate. Left side is incomplete 1/3. Right side is complete with 3mm of segment separation.

Patient 3 (Figure 6): This patient has a grade III bilateral cleft of the secondary palate and a normal primary palate. The evaluation of the primary palate is 0. The evaluation of the secondary palate is obtained directly from Table 1. Therefore, Evaluation$_{cleft}$= 55.

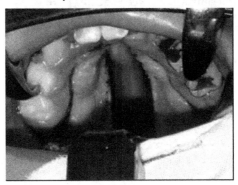

Fig. 6. Bilateral cleft of the secondary palate grade III with a normal primary palate.

	Cleft						Lip				
	x_1	x_2	x_3	x_4	x_5	x_6	x_7	x_8	x_9	x_{10}	x_{11}
P_1	16	0	no	no	no	no	no	no	no	no	no
P_2	29	0	no	no	no	no	no	no	no	no	no
P_3	0	55	yes	yes	yes	yes	yes	yes	yes	yes	yes

Table 4. Complete description of the cleft/lip of the three patients.

	Cleft					Nose			
	x_1	x_2	x_{12}	x_{13}	x_{14}	x_{15}	x_{16}	x_{17}	x_{18}
P_1	16	0	no	no	no	no	barely	barely	barely
P_2	29	0	no	barely	no	barely	no	absent	greater
P_3	0	55	yes	yes	yes	yes	yes	normal	normal

Table 5. Complete description of the cleft/nose of the three patients.

Cleft similarity. Using equation (1) and considering the cleft description of patients P_1 and P_2 (Table 4), the similarity result is given by:

$$\beta_{cleft}(I(P_1), I(P_2)) = 1 - \left[0.65\left(\left|\frac{x-y}{100}\right|\right) + 0.35\left(\left|\frac{x-y}{55}\right|\right)\right] = 1 - \left[0.65\left(\left|\frac{16-29}{100}\right|\right) + 0.35\left(\left|\frac{0-0}{55}\right|\right)\right]$$

$$\beta_{cleft}(I(P_1), I(P_2)) = 1 - [0.65(0.13)] = 1 - 0.085 \approx 0.92$$

Lip similarity. Using equation (2) and considering lip description of patients P_1 and P_2 (Table 4), the similarity result is given by:

$$\beta_{lip}(I(P_1), I(P_2)) = 1 - \left[\begin{matrix}0.16(0) + 0.15(0) + 0.14(0) + 0.15(0) + 0.08(0) \\ +0.12(0) + 0.10(0) + 0.05(0) + 0.05(0)\end{matrix}\right] = 1$$

Nose similarity. Using equation (3) and taking into account nose description of patients P_1 and P_2 (Table 5), the similarity result is given by:

$$\beta_{nose}\big(I(P_1), I(P_2)\big) = 1 - \begin{bmatrix} 0.17(0) + 0.25(0.33) + 0.10(0) + 0.10(0.33) + 0.11(0.33) \\ +0.15(0.33) + 0.12(0) \end{bmatrix} \simeq 0.84$$

Using equation (4) the total similarity between patients P_1 and P_2 is given by:

$$\beta_{TC}\big(I(P_1), I(P_2)\big) = [0.60(0.92) + 0.20(1) + 0.20(0.84)] \simeq 0.93$$

The total similarity between patients (P_1, P_3) y (P_2, P_3) was calculated in the same form as in the case showed above. These total similarities are given by:

$$\beta_{TC}\big(I(P_1), I(P_3)\big) = [0.60(0.55) + 0.20(0) + 0.20(0.15)] \simeq 0.36$$

$$\beta_{TC}\big(I(P_2), I(P_2)\big) = [0.60(0.47) + 0.20(0) + 0.20(0.15)] \simeq 0.31$$

The similarity found in the case of patients 1 and 2 clearly reflect that there is a great likelihood between them. This is clear because both present a cleft in the primary palate (palate, lips and nose). Notice in the case of the lips, that the likelihood resulted 1 because of the fact that it is a structure affected by the cleft, the description of the lips of the patients is identical. In the case of the nose even though, evidently, the deformation is larger in patient 2 because we are dealing with a bilateral cleft, the nose in both cases is deformed, hence, the likelihood between noses turned out to be high (>0.8).

In the case of the cleft of patient 3, since it occurs on the secondary palate, it means that the lip and the nose have a normal condition and, thus, the likelihood in this structures with patients 1 and 2 is null ($\beta = 0$) and, therefore, the full likelihood between patient 3 and the other two is low. As we mention, these three patients were evaluated in order to illustrate the proposed similarity function.

5.2 Orthodontics mathematical model

5.2.1 Variables and comparison criteria

A set of 12 variables were defined for bilateral clefts description and just a subset of 9 of them were considered for the unilateral fissures. These 12 variables with their respective domains, were defined taking into account the condition of the maxilla, premaxilla, mandible and the patient's bite (Table 6). Dental malocclusion can be produced through maxillary retrusion or mandibular protusion. The segments (bones that form the premaxilla) are evaluated in terms of their contact. Maxillary collapse can be present unilaterally (left or right) or anteroposterior. Dental occlusion and overbite are related to the bite on different planes. The condition of the premaxilla is also evaluated on three different planes (see variables 10–12): that is, whether it is protrusive or retrusive, deviated, or if there is some discrepancy in the vertical plane (Ortiz-Posadas et al, 2004).

Likewise, the domain of each of the variables was defined: malocclusion takes only the two logical values "yes" or "no". Segment contact is evaluated in terms of the millimeters of separation in the interval [0, 30] mm. The domain of the maxillary collapse variable is 4-valent (no, barely, moderate, severe). The dental occlusion variable can take the three Angle classification values (C1, C2 and C3). In the case of overbite, its domain is defined in the interval [20, 6] mm. The premaxillary variable has three domains, depending on the plane that is being evaluated: bivalent (central or deviated), trivalent (normal, protrusive and retrusive) and the interval [10, 10] mm. It should be mentioned that not all the variables are evaluated in all cleft palates. This will depend on the characteristics of the fissure in terms of whether it is unilateral or bilateral, as will be seen later.

x_i	M_i	C_i
1. Malocclusion by maxillary retrusion	Yes, no	<table><tr><td></td><td>yes</td><td>no</td></tr><tr><td>yes</td><td>0</td><td>1</td></tr><tr><td>no</td><td></td><td>0</td></tr></table>
2. Malocclusion by protrusive mandible	Yes, no	
3. Contact of the segments	[-30,0] mm	$\begin{cases} 0 & si\ |x-y| \le 1 \\ |x-y|/20 & si\ 1 < |x-y| \le 20 \\ 1 & si\ |x-y| > 20 \end{cases}$
4, 5, 6. Collapse of the maxillary (left, right and antero-posterior)	no (N), barely (B), moderate (M) severe (S)	<table><tr><td></td><td>N</td><td>B</td><td>M</td><td>S</td></tr><tr><td>N</td><td>0</td><td>0.25</td><td>0.57</td><td>1</td></tr><tr><td>B</td><td></td><td>0</td><td>0.32</td><td>0.75</td></tr><tr><td>M</td><td></td><td></td><td>0</td><td>0.43</td></tr><tr><td>S</td><td></td><td></td><td></td><td>0</td></tr></table>
7. Dental occlusion	Angle C1, C2, C3	Boolean
8, 9. Overbite (vertical and horizontal)	[-20,6] mm	$|x-y|/26$
10. Premaxilla (horizontal plane)	normal, protusive, retrude	Boolean
11. Premaxilla (centric)	central, deflect (left, right)	Boolean
12. Premaxilla (vertical discrep)	[-10,10] mm	$|x-y|/20$

Table 6. Variables, domains and comparison criteria for orthodontics

Regarding the comparison criteria defined for each variable, it can be observed that the segment contact, overbite and vertical discrepancy premaxilla variables have the relative difference between two values as their comparison criterion. In particular, for segment contact, if the absolute difference between the values being compared is less or equal than 1, then the values are similar (the result of their comparison is 0). On the opposite, if the difference is greater or equal than 20 mm, then the values are different because the result of comparison is the maximum. As the malocclusion variable is bivalent, it has a Boolean comparison criterion and, in the case of the dental occlusion variable, it can take three independent and non-ordered values, that is, different from one another; that is why the comparison criterion is also Boolean. However, in the case of the maxillary collapse variable, a fuzzy criterion is defined because it does not have a homogeneous scale, or rather; the difference between two consecutive values is not equivalent, according to the criterion of the orthodontist. In the case of overbite, a fuzzy criterion was defined as a result of the absolute difference of values over 26, which is the maximum difference that can arise according to the defined interval. With respect to the premaxilla, a Boolean comparison criterion was defined for its bivalent and trivalent domains. A fuzzy criterion was defined for the interval as a result of the absolute difference of values over 20, which is the maximum difference possible. It must be stressed that the criteria for each of the variables were defined together with the orthodontist, taking into account his/her clinical knowledge and experience.

It should be mentioned that all the variables considered do not have the same importance for the orthodontist. Hence, informational importance (relevance) was assigned to each of them with the support of the clinical model, the specialist experience and the type of fissure. The relevance is shown in Table 7.

Variable	Relevance (ρ)	
	Unilateral cleft	Bilateral cleft
1. Malocclusion by maxillary retrusion	0.10	0.04
2. Malocclusion by protrusive mandible	0.05	0.04
3. Contact of the segments	0.16	0.05
4, 5. Collapse of the maxillary (left, right)	0.20	0.08
6. Collapse of the maxillary (antero-posterior)	0.20	0.09
7. Dental occlusion	0.17	0.07
8. Overbite (vertical)	0.12	0.04
9. Overbite (horizontal)	0.10	0.04
10. Premaxilla (horizontal plane)	Cannot be evaluated	0.10
11. Premaxilla (centric)	Cannot be evaluated	0.10
12. Premaxilla (vertical discrepancy	Cannot be evaluated	0.10

Table 7. Relevance of each variable for orthodontics

5.2.2 Similarity function

The orthodontics similarity function was defined taking into account if there is a unilateral or bilateral cleft. So we defined two functions:

Definition 6. Let $\beta_{U\,orthodontics}$ be the similarity function for unilateral clefts defined by:

$$\beta_{Uorthodontics}\left(I(P_i), I(P_j)\right) = 1 - \frac{\sum_{t=1}^{9} \rho_t C_t\left(x_t(P_i), x_t(P_j)\right)}{1.1} \tag{5}$$

Definition 7. Let $\beta_{B\,orthodontics}$ be the similarity function for bilateral clefts defined by:

$$\beta_{Borthodontics}\left(I(P_i), I(P_j)\right) = 1 - \frac{\sum_{t=1}^{12} \rho_t C_t\left(x_t(P_i), x_t(P_j)\right)}{0.75} \tag{6}$$

5.2.3 Evaluation of orthodontics similarity

To further illustrate the evaluation of the orthodontic similarity, four patients with different clefts were evaluated with the proposed function. The descriptions of the patients are shown in Table 8. The number of each column represents the variable corresponding to Table 5.

Each row is the description of the patient in terms of the domain of each variable. It can be observed that P_1 and P_2 have a similar cleft. For this reason, the expected similarity would be almost the maximum. Patients P_3 and P_4 have very different descriptions, so the expected similarity would be low.

Using Definition 6 and considering patients description, the similarity results are given by:

$$\beta_{Uorthodontics}\big(I(P_1), I(P_2)\big) = 1 - \frac{\left(\begin{array}{c} 0.1(0) + 0.05(0) + 0.16(0) + 0.2(0) + \\ +0.2(0) + 0.17(0) + 0.12(0) + 0.1(0.12) \end{array}\right)}{1.1} = 0.98$$

$$\beta_{Borthodontics}\big(I(P_3), I(P_4)\big) = 1 - \frac{\left(\begin{array}{c} 0.04(1) + 0.04(1) + 0.05(0.1) + 0.08(1) + \\ +0.08(1) + 0.09(1) + +0.07(0.5) + 0.04(0.15) + \\ +0.04(0.19) + 0.1(1) + 0.1(1) + 0.1(0) \end{array}\right)}{0.75} = 0.16$$

It is known that the maximum similarity that can be obtained is equal to 1, and this occurred when comparing two equal fissures (with the same values of the characteristics). In relation to the similarity obtained for patients P_1 and P_2, it can be observed that the similarity was very high, as mentioned earlier. In relation to the similarity for patients P_3 and P_4, it can be observed that the similarity was low. Observe that in both cases, the similarity result was close to the expected one above.

Patient	Variable											
	1	2	3	4	5	6	7	8	9	10	11	12
P_1	yes	no	0	barely	no	barely	C3	-1	-2	cannot be evaluated		
P_2	yes	no	0	barely	no	barely	C3	2	-2	cannot be evaluated		
P_3	no	no	2	no	no	no	C2	2	3	protu	deflected	0
P_4	yes	no	2	barely	barely	barely	C3	0	0	norm	centric	0

Table 8. Four patients described in terms of the orthodontics variables

5.3 Speech mathematical model

To evaluate the speech of these patients, the experts consider two aspects: compensatory articulation and dyslalia. Compensatory articulation is measured through phonemes b, f, p, t, k, ch, s. These are evaluated in specific language (language articulated by repetition) and in spontaneous language (the one spoken naturally). Each one of these phonemes is evaluated as constant, non-constant or omitted. What is evaluated is the number of phonemes with omission or inconstancy in each type of language. We also consider different perturbations in other phonemes, stemming from the variable dyslalia (impairment of the power of speaking, due to a defect of the organs of speech). Eventually, one may consider the result of a nasopharyngeal endoscopy, which measures the velopharyngeal deficiency in a scale of light, moderate and severe. Finally, the variable dysarthria is an exclusion criterion for the patient to receive language therapy, since it represents a neurological problem and no rehabilitation is possible.

5.3.1 Variables and comparison criteria

We defined 5 variables: 1) Omissions in the specific language, 2) Omissions in the spontaneous language, 3) Inconstancies in the specific language, 4) Inconstancies in spontaneous language, and 5) Dyslalia (Ortiz-Posadas MR and Lazo-Cortés MS, 2002). The domain of the first four variables is the set {0, 1, 2, 3, 4, 5, 6, 7} related with the seven evaluated phonemes. The variable dyslalia only takes two possible values (yes/no). We also defined the comparison criteria for each variable. In this case we must calculate the difference in the omissions and inconstancies present in each of the languages. Therefore, the comparison criterion for the phonemes was defined as the absolute difference divided by 7 (the number of phonemes being evaluated). In the case of the variable dyslalia, the criterion is Boolean. (For Boolean criterion form see Table 6, variables x_1 and x_2).

Language	x_i	ρ_i	M_i	C_i
Specific	Omission	0.28	{0, 1, 2, 3, 4, 5, 6, 7}	$|x - y|/7$
	Inconstancy	0.14		
Spontaneous	Omission	0.18	{0, 1, 2, 3, 4, 5, 6, 7}	$|x - y|/7$
	Inconstancy	0.10		
	Dislalia	0.30	yes, no	Boolean

Table 9. Speech variables, domain and comparison criteria

5.3.2 Similarity function

This function allows the comparison between the full descriptions of the languages of two patients. To define the similarity function in this case, it was necessary to change the code in the patient's description. It is important to mention that all phonemes have the same relative importance, so it is irrelevant in which particular phoneme the problem arises. Rather, we detect the total number of omissions and/or inconstancies which the patient displays in every language. We have to stress that if some phoneme is omitted, it is always the case that an inconstancy is present in the same phoneme, but not the inverse. Likewise, if the omissions and/or inconstancies arise in a specific language, they are also present in the spontaneous language. On the other hand, if we start from the domain of these variables {0, 1, ...,7}, the largest number of omissions and inconstancies the patient may display in every language is 7. Considering the elements just mentioned, a change in coding for the patient's description was determined as follows:

- Once each phoneme is evaluated [constant (c), inconstant (i), omission (o)] the amount of phonemes where there were inconstancies is counted in both languages.
- A similar count is recorded for those phonemes where omissions were detected.
- If patient presents a determined number of omissions (which implies a similar number of inconstancies) and a number of inconstancies (in different phonemes from those in which omission was found) to such inconstancies is added the number of omissions. This sum may not be larger than 7.

Example. Let us assume that a patient displays omissions in four phonemes (b, f, p, t) and an inconstancy in phoneme k, evaluated in spontaneous language. He/she displays a total of four omissions and five inconstancies. In specific language he/she displays four omissions and one inconstancy. The patient does not display dyslalia. Changing the codes relative to the initial description, the final description is as shown in Table 10.

Description	Specific L		Spontaneous L		
	o	i	o	i	dyslalia
Initial	(4	1	4	1	0)
Code change	(4	4 + 1	4	4 + 1	0)
Final	**(4**	**5**	**4**	**5**	**0)**

Table 10. Code change of a patient speech description.

Let us now consider the language evaluation of the worst patient (that which displays omissions in all phonemes). For the purpose of code change, we assume that she/he displays inconstancy in all phonemes. In this case, patient is assumed to display dyslalia. The description is shown in Table 11 and final descriptions are shown in Table 12.

	Specific L		Spontaneous L		
	o	i	o	i	dyslalia
Initial	(7	0	7	0	1)
Code change	(7	7 + 0	7	7 + 0	1)
Final	**(7**	**7**	**7**	**7**	**1)**

Table 11. Speech description of worst patient

	Specific L		Spontaneous L		
	o	i	o	i	dyslalia
P_1:	(4	5	4	5	0)
P_2:	(7	7	7	7	1)

Tabla 12. Final speech description of two patients

The speech similarity function was defined taking into account the five variables as follows:

Definition 8. Let β_{speech} be the similarity function for speech defined by:

$$\beta_{speech}(I(P_1), I(P_2)) = 1 - \sum_{k=1}^{5} p_k C_k \left(x_k(P_1), x_k(P_2) \right) \tag{7}$$

5.3.3 Evaluation of speech similarity

Considering both descriptions in Table 11 and using equation (7), similarity between these patients is:

$$\beta_{speech}(I(P_1), I(P_2)) = 1 - \left\{ (0.28)\tfrac{3}{7} + (0.18)\tfrac{3}{7} + (0.14)\tfrac{2}{7} + (0.10)\tfrac{2}{7} + (0.30)1 \right\} \approx 0.44$$

This result clearly reflects that there is a low likelihood between these patients, because language in P_1 is better than in P_2 so, their languages are too different.

5.4 Psychology mathematical model

5.4.1 Variables and comparison criteria

In psychology case, six variables were defined taking into account issues related to patient's home environment: such as grief, a variable related to the shock it has on parents about having a child with a cleft palate; family integration, related to the primary core members of the family (father, mother and children); family dysfunction, with which assesses whether they are meeting the roles of each member of the family; image of the parents, who refers to the perception of parents about their child. Other variables are social integration and self-image, which is directly related to the patient's integration in their social environment (school, family and peer groups) and the perception of himself, respectively.

Likewise, the domain of each variable was defined. Five of the variables take only two logical values: grief (current or sealed), integration family (yes or no), family dysfunction (yes or no), image of the parents (positive or negative) and self-image (positive or negative). The domain of social integration variable is 5-valent (excellent, very good, good, regular and bad). It is noteworthy that some of these variables are evaluated in the initial condition of the patient, i.e., before any treatment. Others may be assessed at any time before or after receiving some treatment and some others can only be assessed after treatment.

Regarding the comparison criteria defined for each variable, as grief, family integration, family dysfunction, image of the parents and self-image variables are bivalent, they have a Boolean comparison criterion (see Table 6). In the case of social integration variable its comparison criterion is of fuzzy type, with a homogeneous scale, or rather, the difference between two consecutive values is equivalent.

It should be mentioned that, as in surgery, orthodontics and language therapy specialties, all the variables considered in psychology do not have the same importance for the psychologist. Hence, informational importance (relevance) was assigned to each of them with the support of the specialist experience. The variables, their domain and the comparison criterion are shown in Table 13.

x_i	ρ_i	M_i	C_i				
1. Grief	0.08	Current or sealed	Boolean				
2. Family integration	0.10	Yes, no	Boolean				
3. Family dysfunction	0.11	Yes, no	Boolean				
4. Image of the parents	0.15	Positive, negative	Boolean				
5. Self-image	0.20	Positive, negative	Boolean				
6. Social integration	0.50	Excellent(E), Very Good(VG) Good(G) Regular(R) Bad(B)		E	VG	G	R	B
			E	0	0.2	0.4	0.8	1
			VG		0	0.2	0.6	0.8
			G			0	0.4	0.6
			R				0	0.2
			B					0

Table 13. Variables, domains, relevance and comparison criteria for psychology

5.4.2 Similarity function

Definition 9. Let β_{Psy} be the similarity function for psychology defined by:

$$\beta_{Psy} = \left(I(P_j), I(P_k)\right) = 1 - \frac{\sum_{i=1}^{6} \rho_i c_i \left(x_i(P_j), x_i(P_k)\right)}{1.14} \tag{8}$$

5.4.3 Evaluation of psychological similarity

To illustrate the evaluation of the similarity function modeled for the psychology specialty, we take the psychological description of the three patients shown in Table 14 and use the equation (8). The similarity result is given by:

$$\beta_{Psy}\left(I(P_1), I(P_2)\right) = 1 - \frac{\left(0.08(0) + 0.1(1) + 0.11(1) + 0.15(0) + 0.2(0) + 0.5(0.4)\right)}{1.14} = 0.64$$

$$\beta_{Psy}\left(I(P_1), I(P_3)\right) = 1 - \frac{\left(0.08(01) + 0.1(1) + 0.11(1) + 0.15(0) + 0.2(1) + 0.5(1.0.4)\right)}{1.14} = 0.13$$

It is clear that the similarity between the first two patients is greater than between P_1 and P_3, since as mentioned the psychological condition of the latter is the worst and when compared with P_1 excellent condition, similarity is obviously minimal. In this sense, the similarity that exists between patients who are located in the same class should be high while the similarity between patients, who are located in very different kinds, should be therefore very low as illustrated.

Patient	Variable					
	1	2	3	4	5	6
P_1	Current	Yes	No	Positive	Positive	Excellent
P_2	Current	No	Yes	Positive	Positive	God
P_3	Sealed	No	Yes	Positive	Negative	Bad

Table 14. Three patients described in terms of the psychologist variables

6. Mathematical model application

Surgical complexity for cleft reconstruction will depend on fissure complexity involving lip, nose and/or palate. Cleft correction translates into a very slow and complex process; because it is related to the growth and development of the patient and it requires least one surgical procedure. The importance of prognosis of the patient's rehabilitation, and subsequent evaluation of the surgical result, is the physician's self-feedback during all the rehabilitation process. The physician will learn if the work patient rehabilitation is adequate, or if it can be improved. This has a direct consequence in the future quality of patient's life.

6.1 Rehabilitation prognosis

The rehabilitation prognosis of patients with cleft palate is carried out by considering the original condition of the patient and taking into account the degree of rehabilitation attained by previous patients cared for in the hospital. Prognosis is conceived as a result from a supervised classification problem, and it uses a training matrix made from: cleft descriptions from patients already finished their rehabilitation, and a classification algorithm (voting algorithm). The training matrix is divided into three post-surgical classes (excellent, very good and good). These classes were determined from the evaluation of each patient's surgical result. These classes provide the expert criterion for evaluation (classification) of the degree of rehabilitation accomplished by the patient. Each patient is prognosticated (classified) by comparing his/her initial description with the initial descriptions of patients already included in the training matrix. The most relevant patients for the prognosis will be those who are most similar to the patient one is about to classify. This means that the prognosis corresponds to the class that includes the patients most similar to the subject that will be classified. In this way, a patient will be predicted as very good if his/her description is most similar to patients from the training matrix that was included in the very good class. In the same way, evaluation of rehabilitation advance is made using the patient's post-surgical description, and applying the expert criteria which defined post-surgical classes mentioned above. The classification will correspond to the patient's rehabilitation advance.

6.2 Data acquisition

The methodology was tested with a sample of 95 patients cared for by the cleft palate team at the reconstructive surgery service of the Pediatric Hospital of Tacubaya, which belongs to the Health Institute of the Federal District in Mexico City. For acquiring patient data we designed a patient's registration form Figs. 7 and 8 given to the surgeons in order to fill it out with the cleft description by the variables defined for.

6.3 Results

With the 95 patient's data two matrices were made: learning and control. The learning matrix consisted of 32 patients, distributed in the following way: 10 in the excellent (E) class, 14 in the very good (VG) class, and 8 in the good (G) class. Similarly, the control matrix consisted of 63 patients: 19 in E, 29 in VG, and 15 in G. The classification was made with patients from the control matrix and the results obtained are shown in Table 15. The diagonal in the table highlights classification successes. Out of 19 patients in the excellent class, the algorithm correctly classified 17 and the remaining two patients were placed in the very good class. Of 29 patients located in the VG class, 26 were properly classified and three were classified as good. For patients in the good class, 14 stayed in this same class and only one was classified as very good. In general, 57 patients were correctly classified.

Class (algorithm) Class (inference)	E	VG	G	Total
Excellent (E)	17	2	0	19
Very good (VG)	0	26	3	29
Good (G)	0	1	14	15
Total	17	29	17	63

Table 15. Classification results for 63 cleft palate patients

However, 63 patients were evaluated with this similarity function for classifying the surgical complexity of their clefts. The efficiency of the similarity function was 90%, according to the complexity defined by the surgeons' team. This means that the similarity function, as well as the cleft description with the 18 variables defined, well modeled the complexity of the unilateral and bilateral clefts according to the surgeons expertise.

Date:	Initial assessment:	Folow-up :
Patient's name:		Birth date:
Phycisian's name:		Exp No.

Primary palate						
Variables	Left			Right		
Incomplete	microform	1/3	2/3	microform	1/3	2/3
Complete	mm			mm		

Secondary palate						
Variables	Left			Right		
Incomplete	1/3		2/3	1/3		2/3
Complete	GI	GII	GIII	GI	GII	GIII
Submucous	Without bifid uvula			With bifid uvula		

Lip				
Variables	Yes	Almost	Barely	No
Symetry of lip height				
Normal lip height				
Muscular integrity				
Skin integrity				
Mucous membrane integrity				
Symmetry of lip thickness				
Normal sulcus depth				
Symmetry of philtral ridges				
Presence of cupid arch				

Nose				
Variables	Yes	Almost	Barely	No
Symmetry of nasal floor				
Symmetry of nostril archs				
Symmetry of notrils (vertical plane)				
Symmetry of nostrils (anteropost plane)				
Nasal septum deviation				
Length of columella	Normal	Almost	Barely	Abscent
Width of nasal base	Greater	Normal	minor	

Fig. 7. Patient's registration form

Orthodontics			
Malocclusion by maxillary retrusion	Yes		No
Malocclusion by protrusive mandible	Yes		No
Contact of the segments	mm		
Collapse of the maxillary	Left	Right	Antero-post
Dental occlusion	C1	C2	C3
Overbite	mm vertical		mm horizontal
Premaxilla (horizontal plane)	Normal	Protusive	Retrude
Premaxilla (centric)	Central	Left deflect	Right deflect
Premaxilla (vertical discrepancy)	mm		
Dentadura type	Decidua	Mixed	Permanent

Speech and language														
Phoneme	B		F		P		T		K		CH		S	
Specific language	o	i	o	i	o	i	o	i	o	i	o	i	o	i
Spontaneous language	o	i	o	i	o	i	o	i	o	i	o	i	o	i
Dyslalia	Yes			No										
Velopharyngeal deficiency	Light			Moderate			Severe							
Nasopharyngeal endoscopy	Date:													

Psychology		
Grief	Current	Sealed
Family integrat	Yes	No
Family dysfunct	Yes	No
Parent´s image	Positive	Negative
Self-image	Positive	Negative
Social integration	E, VG, G, R, B	

Observations

Fig. 8. Patient's registration form

7. Conclusion

In this work we developed a mathematical model that makes possible a full description of cleft lip and palate. In all we defined forty one variables with their domains, and thirteen comparison criterion of different nature (Boolean, fuzzy, absolute difference, etc.). The model includes, further, the importance of every variable as well as a weight which reflects the complexity of the cleft. Likewise we defined a function to evaluate the similarity between the clefts. The usefulness of having one such function is that allows evaluating the likelihood not only of different patients, but of the same patient in different points in time. Compare, for example, her/his original condition with her/his condition after a given surgical procedure, yielding information to the surgeon relative to the change in the patient and, therefore, the effect in her/his rehabilitation from the surgical point of view. Furthermore, it is possible to compare clefts which present themselves in different palates with different characteristics (unilateral, bilateral).

We present relevant applications in the four clinical specialties that form the multidisciplinary cleft lip and palate team, and show that the result of the similarity between patients was very close to the expected one; as well as the application of voting algorithm classifying 63 patients, with an efficiency of 90%.

It is important to mention that the methodology used in the mathematical modeling of the clinical problem, was successfully used in the evaluation of surgical complexity of cleft, orthodontic and psychology condition and in the evaluation of speaking of patients with this kind of malformations. The method has been of great value for the different specialists, since it allows them to make the description of the patient during their rehabilitation, and enables them to compare the change in the patient's status. With this information they have been able to ascertain the efficacy of the therapy applied to their patients. They have the opportunity to modify or continue the therapeutic strategy. Hence, once again, the usefulness of the mentioned approach in problems associated to the medical practice has been shown. The evaluation doing by the Cleft Palate Team (surgeons, orthodontists, speech therapists and psychologists) of the patient with cleft lip or palate provides an integral approach of the patient condition at any time of the rehabilitation.

8. References

Children's Hospital of Wisconsin. Cleft lip and/or palate. Feb 2009, Available from <http://www.chw.org/display/PPF/DocID/35472/Nav/1/router.asp>

Coy K, Spelz M, JonesK. (2002). Facial appearance and attachment in infantswith orofacial clefts: a replication. *Cleft Palate-Craniofac J.* Vol. 39, pp. 66–72.

Fox VA, Dodd B, Howard D. (2002). Risk factors for speech disorders in children. *Int J Lang Commun Dis.* Vol. 37, pp. 117–31.

Friede H, Figueroa AA, Naegele ML, Gould HJ, Kay CN, Aduss H. (1986). Craniofacial growth data for cleft lip patients infancy to 6 years of age: potential applications. *Am J Orthodont.* Vol. 90, pp. 388–409.

Health Ministry of Mexico. (2008). Cleft lip and palate incidence by age. In: *Unique Information System for Epidemiology Vigilance*, May 2011, Available from: <http://www.dgepi.salud.gob.mx/anuario/html/anuarios.html (In Spanish)

Hodgkinson PT, Brown S, Duncan D, Grant C, McNaughton A, Thomas P, Mattick CR. (2005). Management of children with cleft lip and palate: A review describing the application of multidisciplinary team working in this condition based upon the experiences of a regional cleft lip and palate centre in the united Kingdom. *Fetal and Maternal Medicine Review.* Vol. 16, No. 1, pp. 1-27.

Kernahan DA, Stark RB. (1958). A new classification for cleft lip and cleft palate. *Plastic Reconstructive Surgery,* Vol. 22, pp. 435-439.

Kerr WJ, Miller S, Dawber JE. (1992). Class III malocclusion: surgery or orthodontics? *Br J Orthod.* Vol. 19, pp. 21-4.

Langlois J. (1995). Infant attractiveness predicts maternal behaviors and attitudes. *Dev Psychol.* Vol. 31, pp. 464–72.

Martínez-Trinidad JF and Guzmán-Arenas A. (2001). The logical combinatorial approach to pattern recognition, an overview through selected works. *Pattern Recognition,* Vol. 34, pp. 741-751.

Ortiz-Posadas MR and Lazo-Cortés MS. (2002). A Mathematical Model to Evaluate the Speaking of Patients with Cleft Palate. *Proceedings of 2nd European Medical and Biological Engineering Conference.* Vienna Austria, September 2002.

Ortiz-Posadas MR, Vega-Alvarado L and Toni B. (2004). A similarity function to evaluate the orthodontic condition in patients with cleft lip and palate. *Medical Hypotheses,* Vol. 63, No. 1, pp. 35-41.

Ortiz-Posadas MR, Vega-Alvarado L and Toni B. (2009). A Mathematical Function to Evaluate Surgical Complexity of Cleft Lip and Palate. *Computer Methods and Programs in Biomedicine,* Vol. 94, pp. 232-238.

Parker SE, Mai CT, Canfield MA, Rickard R, Wang Y, Meyer RE, Anderson P, Mason CA, Collins JS, Kirby RS, Correa A. (2010). Updated National Birth Prevalence Estimates for Selected Birth Defects in the United States, 2004–2006. *Birth Defects Research Part A: Clinical and Molecular Teratology,* Vol. 88, No. 12 (Dec), pp. 1008-16.

Pelchat D, Bisson J, Bois C, Saucier J. (2003). The effects of early relational antecedents and other factors on the parental sensitivity of mothers and fathers. *Inf Child Dev.* Vol. 12, pp. 27–51.

Pruzinsky T. (1992). Social and psychological effects of major craniofacial deformity. *Cleft Palate-Craniofac J.* Vol. 29, pp. 578–84.

Semb G. (1991). A study of facial growth in patients with unilateral cleft lip and palate treated by the Oslo CLP team. *Cleft Palate Craniofac J.* Vol. 28, pp. 1–21.

Stellzig-Eisenhauer A, Lux CJ, Schuster G. (2002). Treatment decision in adult patients with Class III malocclusion: orthodontic therapy or orthognathic surgery? *Am J Orthod Dentofacial Orthop.* Vol. 122, pp. 27-37.

Sze – Van F, Bendeus M, Wing – Kit R. (2007). A multidisciplinary team approach of cleft lip and palate management. *Hon Kong Dental Journal,* Vol. 4, pp. 38:45.

World Health Organization. (Feb, 2007). Oral Health, Fact sheet No. 318. In: *WHO Media Centre.* June 2011. Available from
<http://www.who.int/mediacentre/factsheets/fs318/en/>

Witzel MA, Salyer KE, Ross RB. (1984). Delayed hard palate closure: the philosophy revisited. *Cleft Palate J.,* Vol. 21, pp. 263-69.

Witzel MA. (1991). Speech evaluation and treatment. *Oral Maxillofacial Surgery Clinical North America,* Vol. 3, pp. 501–516.

10

Stem Cell Research:
A New Era for Reconstructive Surgery

Qingfeng Li[1] and Mei Yang[2]
*[1]Shanghai Jiaotong University, Department of Plastic
and Reconstructive Surgery, Shanghai*
[2]Division of Plastic Surgery, Southern Illinois University School of Medicine, Illinois
[1]China
[2]USA

1. Introduction

Reconstructive Surgery has gained tremendous development due to the emergence of flap techniques, since last century. However, many defects and deformities still cannot be cured satisfactorily, such as severe facial defects, or deformity caused by burns, tumor resection, or trauma. It can be more complicated if the injury involves the loss of bone or cartilage. The allotransplantation of composite tissue has been used for such cases, however, such technique is limited in a lack of source of tissue, complicated surgical process, and severe morbidity left at the donor site. Composite tissue allotransplantation is also regarded as one of the possible resolutions. Nevertheless, immunological rejection, lack of proper donors, and more importantly, psychological rejection, making such transplantation difficult to be a common or routine treatment. [1-6]

The exploration of unlimited tissue engineering sources has been considered to be a promising alternative for such cases. Significant advances have been achieved in this area, especially after various adult stem cells have been found to contribute to the regeneration of various tissues in the body. This chapter begins with an introduction of progress of tissue engineering in plastic surgery. Three types of tissues, which are of specific interest in plastic and reconstructive surgery including skin, cartilage and bone, are addressed in this chapter. Based on these studies, a new concept of "*in vivo* tissue fabrication" is proposed and its clinical perspective in the field of reconstructive surgery is also discussed.

2. Stem cells and skin regeneration

The repair of skin defects resulting from wound, burn or tumor surgery has remained a challenge to clinical surgeons. Autologous skin graft has been the "golden standard" for the replacement of lost skin. However, the source of the skin becomes a problem, especially for patients with large-area burn injury. Moreover, problems, like the morbidity at the donor site, scaring, and the graft failure, also put the doctors in dilemma. Looking for skin substitutes has been a focus in plastic surgery.

Skin is the largest organ of the integumentary system in the body, which plays a key role in protecting the body against pathogens and excessive water loss. Its other functions involves insulation, temperature regulation, and sensation. Normal skin is composed of two primary layers: the epidermis, which provides waterproofing and serves as a barrier to infection, and dermis, which connects with subcutaneous tissue and support the structure of epidermis. Another function of dermis is related with various glands and follicles located in it. Deep damage at dermis level, can not only cause the exposure of deep tissue, but also result in the function damage of the skin.

Skin tissue engineering begins with epidermal cell culture, however, such technique is limited by a fragile texture of the skin, which can be easily torn away from dermis. Moreover, without hair follicles and glands, such cultured skin doesn't have other functions as normal skin either. [1-3] Great development has been achieved in skin engineering with the finding of various stem cells, especially adult stem cells. Mesenchymal stem cells (MSCs), first isolated by Friedenstein et al. in 1966, are multipotent stem cells, which are able to differentiate into adipocytes, osteoblasts, and chondrocytes. [4] They are good source of cell transplantation because of their multi-directional differentiation, easy collection, and weak immunogenicity. It was later found that such heterogeneous group of multipotent progenitor cells can be harvested from several tissues, including bone marrow (BM), adipose tissue, skeletal muscle, fat, (umbilical cord) blood, amniotic fluid, and different fetal tissues. [5] MSCs therapy has provided alternative solutions for the repair and regeneration of various tissues and organs. Many studies have shown that BM-MSCs can promote wound healing by transdifferentiating into skin components. [6, 7] An important role of BM-MSCs has been found in recent study by Yang et al. that BM-MSCs can strengthen cell proliferation, collagen synthesis, vascularization, and growth factor release during skin regeneration. [8] Besides, some recent researches have shown that somatic cells can also be reprogrammed to an embryonic like state. Induced Pluripotent Stem Cells (IPSCs) are one of the examples. By being exposed to a defined set of transcription factors — Oct4, Sox2, Klf4, and c-Myc — and embryonic stem cell culture conditions, a differentiated cell type (e.g., fibroblast) can be reprogrammed to a pluripotent state and are capable of directed differentiation into various tissue types. One of the most exciting findings about these cells is that they can differentiate into a multi-potent keratinocyte lineage capable of forming a fully differentiated epidermis, hair follicles, and sebaceous glands in a reconstituted *in vivo* environment. [9]

Now the cell-based therapy has been further expanded with the use of various synthetic or natural engineered extracellular matrices. It has been reported that such matrices can improve cell survival and functions compared with the injection of isolated cells into the defect sites, by providing cells with suitable microenvironments. Lee et al. [10] dissociated epidermal and dermal cells in high-density suspension and let these cells reconstitute *in vitro* to generate its own matrix. After transplanted with a wound matrix, there cells went through a process similar as embryonic skin development and formed skin with full function. Despite of these encouraging results from the lab, many issues still remain to be settled, like the source of cells especially for those without enough skin on the body, the immune reaction if allogeneic cell source is used, the long *in vitro* expansion time to acquire enough cells, and the directional induced differentiation of stem cell to form a functional skin *in vivo*.

3. Stem cells and bone regeneration

The development of bone tissue engineering has brought great progress in the reconstruction of bone defects. Successful clinical application of tissue engineered bones have been found in various reports from craniofacial reconstruction in areas such as calvarial, orbital, and palatal bone defects to repair of long bone defects in the femur and articular osteochondral defects. [11]

During the early phase of bone tissue engineering, differentiated somatic cells, like osteoblasts from periosteum, have been seeded on a degradable scaffold to generate bone tissue. [12, 13] Such technique was later found to be limited in the source of cells and the morbidity at the donor site. According to the published literature, bone marrow derived mononuclear cells (BM-MNCs), BM-MSCs, adipose derived mesenchymal cells (ADSCs), stem cells from skeletal muscle and the stromal vascular fraction (SVF) have all been proved to have bone regeneration promoting effects and have been used for bone tissue engineering *in vit*ro or *in vivo*. [14-16] However, there is no consensus which type of cells is associated with better bone regeneration potential. Some studies have suggested that the osteogenic potential is similar between BM-MSCs and ADSCs, however, ADSCs might be a better alternative due to the lack of morbidity at the donor site. [17] Other studies also claimed that the avoidance of *in vitro* expansion might make SVF more suitable for clinical application. [15, 17]

Besides, various scaffolds, both biological and synthetic, have also been studied in this field. Bruder et al. used porous ceramic cylinders consisting of hydroxyapatite (65 per cent) and beta-tricalcium phosphate ceramic (35 per cent) with BM-MSCs for bone regeneration. [18] Arca et al. used acellular crosslinked porcine-derived cancellous bone graft with BM-MSCs for *in vitro* bone tissue engineering and an osteoinductive capacity was found in such material. [19] The choosing of scaffold material is largely determined by the bone defect itself. Fast resorbing materials, like tricalcium phosphates (TCP) can be used in a wound without special requirements of mechanical support, and slower degradation can be achieved by using materials like hydroxyapatite (HA) or through a combination of different materials, such as TCP and HA, or polyglycolic acid (PGA) and polylactic acid (PLA). [20]

Another progress in bone tissue engineering is using stem cells as gene therapy vector. Hao et al. found that osteogenic potency of ADSCs was enhanced by transfection with bone morphogenetic protein 2 (Ad-hBMP2). [16] In another study, ADSCs encoding VEGF was found to have a greater osteogenic capacity both *in vitro* and *in vivo*. [21] Moreover, enhanced vascularization was also observed by such genetically modified stem cells. Such combination of stem cells, scaffold, and gene therapy, not only extend the bone regeneration capacity of stem cells, but also help to improve the microenvironment for wound healing. [16, 20] Clinical success was also achieved by using cell-based tissue-engineering approach to treat patients with large bone defects. [22] Despite of great progress of bone tissue engineering has been made both from research and from clinical practice, further studies are still need to improve the isolation of cells, the construct of the scaffold, and the whole cell processing process to make it more suitable for clinical application.

4. Cartilage tissue engineering

Cartilage tissue engineering typically involves the combination of a biodegradable scaffold material with a certain type of cells to differentiate into chondrocytes. Previously, autologous chondrocytes were applied to generate cartilage *in vitro* as substitute of the injured cartilage tissue. Such technique constituted the early cartilage tissue engineering, however, it is also limited by the source of cells as well as the morbidity left at the donor site. [23, 24] The progress of regenerative medicine has provided more alternatives for cartilage tissue engineering. Mesenchymal stem cells isolated from many tissues, including bone marrow, adipose tissue, synovium, and umbilical cord, have all been found to have a chondrogenic potential and can be applied for cartilage tissue engineering. According to a recent study, the chondrogenic potential is similar between BM-MSCs and ADSCs. [25] Besides, adipose stromal vascular fraction has also been proven to be a good alternative for cartilage tissue engineering. Without *in vitro* expansion, such cells are more practical for clinical application. [26] A variety of materials have also been proposed as scaffolds, which constitute another important factor of tissue engineering of cartilage. These scaffolds not only act as protection during cell delivery, but also provide structural support for the growth of cells. Now many scaffolds are also modified to recreating an extracellular environment that is similar to that *in vivo*. [27] With the limited source of natural scaffold, synthetic materials have gained tremendous development in the recent years. Instead of using single-element material, such as collagen, silk or hydrogel scaffold in the past, now more and more studies tend to use combined materials to adjust an optimal mechanical strength or degradation for better *in vivo* tissue formation, like silk-fibrin/hyaluronic acid composite gels or silk fibroin-chitosan combination. Such combinations have also been used to create a 3-D structure with spatially-varying mechanical properties to mimic the native extra cellular matrix (ECM) composition. [27-30]

Great progress has been achieved in cartilage tissue engineering during the past decades, however, some issues still remain in this area, for example the directed differentiation of stem cells, the simulation of actual physiological condition into the body, the integration of tissue engineered cartilage to the body, and so on. Growth factors have been found to be promising in the directed differentiation of stem cells. A combination of FGF-2 or FGF-6 with TGFβ2 has been proven by Bosetti et al. to be effective to induce the chondrogenic differentiation of MSCs. Similarly, TGF-beta3, BMP-6, and IGF-1 have all been found to have such effects. [31, 32] Studies have also been performed to address the issue of adjusting tissue engineered cartilage to the actual condition *in vivo*. Ronzière et al. found that reduced oxygen was associated with higher chondrogenic protential for both cultured BM-MSCs and ADSCs. [33] Besides, various bioreactors have also been introduced to increase the mechanical property of the tissue engineered cartilage. Tarng et al. found in their study that the composition of the engineered cartilage, including their ECM composition, cell distribution, zonal organization and mechanical properties, resembles native cartilage if shear stress and hydrodynamic pressure were provided simultaneously. [34]

Engineered cartilage has also become an alternative for auricular reconstruction in plastic and reconstructive surgery. Ruszymah et al. has constructed a human external ear with human cartilage cells and skin cells seeded on a high density polyethylene. [35] Positive clinical results have also been achieved by such technique. Neumeister et al. combined the techniques of vascular prefabrication, tissue culturing, and capsule formation to fabricate ear construct that is reliably transferable on its blood supply. [36] Despite of the encouraging progress, many improvements are still needed for its clinical application, such as to shorten the *in vitro* expansion time, to strengthen the mechanical property of the neocartilage, and to simplify the whole process.

5. Stem cells and vascularization

Flap surgery is often used in reconstructive surgery to repair defects resulting from trauma, congenital defects or cancer excision. Partial or complete flap necrosis is a common postoperative complication, which is mainly due to the lack of adequate nutrient blood flow resulting from vascular compromise. Tissue damage happens during sustained ischemia period and also happens during reperfusion period often initiated by a salvage surgery. [37]

Studies of vascularization process after flap surgery showed that the formation of new blood supply is achieved by two mechanisms: namely, angiogenesis and vasculogenesis. Angiogenesis refers to the sprouting of microvessels through a preexisting capillary network, whereas vasculogenesis refers to vascular formation from endothelial progenitor cells that differentiate or endothelia cells that proliferate *in situ*. With both mechanisms associated with the vascularization of flap postoperatively, a therapy focused on both mechanisms is supposed to be the most effective. [38, 39]

Cell-based therapy has become a new focus in this area. Previously, Park et al. injected endothelial progenitor cells (EPCs) into the systemic circulation of nude mice with cranially based random-pattern skin flap. [40] Three days after the treatment, EPCs began to appear around ischemia site and the vascular density increased significantly after EPCs administration. Later, better vascularization promoting effect was also verified by Yi et al. with EPCs encoding VEGF as gene therapy. [41] They found these gene-engineered EPCs not only showed greater ability of adhering and incorporating into newly formed vessels, but also enhanced native angiogenesis. According to these studies, EPCs not only showed great potential of incorporating into newly formed vessels, but also enhanced native angiogenesis.

Mesenchymal stem cells like BM-MSCs and ADSCs have also been proven to contribute to vascularization of ischemic tissue. [42, 43] On a random skin flap model, Lu et al. found that the transplantation of ADSCs can significantly increase the flap viability by differentiating into endothelial cells. [44] Other studies also show that ADSCs can promote endothelial cell proliferation and blood vessel formation through paracrine secretion of growth factors, including vascular endothelial growth factor (VEGF), basic fibroblast growth factor (bFGF), transforming growth factor (TGF)-b1, TGF-b2, hepatocyte growth factor (HGF), platelet-derived growth factor (PDGF)-AA and et al. [45] Such effects have also been found in BM-MSCs. The regenerative stem cells not only act as a cell source for angiogenesis, but also secrete multiple growth factors to support angiogenesis. Besides, they can also be used as a vector for gene therapy without the problem of immune reaction or other problems that can be caused by a viral vector. [45, 46]

However, in most clinical settings, the occurrence of ischemia is unpredictable with rapid aggravation. There is no time for *in vitro* expansion the aforementioned stem cells. In the recent studies, both BM-MNCs and SVF, have been found to promote the survival of ischemic flaps. [47] With great progress in stem cell therapy, more optimal choices will appear for the treatment of ischemia flaps. But still what is known from these cells is not enough, lots of work have to be done to explore the mechanism of cell therapy, and to improve the survival of transplanted cells as well as their therapeutic effects.

6. Stem cells and breast tissue engineering

The removal of a breast has implications for the psychologic, social, and sexual well-being of the patient, establishing the essential need for breast reconstruction after mastectomy. Now breast reconstruction has been involved as an important part in the management of breast cancer. However, most of breast reconstruction has been achieved by autologous tissue transplantation, such as transverse rectus abdominis myocutaneous and deep inferior epigastric perforator flap. Although such autologous tissue reconstruction could bring great improvement in both appearance and texture to the defects, they are also associated with certain side effects, like great morbidity at the donor site, longer operation process, and the risk of flap failure. Looking for a safe and effective technique with less trauma to the body has been a key issue in breast reconstruction. [48]

Fat tissue has been considered as a good source of tissue for breast reconstruction and lipofilling has therefore been used frequently for the reconstruction of breast after mastectomy. However, large sum of lipofilling is associated with problems, like necrosis, cysts formation, and microcalcification formation. Some scientists have tried to solve this problem through tissue engineering. [49] Coleman et al have tried to enhance the nutrient supply as well as the survival of the fat tissue by microinjection. [50] Patrick et al., however, combined preadipocytes with porous scaffold of poly (L-lactic-co-glycolic) acid (PLGA) for fat transplantation. During the initial phase of the study, satisfactory results were observed by such method, however, after long-term observation fat tissue was found absorbed with the degradation of PLGA. [51] Based on these studies, Lin et al have further tried to combine ADSCs with a composite scaffold, made by a mix of gelatin sponges, polyglycolic acid, and polypropylene. Scaffolds were found to be filled with newly formed adipose tissue and had retained their predefined shape and dimensions after 6 months' *in vivo* transplantation. [52]

Despite of great success achieved in breast tissue engineering as proven in many publications, great concern has been arisen about the oncological safety about these techniques. More and more studies have shown ADSCs may either present as a source of tumor or provide an environment for the growth of the tumor, lipofilling combined with ADSCs and ADSCs based breast tissue engineering has been greatly impeded. [53-55] Another type of cells in the adipose tissue, SVF, may present as an alternative, however, studies are still needed to verify its safety. [56] Since still there has not been enough evidence showing that these techniques can indeed cause tumor clinically and great progress is still achieving in the understanding of cancer and stem cells, breast tissue engineering may still regain its prospect in the future. [57]

7. *In vivo* tissue prefabrication

With various flap surgeries in reconstructive surgery, soft tissue defects can now be repaired with better appearance and function, which cannot be achieved by skin graft. However, flap surgery is still challenged when there is composite tissue defect, including cartilage or bone. Autologous composite tissue transplantation has been used for such cases, but the great morbidity at the donor site often makes the doctor retreat from it. Allotransplantation of composite tissue has also been considered as a possible solution.

However, it is limited by immunological rejection, lack of proper donors, and some kind of psychological resistance.

Base on the traditional prefabricated flap technique in plastic surgery and tissue engineering, a new concept of "*in vivo* tissue prefabrication" has been proposed here. Prefabricated flap technique (or preliminited flap technique in some literature), first introduced in 1980s, refers to implanting the vessels and vessel carrier within multiple autologous tissues (bones or cartilage) and/or artificial material in the donor site that does not possess an axial blood supply. [58, 59] It potentially allows any defined tissue volume or components to be transferred to any specified recipient site, providing ideal solution to the repair of complex tissue defects. Using such technique, Kobayashi et al. has achieved successful total lower eyelid reconstruction on patients. [60] Besides, more complicated structures, like nose and ear, have also been successfully prefabricated. [61, 62]

Now with the progress of tissue engineering, many tissues, such as cartilage and bone, can be created by *in vivo* tissue engineering. Such tissue engineered cartilage or bone can be fabricated with skin, subcutaneous tissue, and blood vessel to be a composite tissue for defects repair. Okuda et al. has created tissue engineered bone by culturing adipose-derived stem cells with porous beta-tricalcium phosphate. After transplanted into superficial inferior epigastric artery flap, angiogenesis was successfully induced into the tissue engineered bone tissue and a compsite tissue flap including bone and muscle was also successfully prefabricated. [63] Similarly, Feucht et al. induced tissue engineered cartilage *in vitro* with chondrocytes from auricular biopsies. The cartilage-engineered constructs was then implanted beneath a random-pattern skin flap for prefabrication. 6 weeks later, the flap was elevated and transferred as a free composite flap. [64] Neovascularization was achieved in the tissue engineered cartilage and its growth was also maintained. The aforementioned studies have tried an *in vitro* way to generate tissue for later prefabrication, however, *in vivo* tissue engineering actually provides a better solution to the problem. By introducing cell embedded scaffold directly into the body, the process of tissue engineering and flap prefabrication can be combined, which not only reduce the time for both procedures, but also leads to more effective tissue engineering. For example, the *in vivo* environment can provide optimal conditions to facilitate functional tissue engineering. Moreover, with better vascularization *in vivo*, lager size tissue engineering can be achieved. [65]

8. Conclusions

In vivo tissue prefabrication technique, combining traditional prefabricated flap technique and tissue engineering, not only brings vascular supply to the engineered tissue, but also greatly reduce the morbidity at the donor site during traditional flap prefabrication. With the development of tissue engineering, many tissues can be generated *in vitro* or *in vivo*. Combined with prefabrication with various tissue types or with better blood supply technique, such cultured tissues can be prefabricated for repair and reconstruction. In the future, more complicated parts on the body, like ear, nose or thumb, may also be prefabricated. Moreover, according to the recent studies, neovascularization, the key to a successful prefabrication, can be enhanced and greatly speeded with stem cells transplantation, which means a perfect substitute of the lost body part can be generated in shorter time in the future.

9. References

[1] Ebeling AH, Fischer A. Mixed cultures of pure strains of fibroblasts and epithelial cells. J Exp Med. 1922 Aug 31;36(3):285-9.

[2] Freeman AE, Igel HJ, Waldman NL, Losikoff AM. A new method for covering large surface area wounds with autografts. I. In vitro multiplication of rabbit-skin epithelial cells. Arch Surg. 1974 May;108(5):721-3.

[3] Green H, Kehinde O, Thomas J. Growth of cultured human epidermal cells into multiple epithelia suitable for grafting. Proc Natl Acad Sci U S A. 1979 Nov;76(11):5665-8.

[4] Friedenstein AJ, Piatetzky-Shapiro II, Petrakova KV. Osteogenesis in transplants of bone marrow cells. J Embryol Exp Morphol. 1966 Dec;16(3):381-90.

[5] Ding DC, Shyu WC, Lin SZ. Mesenchymal stem cells. Cell Transplant. 2011;20(1):5-14.

[6] Luo G, Cheng W, He W, Wang X, Tan J, Fitzgerald M, Li X, Wu J. Promotion of cutaneous wound healing by local application of mesenchymal stem cells derived from human umbilical cord blood. Wound Repair Regen. 2010 Sep-Oct;18(5):506-13. doi: 10.1111/j.1524-475X.2010.00616.x.

[7] Wu Y, Zhao RC, Tredget EE. Concise review: bone marrow-derived stem/progenitor cells in cutaneous repair and regeneration. Stem Cells. 2010 May;28(5):905-15.

[8] Yang M, Li Q, Sheng L, Li H, Weng R, Zan T. Bone marrow-derived mesenchymal stem cells transplantation accelerates tissue expansion by promoting skin regeneration during expansion. Ann Surg. 2011 Jan;253(1):202-9.

[9] Uitto J. Regenerative medicine for skin diseases: iPS cells to the rescue. J Invest Dermatol. 2011 Apr;131(4):812-4.

[10] Lee LF, Jiang TX, Garner W, Chuong CM. A simplified procedure to reconstitute hair-producing skin. Tissue Eng Part C Methods. 2011 Apr;17(4):391-400.

[11] Quarto R, Mastrogiacomo M, Cancedda R, Kutepov SM, Mukhachev V, Lavroukov A, Kon E, Marcacci M. Repair of large bone defects with the use of autologous bone marrow stromal cells. N Engl J Med. 2001 Feb 1;344(5):385-6.

[12] Breitbart AS, Grande DA, Kessler R, Ryaby JT, Fitzsimmons RJ, Grant RT. Tissue engineered bone repair of calvarial defects using cultured periosteal cells. Plast Reconstr Surg. 1998 Mar;101(3):567-74; discussion 575-6.

[13] Crane GM, Ishaug SL, Mikos AG. Bone tissue engineering. Nat Med. 1995 Dec;1(12):1322-4.

[14] Griffin M, Iqbal SA, Bayat A. Exploring the application of mesenchymal stem cells in bone repair and regeneration. J Bone Joint Surg Br. 2011 Apr;93(4):427-34.

[15] Jurgens WJ, Kroeze RJ, Bank RA, Ritt MJ, Helder MN. Rapid attachment of adipose stromal cells on resorbable polymeric scaffolds facilitates the one-step surgical procedure for cartilage and bone tissue engineering purposes. J Orthop Res. 2011 Jan 18. doi: 10.1002/jor.21314. [Epub ahead of print]

[16] Hao W, Dong J, Jiang M, Wu J, Cui F, Zhou D. Enhanced bone formation in large segmental radial defects by combining adipose-derived stem cells expressing bone morphogenetic protein 2 with nHA/RHLC/PLA scaffold. Int Orthop. 2010 Dec;34(8):1341-9. Epub 2010 Feb 7.

[17] Rhee SC, Ji YH, Gharibjanian NA, Dhong ES, Park SH, Yoon ES. In vivo evaluation of mixtures of uncultured freshly isolated adipose-derived stem cells and

demineralized bone matrix for bone regeneration in a rat critically sized calvarial defect model. Stem Cells Dev. 2011 Feb;20(2):233-42. Epub 2010 Oct 12.

[18] Bruder SP, Kraus KH, Goldberg VM, Kadiyala S. The effect of implants loaded with autologous mesenchymal stem cells on the healing of canine segmental bone defects. J Bone Joint Surg Am. 1998 Jul;80(7):985-96.

[19] Arca T, Proffitt J, Genever P. Generating 3D tissue constructs with mesenchymal stem cells and a cancellous bone graft for orthopaedic applications. Biomed Mater. 2011 Feb 28;6(2):025006. [Epub ahead of print]

[20] Janicki P, Schmidmaier G. What should be the characteristics of the ideal bone graft substitute? Combining scaffolds with growth factors and/or stem cells. Injury. 2011 Jul 1. [Epub ahead of print]

[21] Behr B, Tang C, Germann G, Longaker MT, Quarto N. Locally Applied VEGFA Increases the Osteogenic Healing Capacity of Human Adipose Derived Stem Cells by Promoting Osteogenic and Endothelial Differentiation. Stem Cells. 2010 Dec 23. [Epub ahead of print]

[22] Warnke PH, Springer IN, Wiltfang J, Acil Y, Eufinger H, Wehmöller M, Russo PA, Bolte H, Sherry E, Behrens E, Terheyden H. Growth and transplantation of a custom vascularised bone graft in a man. Lancet. 2004 Aug 28-Sep 3;364(9436):766-70.

[23] Moskalewski S, Kawiak J. Cartilage formation after homotransplantation of isolated chondrocytes. Transplantation. 1965 Nov;3(6):737-47.

[24] Keeney M, Lai JH, Yang F. Recent progress in cartilage tissue engineering. Curr Opin Biotechnol. 2011 Apr 28. [Epub ahead of print]

[25] Havlas V, Kos P, Jendelová P, Lesný P, Trč T, Syková E. Comparison of chondrogenic differentiation of adipose tissue-derived mesenchymal stem cells with cultured chondrocytes and bone marrow mesenchymal stem cells. Acta Chir Orthop Traumatol Cech. 2011;78(2):138-44.

[26] Chlapanidas T, Faragò S, Mingotto F, Crovato F, Tosca MC, Antonioli B, Bucco M, Lucconi G, Scalise A, Vigo D, Faustini M, Marazzi M, Torre ML. Regenerated silk fibroin scaffold and infrapatellar adipose stromal vascular fraction as feeder-layer: a new product for cartilage advanced therapy. Tissue Eng Part A. 2011 Jul;17(13-14):1725-33.

[27] Egli RJ, Wernike E, Grad S, Luginbühl R. Physiological cartilage tissue engineering effect of oxygen and biomechanics. Int Rev Cell Mol Biol. 2011;289:37-87.

[28] Park S, Cho H, Gil ES, Mandal B, Min BH, Kaplan DL. Silk-fibrin/hyaluronic acid composite gels for nucleus pulposus (NP) tissue regeneration. Tissue Eng Part A. 2011 Jul 7. [Epub ahead of print]

[29] Sá-Lima H, Tuzlakoglu K, Mano JF, Reis RL. Thermoresponsive poly(N-isopropylacrylamide)-g-methylcellulose hydrogel as a three-dimensional extracellular matrix for cartilage-engineered applications. J Biomed Mater Res A. 2011 Jun 30. doi: 10.1002/jbm.a.33140. [Epub ahead of print]

[30] Bhardwaj N, Nguyen QT, Chen AC, Kaplan DL, Sah RL, Kundu SC. Potential of 3-D tissue constructs engineered from bovine chondrocytes/silk fibroin-chitosan for in vitro cartilage tissue engineering. Biomaterials. 2011 Sep;32(25):5773-81. Epub 2011 May 20.

[31] Bosetti M, Boccafoschi F, Leigheb M, Bianchi AE, Cannas M. Chondrogenic induction of human mesenchymal stem cells using combined growth factors for cartilage tissue engineering. J Tissue Eng Regen Med. 2011 Feb 28. doi: 10.1002/term.416. [Epub ahead of print]

[32] Freyria AM, Mallein-Gerin F. Chondrocytes or adult stem cells for cartilage repair: The indisputable role of growth factors. Injury. 2011 Jun 20. [Epub ahead of print]

[33] Ronzière MC, Perrier E, Mallein-Gerin F, Freyria AM. Chondrogenic potential of bone marrow- and adipose tissue-derived adult human mesenchymal stem cells. Biomed Mater Eng. 2010 Jan 1;20(3):145-58.

[34] Tarng YW, Huang BF, Su FC. A novel recirculating flow-perfusion bioreactor for periosteal chondrogenesis. Int Orthop. 2011 Jun 15. [Epub ahead of print]

[35] Ruszymah BH, Chua KH, Mazlyzam AL, Aminuddin BS. Formation of tissue engineered composite construct of cartilage and skin using high density polyethylene as inner scaffold in the shape of human helix. Int J Pediatr Otorhinolaryngol. 2011 Jun;75(6):805-10. Epub 2011 Apr 11.

[36] Neumeister MW, Wu T, Chambers C. Vascularized tissue-engineered ears. Plast Reconstr Surg. 2006 Jan;117(1):116-22.

[37] Novakovic D, Patel RS, Goldstein DP, Gullane PJ. Salvage of failed free flaps used in head and neck reconstruction. Head Neck Oncol. 2009 Aug 21;1:33.

[38] Folkman J, Shing Y. Angiogenesis. J Biol Chem. 1992 Jun 5;267(16):10931-4.

[39] Asahara T, Murohara T, Sullivan A, Silver M, van der Zee R, Li T, Witzenbichler B, Schatteman G, Isner JM. Isolation of putative progenitor endothelial cells for angiogenesis. Science. 1997 Feb 14;275(5302):964-7.

[40] Park S, Tepper OM, Galiano RD, Capla JM, Baharestani S, Kleinman ME, Pelo CR, Levine JP, Gurtner GC. Selective recruitment of endothelial progenitor cells to ischemic tissues with increased neovascularization. Plast Reconstr Surg. 2004 Jan;113(1):284-93.

[41] Yi C, Xia W, Zheng Y, Zhang L, Shu M, Liang J, Han Y, Guo S. Transplantation of endothelial progenitor cells transferred by vascular endothelial growth factor gene for vascular regeneration of ischemic flaps. J Surg Res. 2006 Sep;135(1):100-6.

[42] Szöke K, Beckstrøm KJ, Brinchmann JE. Human adipose tissue as a source of cells with angiogenic potential. Cell Transplant. 2011 Jun 7.

[43] Bhang SH, Cho SW, La WG, Lee TJ, Yang HS, Sun AY, Baek SH, Rhie JW, Kim BS. Angiogenesis in ischemic tissue produced by spheroid grafting of human adipose-derived stromal cells. Biomaterials. 2011 Apr;32(11):2734-47.

[44] Lu F, Mizuno H, Uysal CA, Cai X, Ogawa R, Hyakusoku H. Improved viability of random pattern skin flaps through the use of adipose-derived stem cells. Plast Reconstr Surg. 2008 Jan;121(1):50-8.

[45] Wagner W, Wein F, Seckinger A, Frankhauser M, Wirkner U, Krause U, Blake J, Schwager C, Eckstein V, Ansorge W, Ho AD. Comparative characteristics of mesenchymal stem cells from human bone marrow, adipose tissue, and umbilical cord blood. Exp Hematol. 2005 Nov;33(11):1402-16.

[46] Yang M, Sheng L, Li H, Weng R, Li QF. Improvement of the skin flap survival with the bone marrow-derived mononuclear cells transplantation in a rat model. Microsurgery. 2010 May;30(4):275-81.

[47] Sheng L, Yang M, Li H, Du Z, Yang Y, Li Q. Transplantation of adipose stromal cells promotes neovascularization of random skin flaps. Tohoku J Exp Med. 2011;224(3):229-34.

[48] Yoshimura K, Sato K, Aoi N, Kurita M, Hirohi T, Harii K. Cell-assisted lipotransfer for cosmetic breast augmentation: supportive use of adipose-derived stem/stromal cells. Aesthetic Plast Surg. 2008 Jan;32(1):48-55; discussion 56-7. Epub 2007 Sep 1.

[49] Patrick CW. Breast tissue engineering. Annu Rev Biomed Eng. 2004;6:109-30.

[50] Coleman SR. Structural fat grafting: more than a permanent filler. Plast Reconstr Surg. 2006 Sep;118(3 Suppl):108S-120S.

[51] Patrick CW Jr, Chauvin PB, Hobley J, Reece GP. Preadipocyte seeded PLGA scaffolds for adipose tissue engineering. Tissue Eng. 1999 Apr;5(2):139-51.

[52] Lin SD, Wang KH, Kao AP. Engineered adipose tissue of predefined shape and dimensions from human adipose-derived mesenchymal stem cells. Tissue Eng Part A. 2008 May;14(5):571-81.

[53] Pearl RA, Leedham SJ, Pacifico MD. The safety of autologous fat transfer in breast cancer: Lessons from stem cell biology. J Plast Reconstr Aesthet Surg. 2011 Aug 3.

[54] Razmkhah M, Jaberipour M, Erfani N, Habibagahi M, Talei AR, Ghaderi A. Adipose derived stem cells (ASCs) isolated from breast cancer tissue express IL-4, IL-10 and TGF-β1 and upregulate expression of regulatory molecules on T cells: do they protect breast cancer cells from the immune response? Cell Immunol. 2011;266(2):116-22.

[55] Razmkhah M, Jaberipour M, Hosseini A, Safaei A, Khalatbari B, Ghaderi A. Expression profile of IL-8 and growth factors in breast cancer cells and adipose-derived stem cells (ASCs) isolated from breast carcinoma. Cell Immunol. 2010;265(1):80-5.

[56] Lin SD, Huang SH, Lin YN, Wu SH, Chang HW, Lin TM, Chai CY, Lai CS. Engineering adipose tissue from uncultured human adipose stromal vascular fraction on collagen matrix and gelatin sponge scaffolds. Tissue Eng Part A. 2011 Jun;17(11-12):1489-98.

[57] Tiryaki T, Findikli N, Tiryaki D. Staged Stem Cell-enriched Tissue (SET) Injections for Soft Tissue Augmentation in Hostile Recipient Areas: A Preliminary Report. Aesthetic Plast Surg. 2011 Apr 13.

[58] Yao ST. Microvascular transplantation of prefabricated free thigh flap. Plast Reconstr Surg. 1982 Mar;69(3):568.

[59] Burget GC, Walton RL. Optimal use of microvascular free flaps, cartilage grafts, and a paramedian forehead flap for aesthetic reconstruction of the nose and adjacent facial units. Plast Reconstr Surg. 2007 Oct;120(5):1171-207; discussion 1208-16.

[60] Kobayashi K, Ishihara H, Murakami R, Kinoshita N, Tokunaga K. Total lower eyelid reconstruction with a prefabricated flap using auricular cartilage. J Craniomaxillofac Surg. 2008 Mar;36(2):59-65. Epub 2008 Feb 6.

[61] Akin S. Burned ear reconstruction using a prefabricated free radial forearm flap. J Reconstr Microsurg 2001;17:233-236.

[62] Ozdemir R, Kocer U, Tiftikcioglu YO, Karaaslan O, Kankaya Y, Cuzdan S, Baydar DE. Axial pattern composite prefabrication of high-density porous polyethylene: experimental and clinical research. Plast Reconstr Surg. 2005 Jan;115(1):183-96.

[63] Okuda T, Uysal AC, Tobita M, Hyakusoku H, Mizuno H. Prefabrication of tissue engineered bone grafts: an experimental study. Ann Plast Surg. 2010 Jan;64(1):98-104.

[64] Feucht A, Hoang NT, Hoehnke C, Hien PT, Mandlik V, Storck K, Staudenmaier R. Neovascularisation and free microsurgical transfer of cartilage-engineered constructs. HNO. 2011 Mar;59(3):239-47.

[65] Zan T, Li Q, Dong J, Zheng S, Xie Y, Yu D, Zheng D, Gu B. Transplanted endothelial progenitor cells increase neo-vascularisation of rat pre-fabricated flaps. J Plast Reconstr Aesthet Surg. 2010 Mar;63(3):474-81. Epub 2008 Dec 30.

11

Advanced 3-D Biomodelling Technology for Complex Mandibular Reconstruction

Horácio Zenha, Maria da Luz Barroso and Horácio Costa
Plastic, Reconstructive & Maxillofacial Surgery Department
Centro Hospitalar V.N.Gaia/Espinho
Portugal

1. Introduction

Reconstructive surgery of the head and neck is a demanding field. The specific anatomical complexity of the region, and its almost inevitable exposure to the public, demand for highly refined and careful reconstructive procedures. In fact, in the last decades, the trend in reconstructive surgery, as for the general medical field, is to put the standard of care in an extremely high level and this adds an extra perfectionist input in treatment goals.

In the classical principles of treatment in plastic surgery, restoration of function is always regarded as first objective. Regular mastication, swallowing, respiration and speech are the goals to reach when planning facial reconstructive procedures. In the modern principles, this first priority has been caught up by a new priority goal – the aesthetic result. In head and neck reconstruction, this new goal is even more important because of the prime social role this anatomical region sustains. So, it is not enough to restore functions, but we should also seek for facial harmony and the most perfect symmetry.

Facial structure is complex and unique among individuals. The challenge of recreating its 3-dimensional (3-D) morphology is enormous and traditionally a very artistic endeavour. Hard, time-consuming and "eye-match" manual techniques where normally used in order to obtain satisfactory results. This is particularly valid when we focus on severe defects of the head and neck.

Reconstruction with local or regional tissues is normally preferred in general plastic surgery, especially because of the similarity of neighbouring tissues regarding the final result. This concept changes in the facial region due to 2 fundamental reasons: the face is in the cephalic extremity of the human body and there is a relative lack of possible neighbour donor sites; and that option would imply the sacrifice of other areas that are also important to overall function and aesthetic adding unnecessary morbidity to the solution. So, distant free flaps are very often used as the first choice for complex reconstruction of the head and neck. This technique allows us to bring to our "reconstruction site" a much less limited amount of tissue and restore severe compound defects (skin, bone, mucosa...). As counterpart, it has considerable technical, logistic and time-consuming difficulties. The dissection and transfer of free flaps requires specific training and capabilities. Vessels anastomosis are done under microscope and, apart from the surgical team, all the operating room personnel should be used the routines on its manipulation so the time this phase of the surgery lasts can be minimized. Two surgical teams should work together: one at the recipient site, where the extirpation of the tumour or recreation of the previous defect and dissection of recipient vessels is done; while the other dissects the free flap selected, and so time can be spared. Nonetheless, it is not easy to complete these procedures in less than 5-6 hours. The management of osteocutaneous/osteomucosal compound defects and extensive mandibular defects is particularly troublesome, especially the correct modelling of the anatomically "curved" mandibular bone which is unique in the human body. The surgeon, apart from the technical skills, has to apply all his inspiration and art into the cases. Manual measurements and calculations and "eye-match" techniques to evaluate symmetries are often applied in the operating theatre. (Zenha et al., 2011)

2. Biomodelling technology

The advances in medical imaging in recent years have been overwhelming with the possibility of obtaining increasing volumes of complex and extremely precise data from the patient. To explore their full potential is sometimes hard for the surgeon, specially when he is forced to mentally transform 2-D images into a 3-D scenery as the one he is faced within the surgical field (Zenha et al., 2011). Three-dimensional (3-D) imaging has been developed to narrow the communication gap between radiologist and surgeon. It represents a big development for data display, diagnosis and surgical planning and is nowadays ready accessible in most centers but it is not a true 3-D technology, as it is displayed on a flat screen or radiological film only in 2 dimensions (D'Urso et al., 1999a).

Biomodelling is the generic term describing the ability to replicate the morphology of a biological structure in a solid substance (Oliveira et al., 2008). Specifically, biomodelling uses radiant energy to capture morphological data on a biological structure and processes such data by a computer to generate the code required to manufacture the structure by rapid prototyping (RP) (Oliveira et al., 2008). It represents the physical 3-D expression of 3-D imaging technology data. Stereolitography (SL) is a RP process. As almost all RP processes, it is based on layered manufacturing methodology in which objects are built as series of horizontal cross sections, each one being formed individually from the relevant raw materials and bonded to preceding layers until it is completed. Technically, the model-fabrication is by polymerisation of liquid UV-sensitive resin using a UV-laser beam on a horizontal plane, with vertical construction by submerging the model stepwise (Bill et al., 1995). Accuracy of SL has been shown in the range of +/-1mm.

Biomodelling technology with SL is a long established method in industry for the construction of prototypes and cast moulds, namely in the space and aeronautic field. Mankovich *et al.* in 1990 reported the 1st SL anatomical models and Stoker *et al.* in 1992 described the use of SL biomodelling for retrospective assessment of a clinical case. However, it was Arvier et al, in 1994, which described the 1st real clinical use of SL biomodelling techniques, with application in cases of mandibular reconstruction and orthognathic surgery. Since then, the development in the technique has been facilitated by improvements in medical imaging, computer hardware, 3D image processing software and the technology transfer of engineering methods into the field of surgery. Colour SL for planning of maxillofacial tumour surgery was described by Kermer *et al* in 1998. In the same year, Peckitt (1998) opened the field of prosthesis manufacturing through SL biomodelling with its accuracy, flexibility and limitations. Kernan & Wimsatt in 2000 described the use of SL biomodels for accurate preoperative adaptation of a reconstruction plate. The concurrent evolution of other technologies like stereophotogrammetry (Xia et al., 2000) has enriched SL biomodelling techniques enabling the diagnosis, simulation and planning of the soft tissues component of the reconstructive procedure. Surgical navigation technology (Schramm et al., 2000 & Gelrich et al., 2002) is another growing field that augmented, and in some instances substituted (Hohlweg-Majert, 2005), the role of SL in maxillofacial surgery.

In craniomaxillofacial surgery, biomodelling technology with SL has been applied in craniofacial, tumour, orthognathic, trauma and implantology and has been considered a valuable tool in several studies (D'Urso et al., 1999a, 2000a; Bill et al., 1995; Sailer et al., 1998; Xia et al., 2006). Application of biomodeling technology has also been reported in neurosurgery (D'Urso & Redmond, 1999b, 1999c & 2000b; Sinn et al., 2006; Westendorf et al., 2007; Staffa et al., 2007; Wurm et al., 2004), orthopedic surgery (Fukui et al., 2003; Brown et al., 2002 & Gutierres et al., 2007), cardiology and cardio-thoracic surgery (Sodian et al., 2002 & Greil et al., 2007), vascular surgery (Lermusiaux et al., 2001), facial aging (Pessa, 2000 & 2001), alloplasty (Coward et al., 1999), forensic medicine (Dolz et al., 2000 & Vanezi et al., 2000) and fetal medicine (D'Urso & Thompson, 1998).

In fact, biomodelling technology associated with rapid prototyping has become an important tool in reconstructive surgery, especially in head and neck complex cases involving mandible reconstruction. The possibility of creating an highly accurate physical model of the patient's anatomy enables better overall evaluation and a careful and detailed surgical planning with significative surgery-time sparing. Also, virtual simulation of the surgical procedure with the generation of surgical templates has been integrated in the process. This virtual simulation step presents an enormous potential in the field of surgical planning and optimisation.

We developed two new stereolitographic biomodel tools to be used intra-operatively that should optimise the reconstructive procedure: surgical cutting guides that preoperatively define the exact defect to be reconstructed and a template that simultaneously guides the osseous free flap osteotomies and enables reconstruction plate modelling.

2.1 Materials & methods

Between 2008 and 2010, 19 patients, of which 10 male and 9 female, were submitted to complex and compound mandibular reconstruction procedures. Age ranged from 9 to 66 years old (mean – 36,5). The ethiology was neoplastic in the majority - 16 cases, 84% - with 12 tumours origin from the mandible and the remaining 4 from the oral mucosa. Histological analysis of the mandibular tumours revealed 8 ameloblastomas, 1 sarcoma, 1osteoclastoma, 1 giant cell tumour and 1 odontogenic queratocyst. The histological characterization of the oral mucosa tumours treated was oral squamous cell carcinoma (3 cases) and minor salivary gland adenocarcinoma (1 case). Other ethiologies were osteoradionecrosis following radiotherapy (RT) adjuvant treatment for oral squamous cell carcinoma (2 cases) and congenital (1 case of Goldenhar syndrome with severe unilateral mandibular hipoplasia). In approximately ¾ of the patients (14 cases) reconstruction was immediate after surgical extirpation. In the remaining (5 cases), there had been previous surgery or congenital malformation that originated the defect to be reconstructed.

The free flaps selected for reconstruction of the mandibular defects were the iliac crest flap (13 cases) and the fibula flap (6 cases, in association with a radial forearm flap in 3 cases). These flaps were selected because of: their "bone stock" availability; the similarity of contour with the mandible; the relatively good and long vascular pedicle and the possibility to reconstruct oral mucosa and/or facial and cervical skin with a thin and pliable flap (Costa et al., 2011). The iliac crest free flaps were always transferred as osteomuscular flaps. The fibula flaps were all transferred as osteoseptocutaneou flaps with the skin paddle used for cervico-facial skin reconstruction in 3 cases, intra and extra-oral reconstruction in 2 cases and as a facial volume enhancer in a buried flap (after deepithelization) in the case of congenital hemifacial microssomia. In 3 of the fibula flap patients, due to magnitude of the defect, it was necessary to perform a second free flap – radial forearm fasciocutaneous – to be used in a sequentially linked flow-through technique and to which the fibula flap vessels were anastomosed.

2.2 The process

Surgical planning using biomodelling technology starts with a CT scan of the head and neck of the patient (Figure 1). A specialized scanning protocol is required with image slices in the range of 0,5-1mm in order to obtain isotropic data. This 2-D DICOM data is then converted in 3-D data through a specific software, AnatomicsPro®, that automatically generates surface-based STL (Standard Tesselation Language) files and contour-based SLC (Stereolitography) files proper for solid modelling via rapid prototyping. Further image processing is required to identify and separate (segmentation) the anatomy to be modelled.

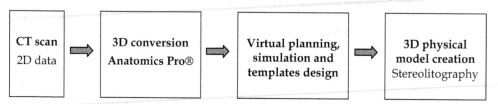

Fig. 1. The dynamic process of biomodelling technology application in complex mandibular reconstruction. The strereolitography models are generated for "hands-on" surgical planning and intra-operative use.

Virtual simulation and rehearsal of the surgical procedure is done through another software, Freeform Modelling®, where, advanced mathematical techniques, enable the exact calculation of the contours, angles, length and morphology of the reconstructive procedure and also the generation of surgical templates to be used intra-operatively. We can plan and simulate with high accuracy all the "osseous phase of the surgery". In immediate reconstructions we define exactly were we want to cut the mandible and design a surgical guide that fits in that area in the original mandible. In secondary reconstructions, we calculate the bone defect with several instrumental techniques like virtual manipulation of the remaining mandible, mirror-imaging and standardized cephalometric mandible measurements (Figure 2). We are able to create different templates that guide: donor-bone harvesting; bone-modelling osteotomies and titanium plate modelling. It is also possible to generate pre-modelled titanium plates by stereolitography but due to the logistics needed and the costs involved it wouldn't be worthwhile. The 3-D physical models are then fabricated by RP and used to optimise planning, with "hands-on" evaluation and training, and are ready to be sterilized for surgical utilization (Figure 3).

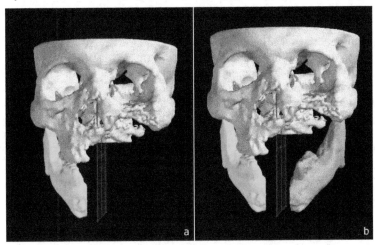

Fig. 2. Virtual manipulation and surgical planning are done through a specific software (Freeform Modelling®). It enables the mobilization of remaining anatomical structures (blue hemimandible) to the correct position and the calculation of the defect to restore through techniques like mirror-imaging (grey left hemimandible).

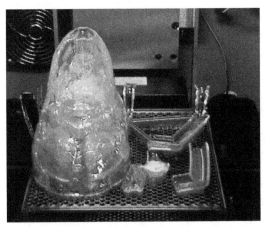

Fig. 3. Fabrication of the acrylic biomodels by stereolitography. The skull and templates are used for detailed surgical planning and intra-operative use.

Intra-operatively the surgical cutting guides are used directly in the mandible and define the exact osteotomies sites. Another SL tool is used for planning the osteotomies of the free flap (fibula or iliac crest) and simultaneously guide the reconstruction titanium plate modelling for the necessary osteosynthesis. The final surgical steps are the microsurgical vascular anastomosis that, in this way, are done without further more "aggressive" osseous manoeuvres that could eventually cause damage.

2.3 Results

Free flaps modelling based on the SL 3-D biomodelling tools accomplished an almost anatomical reconstruction in all the cases (Table 1). The innovative surgical templates were easily used intra-operatively and found to be very efficient. Apart from the flap modelling, where they guided the osteotomies needed in order to mimic the original angulated mandible, they were simultaneously used to mould the reconstruction plate. This surgical step was found to be much easier and quicker than in the regular way. Preoperative planning with virtual simulation of the surgical procedure facilitates a two-team approach from the beginning of the surgical procedure accelerating it. The intra-operative availability of the Surgical Guides enables a more straightforward modelling of the free flap along with much less drawbacks. The operative time is diminished in about 45 minutes, according to surgeons estimation, in comparison to similar cases performed without 3-D biomodels, namely due to optimisation of the flap and reconstruction plate modelling phase.

There where two partial flap necrosis (cases 13 and 18) that needed further surgical revisions with local/regional soft-tissue flaps. Delayed wound healing occurred in 4 cases mainly due to RT-damaged skin.

End-results were evaluated according to functional and aesthetic criteria in 4 different categories: unsatisfactory, satisfactory, good and very good. Restoration of swallowing was considered the first priority, followed by mastication along with the possibility of oral rehabilitation and finally the aesthetic result and facial symmetry (Figs. 4, 5 & 6).

Sex	Age	Ethiology	Mandibular defect	Timing	Free Flap	Bone (cm)	OST	Surgery Time (h)	Result
♀	65	Oral adenocarcinoma	Anterior arch	Primary	Fibula OFC + RFF	15	2	11	Good
♀	15	Ameloblastoma	Hemimandible sparing condyle	Primary	Iliac crest OM	10	0	7	Good
♂	46	Oral SCC	Hemimandible sparing condyle	Secondary	Iliac crest OM	12	1	9	Very Good
♂	11	Goldenhar sdr	Hemimandible	Primary	Fibula OFC	9	1	9	Good
♂	66	ORN	Anterior arch	Primary	Fibula OFC	15	2	10	Good
♀	20	Ameloblastoma	Hemimandible sparing condyle	Primary	Iliac crest OM	9	0	10	Very Good
♀	31	Osteoclastoma	Hemimandible sparing condyle	Primary	Iliac crest OM	10	0	8	Very Good

Sex	Age	Ethiology	Mandibular defect	Timing	Free Flap	Bone (cm)	OST	Surgery Time (h)	Result
♀	35	Ameloblastoma	Anterior arch	Primary	Iliac crest OM	11	1	8	Very Good
♂	41	ORN	Hemimandible sparing condyle	Primary	Fibula OFC	8	0	9	Very Good
♀	26	Sarcoma	Hemimandible sparing condyle	Primary	Iliac crest OM	12	1	8	Very Good
♀	34	Ameloblastoma	Hemimandible sparing condyle	Primary	Iliac crest OM	10	0	5	Very Good
♂	46	Ameloblastoma	Hemimandible sparing condyle	Primary	Iliac crest OM	8,5	0	8	Very Good
♂	54	Oral SCC	Anterior arch	Secondary	Fibula OFC + RFF	15	2	11	Satisfactory
♀	53	Queratocyst	Hemimandible	Primary	Iliac crest OM	12	0	7	Very Good
♂	41	Ameloblastoma	Hemimandible sparing condyle	Primary	Iliac crest OM	8	0	7	Very Good
♂	10	Giant cell granuloma	Anterior arch	Primary	Iliac crest OM	10,5	1	8	Very Good
♂	9	Ameloblastoma	Hemimandible	Primary	Iliac crest OM	10,5	2	5	Very Good
♂	45	Oral SCC	Anterior arch	Secondary	Fibula OFC + RFF	16	2	12	Good
♀	46	Ameloblastoma	Anterior arch	Secondary	Iliac crest OM	12	2	6	Very Good

Table 1. Clinical cases of complex oromandibular reconstruction using advanced 3-D biomodelling technology. (OFC- osteofasciocutaneous; OM- osteomuscular; ORN- osteoradionecrosis; OST- osteotomies; RFF- radial forearm flap; SCC- squamous cell carcinoma)

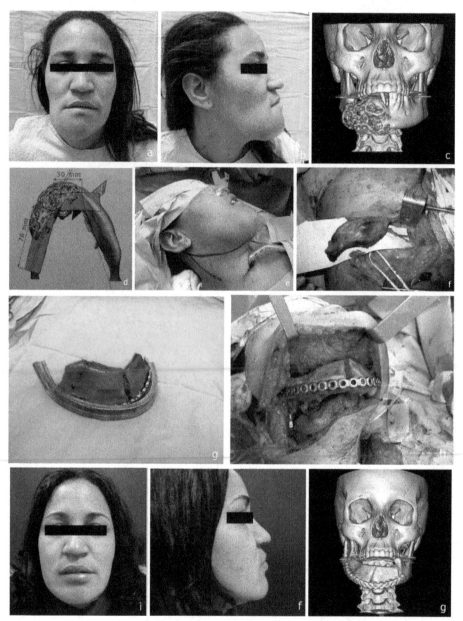

Fig. 4. Female, 35 years old, with a neglected ameloblastoma of the mandible involving the right body and symphisis (a, b & c); Preoperative planning with 3-D biomodelling technology (d); Preoperative markings showing the cervical approach (e); reconstruction with a vascularised iliac crest osteomuscular flap modelled with a 3-D template generated by mirror-imaging and segmentation techniques (f, g & h); 9-month post-operative result showing very good facial contour and bone symmetry (i, f & g).

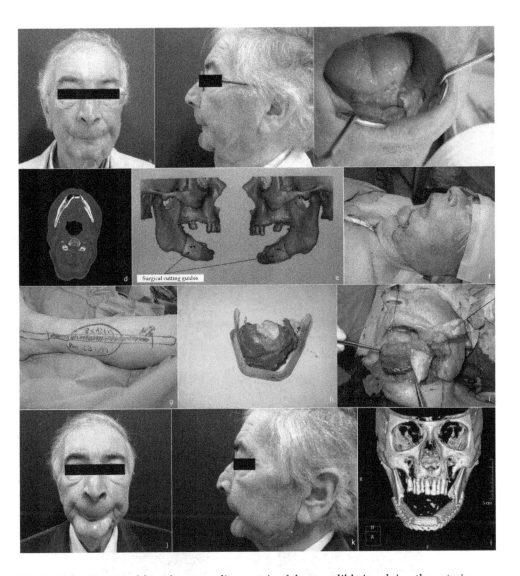

Fig. 5. Male, 66 years old, with osteoradionecrosis of the mandible involving the anterior arch an with orocervical fistulization (a, b, c & d) following radical surgery and RT for an oral squamous cell carcinoma; pre-operative planning with 3-D biomodelling technology showing the surgical cutting guides for bone resection (e); preoperative markings for reconstruction with a osteoseptocutaneous fibula flap (f & g); osteoseptocutaneous fibula flap modelled according to the 3D template that simultaneously guided the titanium plate modelling (h); flap *in situ* (i); Postoperative result at 9 months revealing a good mandibular contour and symmetry. The lack of lower lip projection is due to the temporary removal of the dental plate (j, k & l). Oral rehabilitation with dental implants is in course.

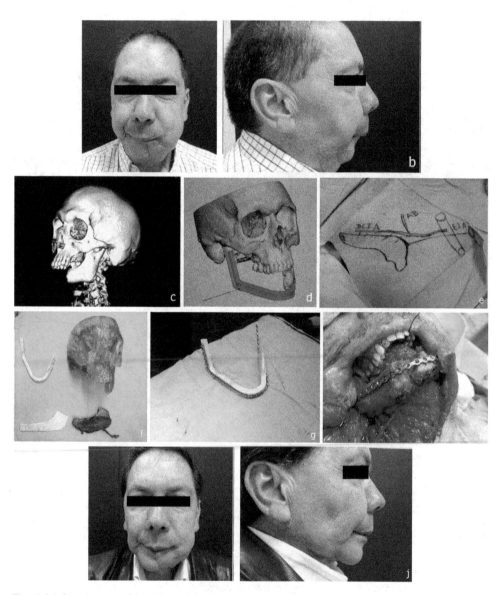

Fig. 6. Male, 46 years old, with an history of oral squamous cell carcinoma submitted to radical excision with left hemimandibulectomy sparing the condyle and RT (a, b & c); pre-operative planning with 3-D biomodelling technology showing the reconstruction plate modelling template generated with mirror-imaging and virtual simulation techniques (d); pre-operative markings for reconstruction with a vascularised iliac crest osteomuscular flap (e); Bone and reconstruction plate modelling based on the surgical 3-D SL templates (f & g); Intra-operative result after osteosynthesis (g); post-operative result at 9 months.

2.4 Advantages

Complex mandible reconstruction cases pose a real challenge. Long and technically demanding procedures are needed and 3-D anatomical reconstruction is very difficult to obtain. Over the last 20 years, Biomodelling technology associated with rapid prototyping has become an important tool in reconstructive surgery (Arvier et al., 1994; Bill et al., 1995 & Sailer et al., 1998). It enables virtual planning and simulation of surgical procedures and the production of very accurate physical models of the patient's anatomy (Winder & Bibb, 2005 & Robiony et al., 2007). It has been applied successfully in several medical fields (Zenha et al., 2011) with particularly interesting results in craniomaxillofacial surgery. We have a 8-year experience in using this technology in complex craniomaxillofacial defects (primary and secondary), with the great majority of the cases involving extensive mandibular defects. We have also applied this technology in craniofacial and maxillary defects. Since the mid-90's, 3-D biomodelling technology is regarded as a valuable tool in congenital malformations (including craniofacial surgery), tumour surgery, traumatology, orthognathic surgery and implantology (Bill et al., 1995). Sailer et al. (1998), indicate its use for craniofacial surgery in cases of hypertelorism, severe asymmetries of the neuro- and viscerocranium, complex cranial synostoses and large skull defects and of less value in cases of consolidated fractures of the periorbital and nasoethmoidal complex. The several studies and clinical applications of this technology by the group of D'Urso et al. (1998a, 1998b, 1999a, 1999b, 1999c, 2000a & 2000b), concluded that biomodelling significatively improved operative planning and diagnosis; reduced operative time and risk, facilitates team communication and also provides patients with a clearer understanding of their pathology and treatment strategy. In a multicentric european study of 466 cases, Wulf et al. (2003) concluded that medical modelling has utility in surgical specialities, especially in the craniofacial and maxillofacial area.

Biomodelling technology represents a whole new era in craniomaxillofacial surgery. The potential that computer surgical simulation of the procedure offers is still to be revealed. After patient image data acquisition by CT, we can pre-operatively and without time-pressure, better define the tumour to extirpate or the defect to reconstruct. We can simulate and rehearse the surgical steps and, with the specific software used, calculate the exact contours, angles, length and morphology of the reconstructive procedure. Finally, it enables the generation of surgical templates to be used intra-operatively. These templates guide the surgical procedure and are used to guide bone harvesting and modelling and also reconstruction plate moulding. This reduces effectively the operative time with major benefits for the patient including lesser wound exposure, decreased anaesthesia time and decreased blood loss (Kernan & Wimsatt, 2000). Team communication is also enhanced and treatment strategies can be discussed in a more detailed and "physical" way.

Patient's original anatomy is more accurately restored by this technology leading to better functional and aesthetic results (Fig 4i,f,g). The final anatomical result is more accurate leading to better functional and aesthetic results. All the patients were found to have at least a satisfactory result, with 94,8% (18 patients) ended with a good and very good end-result. Case 13 was the only considered to have a satisfactory result. This was mainly due to two reasons: the major defect to be reconstructed that needed a combined sequentially linked radial forearm fasciocutaneous flap plus a fibula osteoseptocutameous flap; and to partial flap necrosis that occurred in the fibula flap that forced surgical revision. It is important to point that none of this reaons is directly de+endent on the use of biomodelling technology. More than 2/3 of the patients (68,4%, 13 patients) where judged to have very good results. The differences between patients in the good and in the very good classification are mostly related to external scar appearance and are directly dependent on the pre-operative patient status. This evaluation was parallel to the patient's satisfaction.

2.5 Limitations

Apart from the several advantages that his technology ensures, there are some limitations to consider. The main limitation is the significant economical additional cost to the use of this technology. The virtual planning and manufacturing of the SL surgical templates costs around 1000-1500 €. Cost-effectiveness of this technology has been studied in the literature and is considered worthwhile (Bill et al., 1995; Sailer et al., 1998; D'Urso et al., 1998b & 1999a; Xia et al., 2006) due to the reduction of the operative time (with parallel reduction of potential complications) and to the better anatomical and functional end-results. Also, experience has led us to simplify and refine some steps in the procedure, making it more practical and less time-consuming. Nowadays, we invest more on the virtual planning and simulation phase, and we only generate the surgical guides to be used intra-operatively while at the beginning, we always created the patient's anatomical model. In this way, we define more objectively what is going to be done in the operating room and we spare the extra cost of manufacturing the whole craniofacial skeleton. Another drawback is the higher radiation dosage to which the patient has to be exposed due to the specific CT-scanning protocol that is needed. We consider it be a minor problem when compared to the extra benefits that this technology warrants. More important is the necessary planning and manufacturing time that takes a medium of 2 weeks and can be a troublesome when we are dealing with more urgent cases (oncology and acute trauma). We often still reconstruct the primary oral squamous cell carcinoma with mandibular involvement without the use of this technology.

2.6 Indications

A careful and judicious selection of the patients based on the expected surgical utility is very important. In our opinion, in complex mandible reconstruction, 3-D biomodelling technology is particularly useful in: major secondary defects (oncological, osteoradionecrosis, trauma) with important distortion of craniofacial structure; congenital malformations and primary tumour surgery when the dimensions of the tumour have altered normal anatomy considerably or the resection involves an angled region (genius or angle of the mandible) (Zenha et al., 2011).

3. Conclusion

Complex oromandibular reconstruction is one of the more challenging areas to deal with. The surgical procedures are necessarily long, complex and technically demanding and a satisfactory 3-D anatomical reconstruction is very difficult to obtain. 3-D Biomodelling technology designing of free flaps enables a better pre-operative planning, reduces operative time and significatively improves the aesthetic and biofunctional outcome. These new stereolitographic biomodel tools that exactly define the defect to be reconstructed and guide the osseous free flap osteotomies and also the reconstruction plate modelling are a step forward in the optimisation of the treatment of these cases.

4. Acknowledgments

The authors would like to thank Eng. José Domingos and Eng. Bruno Sá for their technical and scientific support on the conception and development of this technology. The authors would also like to thank all the remaining members of the Plastic, Reconstructive and Maxillofacial Surgery Department of the Centro Hospitalar Vila Nova Gaia/Espinho (medical doctors, nursing staff and secretaries) for their support in the treatment of these patients.

5. References

Arvier JF, Barker TM, Yau YY et al (1994). Maxillofacial biomodelling. *Br J Oral Maxillofac Surg* 1994;32;276-283. ISSN 0266-4356

Bill JS, Reuther JF, Dittmann, W et al (1995). Stereolithography in oral and maxillofacial operation planning. *Int J Oral Maxillofac Surg* 1995; 24;98-103. ISSN 0901-5027.

Brown GA, Milner B & Firoozbakhsh K (2002). Application of computer generated stereolithography and interpositioning template in acetabular fractures: a report of eight cases. *J Orthop Trauma* 2002;16;347-52. ISSN 0890-5339.

Costa H, Zenha H, Azevedo L, Rios L, Luz Barroso M & Cunha C (2011). Flow-through sequentially linked free flaps in head and neck reconstruction *Eur J Plast Surg*, Online first, (May 2011). ISSN 1435-0130.

Coward TJ, Watson RM & Wilkinson IC (1999). Fabrication of a wax ear by rapid-process modelling using stereolithography. *Int J Prosthodont* 1999;12;20-7. ISSN 0893-2174.

Dolz MS, Cina SJ & Smith R (2000). Stereolithography: a potential new tool in forensic medicine. *Am J Forensic Med Pathol* 2000;21;119-23. ISSN 0195-7910.

D'Urso PS & Thompson RG (1998). Fetal biomodelling. *Aust N Z J Obstet Gynaecol* 1998;38;205-7. ISSN 0004-8666.

D'Urso PS, Atkinson RL, Lanigan MW et al (1998b). Stereolithographic (SL) biomodelling in craniofacial surgery. *Br J Plast Surg* 1998;51;522-30. ISSN 0007-1226.

D'Urso PS, Barker TM, Earwaker WJ et al (1999a). Stereolithographic biomodelling in craniomaxillofacial surgery: a prospective trial. *J Craniomaxillofac Surg* 1999; 27; 30-37. ISSN 1010-5182.

D'Urso PS, Thompson RG, Atkinson RL et al (1999b). Cerebrovascular biomodelling: a technical note. *Surg Neurol* 1999;52;490-500. ISSN 0090-3019.

D'Urso PS, Hall BI, Atkinson RL, Weidmann MJ & Redmond MJ (1999c). Biomodel-guided stereotaxy. *Neurosurgery* 1999;44;1084-93. ISSN 0022-3069.

D'Urso PS, Barker TM, Earwaker WJ et al (2000a). Custom cranioplasty using stereolithography and acrylic. *Br J Plast Surg* 2000;53;200-4. ISSN 0007-1226.

D'Urso PS & Redmond MJ (2000b). A method for the resection of cranial tumours and skull reconstruction. *Br J Neurosurg* 2000;14;555-9. ISSN 0268-8697.

Fukui N, Ueno T, Fukuda A & Nakamura K (2003). The use of stereolithography for an unusual patellofemoral disorder. *Clin Orthop Relat Res* 2003;409;169-74. ISSN 0009-921X.

Gellrich NC, Schramm A, Hammer B et al (2002). Computer-assisted secondary reconstruction of unilateral posttraumatic orbital deformity. *Plast Reconstr Surg* 2002 Nov;110;1417-29. ISSN 1529-4242.

Greil GF, Wolf I, Kuettner A et al (2007). Stereolithographic reproduction of complex cardiac morphology based on high spatial resolution imaging. *Clin Res Cardiol* 2007;96;176-85. ISSN 1861-0684.

Gutierres M, Dias AG & Lopes MA (2007). Opening wedge high tibial osteotomy using 3D biomodelling Bonelike macroporous structures: case report. *J Mater Sci Mater Med* 2007;18;2377-82. ISSN 0957-4530.

Hohlweg-Majert B, Schön R, Schmelzeisen R, Gellrich NC & Schramm A (2005). Navigational Maxillofacial surgery using virtual models. *World J Surg* 2005;29;1530-8. ISSN 0364-2313.

Kermer C, Rasse M, Lagogiannis G et al (1998). Colour Stereolithography for planning complex maxillofacial tumour surgery. *J Craniomaxillofac Surg* 1998;26;360-2. ISSN 1010-5182.

Kernan BT & Wimsatt JA (2000). Use of Stereolithography Model for Accurate, Preoperative Adaptation of a Reconstruction Plate. *J Oral Maxillofac Surg* 2000;58;349-51. ISSN 0278-2391.

Lermusiaux P, Leroux C, Tasse JC, Castellani L & Martinez R (2001). Aortic aneurism: construction of a life-sized model by rapid prototyping. *Ann Vasc Surg* 2001;15;131-5. ISSN 0890-5096.

Mankovich NJ, Cheeseman AM & Stoker NG (1990). The display of three-dimensional anatomy with stereolithographic models. *J Digit Imag* 1990;3;200-3. ISSN 0897-1889.

Oliveira M, Hussain NS, Dias AG, Lopes MA, Azevedo L, Zenha H, Costa H & Santos JD (2008). 3-D biomodelling technology for maxillofacial reconstruction. *Materials Science and Engineering* C 28 (2008) 1347–1351, ISSN 0921-5093.

Peckitt NS (1998). Stereolithography and the manufacture of customized implants in facial reconstruction: a flapless surgical technique. *Br J Oral Maxillofac Surg* 1998;36;481. ISSN 0266-4356.

Pessa JE (2000). An algorithm of facial aging: verification of Lambros's theory by three-dimensional stereolithography, with reference to the pathogenesis of midfacial aging, scleral show, and the lateral suborbital trough deformity. *Plast Reconstr Surg* 2000;106;479-88. ISSN 1529-4242.

Pessa JE (2001). The potential role of stereolithography in the study of facial aging. *Am J Orthod Dentofacial Orthop* 2001;119;117-20. ISSN 0889-5406.

Sailer HF, Haers PE, Zollikofer CPE et al (1998). The value of stereolithographic models for preoperative diagnosis of craniofacial deformities and planning of surgical corrections. *Int J Oral Maxillofac Surg* 1998;27;327-333. ISSN 0901-5027.

Schramm A, Gellrich NC, Gutwald R et al (2000). Indications for computer-assisted treatment of cranio-maxillofacial tumours. *Comput Aided Surg* 2000;5(5):342-52. ISSN 1092-9088.

Sinn DP, Cillo JE & Miles BA (2006). Stereolithography for craniofacial surgery. *J Craniofac Surg* 2006;17;869-75. ISSN 1049-2275.

Sodian R, Loebe M, Hein A et al (2002). Application of stereolithography for scaffold fabrication for tissue engineered heart valves. *ASAIO J* 2002;48;12-6. ISSN 1058-2916.

Staffa G, Nataloni A, Compagnone C & Servadei F (2007). Custom made cranioplasty prostheses in porous hydroxy-apatite using 3D design techniques: 7 years experience in 25 patients. *Acta Neurochir* 2007;149;161-70. ISSN 0001-6268.

Stoker NG, Mankovich NJ & Valentino D (1992). Stereolithographic models for surgical planning: a preliminary report. *J Oral Maxillofac Surg* 1992;50;466-71. ISSN 0278-2391.

Robiony M, Salvo I, Costa F et al (2007). Virtual Reality Surgical Planning for Maxillofacial Distraction Osteogenesis: The Role of Reverse Engineering Rapid Prototyping and Cooperative Work. *J Oral Maxillofac Surg* 2007;65;1198-208. ISSN 0278-2391.

Vanezi P, Vanezis M, McCombe G & Niblett T (2000). Facial reconstruction using 3-D computer graphics. *Forensic Sci Int* 2000;108;81-95. ISSN 0379-0738.

Westendorff C, Kaminsky J, Ernemann U, Reinert S & Hoffmann J (2007). Image-guided sphenoid wing meningioma resection and simultaneous computer-assisted cranio-orbital reconstruction: technical case report. *Neurosurgery* 2007;60;173-4. ISSN 0022-3069.

Winder J & Bibb R (2005). Medical Rapid Prototyping Technologies: State of the Art and Current Limitations for Application in Oral and Maxillofacial Surgery. *J Oral Maxillofac Surg* 2005;63;1006-15. ISSN 0278-2391.

Wulf J, Vitt KD, Erben CM, Bill JS & Busch LC (2003). Medical biomodelling in surgical applications: results of a multicentric European validation of 466 cases. Stud Health Technol Inform. 2003;94:404-6. ISSN 0926-9630.

Wurm G, Tomancok B, Pogady P, Holl K & Trenkler J (2004). Cerebrovascular stereolithographic biomodeling for aneurism surgery. Technical note. *J Neurosurg* 2004;100;139-45. ISSN 0022-3085.

Xia J, Wang D, Samman N, Yeung RWK & Tideman H (2000). Computer-assisted three-dimensional surgical planning and simulation: 3D color facial model generation. *Int J Oral Maxillofac Surg* 2000;29;2-10. ISSN 0901-5027.

Xia JJ, Phillips CV, Gateno J et al (2006). Cost-effectiveness analysis for computer-aided surgical simulation in complex cranio-maxillofacial surgery. *J Oral Maxillofac Surg* 2006;64;1780-4. ISSN 0278-2391.

Zenha H, Azevedo L, Rios L, Pinto A, Luz Barroso M, Cunha C & Costa H (2011). The application of 3-D biomodelling technology in complex mandibular reconstruction – experience of 47 clinical cases. *Eur J Plast Surg*, Vol. 34, No. 4, (August 2011), pp. 257-265, ISSN 0930-343X.

Permissions

The contributors of this book come from diverse backgrounds, making this book a truly international effort. This book will bring forth new frontiers with its revolutionizing research information and detailed analysis of the nascent developments around the world.

We would like to thank Dr. Stefan Danilla, for lending his expertise to make the book truly unique. He has played a crucial role in the development of this book. Without his invaluable contribution this book wouldn't have been possible. He has made vital efforts to compile up to date information on the varied aspects of this subject to make this book a valuable addition to the collection of many professionals and students.

This book was conceptualized with the vision of imparting up-to-date information and advanced data in this field. To ensure the same, a matchless editorial board was set up. Every individual on the board went through rigorous rounds of assessment to prove their worth. After which they invested a large part of their time researching and compiling the most relevant data for our readers. Conferences and sessions were held from time to time between the editorial board and the contributing authors to present the data in the most comprehensible form. The editorial team has worked tirelessly to provide valuable and valid information to help people across the globe.

Every chapter published in this book has been scrutinized by our experts. Their significance has been extensively debated. The topics covered herein carry significant findings which will fuel the growth of the discipline. They may even be implemented as practical applications or may be referred to as a beginning point for another development. Chapters in this book were first published by InTech; hereby published with permission under the Creative Commons Attribution License or equivalent.

The editorial board has been involved in producing this book since its inception. They have spent rigorous hours researching and exploring the diverse topics which have resulted in the successful publishing of this book. They have passed on their knowledge of decades through this book. To expedite this challenging task, the publisher supported the team at every step. A small team of assistant editors was also appointed to further simplify the editing procedure and attain best results for the readers.

Our editorial team has been hand-picked from every corner of the world. Their multi-ethnicity adds dynamic inputs to the discussions which result in innovative outcomes. These outcomes are then further discussed with the researchers and contributors who give their valuable feedback and opinion regarding the same. The feedback is then collaborated with the researches and they are edited in a comprehensive manner to aid the understanding of the subject.

Apart from the editorial board, the designing team has also invested a significant amount of their time in understanding the subject and creating the most relevant covers. They scrutinized every image to scout for the most suitable representation of the subject and create an appropriate cover for the book.

The publishing team has been involved in this book since its early stages. They were actively engaged in every process, be it collecting the data, connecting with the contributors or procuring relevant information. The team has been an ardent support to the editorial, designing and production team. Their endless efforts to recruit the best for this project, has resulted in the accomplishment of this book. They are a veteran in the field of academics and their pool of knowledge is as vast as their experience in printing. Their expertise and guidance has proved useful at every step. Their uncompromising quality standards have made this book an exceptional effort. Their encouragement from time to time has been an inspiration for everyone.

The publisher and the editorial board hope that this book will prove to be a valuable piece of knowledge for researchers, students, practitioners and scholars across the globe.

List of Contributors

Michael J. Brenner
Director of Facial Plastic & Reconstructive Surgery, USA
Division of Otolaryngology, Department of Surgery, Southern Illinois University School of Medicine, USA

Jennifer L. Nelson
Division of Otolaryngology, Department of Surgery, Southern Illinois University School of Medicine, USA

Alessandro Bonanno
Texas State University System Regents Professor of Sociology, Department of Sociology, Sam Houston State University, USA

Stefanos Tsourvakas
Orthopedic Department, General Hospital of Trikala, Greece

Ron Israeli
Hofstra North Shore-LIJ School of Medicine, USA

J.J. Vranckx and P. Delaere
KU Leuven University Hospitals, Department of Plastic & Reconstructive Surgery, Department of Otorhinolaryngology, Head and Neck Surgery, Belgium

J.J. Vranckx
Dept. of Plastic & Reconstructive Surgery, KUL Leuven University Hospitals, Leuven, Belgium

A. D'Hoore
Dept. Abdominal Surgery, KUL Leuven University Hospitals, Leuven, Belgium

Nicola S. Russell, Marion Scharpfenecker, Saske Hoving and Leonie A.E. Woerdeman
The Netherlands Cancer Institute – Antoni van Leeuwenhoek Hospital, Amsterdam, The Netherlands

Sarah Nietzer, Gudrun Dandekar, Milena Wasik and Heike Walles
Chair of Tissue Engineering and Regenerative Medicine, University Wuerzburg/Fraunhofer Institute for Interfacial Engineering and Biotechnology IGB, Germany

Martha R. Ortiz-Posadas
Electrical Engineering Department, Universidad Autónoma Metropolitana-Iztapalapa, Mexico

Leticia Vega-Alvarado
Centro de Ciencias Aplicadas y Desarrollo Tecnológico, Universidad Nacional Autónoma de México, México

Qingfeng Li
Shanghai Jiaotong University, Department of Plastic and Reconstructive Surgery, Shanghai, China

Mei Yang
Division of Plastic Surgery, Southern Illinois University School of Medicine, Illinois, USA

Horácio Zenha, Maria da Luz Barroso and Horácio Costa
Plastic, Reconstructive & Maxillofacial Surgery Department, Centro Hospitalar V.N.Gaia/Espinho, Portugal